Ophthalmology

Concise
Medical
Textbooks

Ophthalmology

Kenneth Wybar

M.D., CH.M., F.R.C.S.

*Ophthalmic Surgeon, The Hospital for Sick Children, Great
Ormond Street, and the Royal Marsden Hospital. Surgeon,
Moorfields Eye Hospital. Lecturer in Ophthalmology, University of
London. Civilian Consultant in Ophthalmology, The Royal Navy*

BAILLIÈRE TINDALL LONDON

BAILLIÈRE TINDALL
7 & 8 Henrietta Street, London WC2E 8QE

Cassell & Collier Macmillan Publishers Ltd., London
35 Red Lion Square, London WC1R 4SG
Sydney, Auckland, Toronto, Johannesburg

The Macmillan Publishing Company Inc
New York

First published 1966
Second edition 1974

ISBN 0 7020 0472 3

*Published in the United States of America by
The Williams and Wilkins Company, Baltimore*

*Printed in Great Britain by
Cox & Wyman Ltd,
London, Fakenham and Reading*

Contents

List of Plates

Preface

The necessity for a second edition of this concise textbook within a relatively short time provides an opportunity to make sweeping changes. It has been decided, however, to amend the text only to maintain an up-to-date approach without making any obvious alterations in its general pattern and original purpose: to provide a factual and concise account of ophthalmology with particular regard for the medical student without previous experience of the subject, the general practitioner concerned with the recognition of eye disease in its early stages and the day-to-day care of the more common of these conditions, and the specialist in some other branch of medicine or surgery who is aware of the importance of an ophthalmic examination in an adequate assessment of many forms of systemic disease. Certain sections are included which are scarcely within the province of the medical student and general practitioner, but it seems reasonable to try to provide an account (however brief) of most aspects of ophthalmology, and I have been encouraged in this by the knowledge that the value of a comprehensive and yet concise account of the subject is appreciated by those working for a higher examination and even by the established ophthalmic surgeon.

The diseases which occur in different parts of the eye and its related structures are described in separate chapters, and each of these descriptions is preceded by a brief account of the functional anatomy of the individual structures because this forms the essential basis for a proper understanding of the pathological events which are liable to occur in these tissues. There are, of course, many diseases which affect more than one structure and, to avoid needless repetition, their description is limited to one chapter only. The new features that have been incorporated include: the accommodative convergence and accommodation relationship (AC/A ratio) the A and V phenomena; a modified classification of amblyopia; blow-out fracture of the orbit; the application of fluorescein angiography in a wide range of disorders of the optic nerve-head, the retina and the choroid; the battered-baby syndrome, and the anterior chamber cleavage syndrome.

Acknowledgements

I am most grateful to Dr. P. Hansell, Director of the Medical Illustration Department of the Institute of Ophthalmology, and to Mr. T. Tarrant of that department who so skilfully prepared the original illustrations and diagrams from my rough sketches. Many of these have been used by me in the first edition and in other publications, and I should like to thank the following publishers for permission to use them again: H. K. Lewis and Co. Ltd., for Figs. 40–47 from Lyle and Jackson's *Practical Orthoptics in the Treatment of Squint*; The National Society of Children's Nurseries for Figs. 1 and 48 from *The Eyes in the Early Years of Life* (1963); The Opthalmological Society of the United Kingdom, for Figs. 60–65 and 68–76 from *The Functional Anatomy of the Afferent Visual Pathways* (1962).

I should also like to thank Mr. Tarrant for having supplied the drawings for Figs. 20, 28, 29, 31, 32, 33, 36, 37, 39 and 56, and the Institute for prints of Plate I and Plate III; Messrs Theodore Hamblin for Figs. 4 and 5; Dr. R. Leishman and the *British Journal of Ophthalmology* for the basis for Plate IV; and Mr. S. J. H. Miller and *The Practitioner* for Figs. 57 and 59. Plate V is reproduced with kind permission of Clement Clarke and Plates II, VI, VII and VIII by courtesy of C. Davis Keeler Ltd. Figures 9, 11, 12 and 39 are from May and Worth's *Manual of Diseases of the Eye* by Mr. Keith Lyle and Mr. A. G. Cross and are reproduced with permission of the publishers, Baillière Tindall.

March 1974   *Kenneth Wybar*

1 | Basic Methods of Examination

A distinctive feature of the art and science of ophthalmology is the comparative ease with which many parts of the eye may be examined in detail with relatively simple techniques. It follows that the ophthalmologist is frequently able to come to precise conclusions on the state of health or disease of the various parts of the eye during a purely routine examination, and for this reason it is essential to adopt systematic methods of examination at all times. Indeed it is likely that more errors in diagnosis are made as a result of an inadequate method of examination leading to a failure to detect the true nature of the lesion rather than as a result of an ignorance of its exact significance.

Most of the special methods of examination which are applied to the different parts of the eye are described in the separate chapters dealing with the diseases of these structures, but there are various more general methods of examination which are conveniently considered now.

General Assessment of the Patient

Before proceeding to an examination of the eyes it is important to make an assessment of the patient as a whole, including the general physique, the state of well-being, the facial expression and complexion, the position of the head, and the gait.

Methods of Illumination

DIFFUSE ILLUMINATION

This is a diffuse and even type of illumination which is achieved by daylight from a conveniently situated window or by artificial light from an electric light source, such as a pocket torch, and it provides a

general view of the patient and of the eye, thus obviating the danger
of overlooking some fairly obvious defect by concentrating too rapidly
on the more localized methods of illumination.

FOCAL ILLUMINATION

This is a concentrated and usually bright type of illumination
which is directed to particular parts of the eye so that they are revealed with great clarity against the relatively dark background of
the other structures. It is achieved by the use of a projection lamp
which incorporates a condensing lens within its own case, such as the
'pen' torch or ophthalmoscope which is held by the examiner so that
a focused beam of light is directed to a certain part of the eye.

The examination of the eye by focal illumination is enhanced by
the use of some form of magnification. For many years emphasis was
placed on the use of the *uniocular loupe*, as illustrated in Plate I.
However, this particular method of eye examination, at one time
an essential part of the expertise and art of the budding ophthalmic surgeon, has largely fallen into abeyance as the result of the ready
availability of the *slit-lamp microscope* (see below), which obviously
provides a much more precise examination. It has superseded the
binocular ophthalmic loupe which is maintained directly over the eyes
by a headband which leaves both hands free to control, the lamp
providing focal illumination and to keep the eyelids open, despite
its obvious advantage over the uniocular loupe in providing an
impression of depth.

Slit-lamp Microscope

This is a specialized type of apparatus which is available also with
extra attachments (Plate V) providing facilities for a detailed examination of the region of the filtration angle (gonioscopy) and for a precise
measurement of the intraocular pressure (applanation tonometry)
(pp. 280 and 281). It is also available in portable and hand-held form
(Plates II and VI), hence the gradual decline in the use of the uniocular and binocular ophthalmic loupes.

The beam of light from the slit lamp is maintained accurately in
focus on different parts of the eye by means of a movable mechanical
arm which houses the projection lamp, and the light may be varied in
intensity and in shape (circular, vertical slit or horizontal slit beams).
Such a beam is usually narrow so that it passes through the optical
media of the eye (cornea, anterior chamber, lens and anterior part of
vitreous) without much diffusion, and a section of these structures

(Plate III, *upper*) is readily viewed by the microscope; this is capable of being adjusted to provide varying magnifications and is maintained accurately in different positions by its attachment to a second movable mechanical arm. It is customary in modern slit-lamp microscopes for the light source and the microscope arms to be mounted together so that each is maintained in focus on different

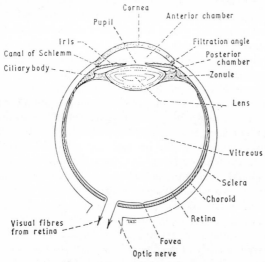

Fig. 1. *The normal eye in horizontal section*

parts of the eye by the movement of a single controlling lever, thus leaving one hand free to control the eyelids of the patient. During this examination the patient's head is fixed in a steady position by a chin rest which is attached to the table, supporting the microscope and projection lamp, and the patient and examiner sit on stools at opposite ends of the table. The slit-lamp microscope is an essential instrument in the critical examination of fine structural changes of the anterior segment of the eye.

Ophthalmoscopic Examination

DIRECT OPHTHALMOSCOPE

Light from the projection lamp of the ophthalmoscope (see Plate VIII, *left*) is reflected into the eye of the patient by an angled mirror and the light which emerges from the eye is viewed by the observer through a small hole in the centre of the mirror. An inverted image (which appears to the observer as an erect one) of the illuminated part of the eye, in particular the fundus (retina, choroid and optic nerve), is formed. The image is focused clearly by a system of lenses mounted on a movable circular disc in the head of the ophthalmoscope to compensate for any errors in the refraction of different parts of the fundi. The ophthalmoscope provides a magnified view of the fundus, usually of about × 15 (Plate III, *lower*). It is held close to the eye of the patient and to the eye of the observer during this examination, The observer's right eye should be used in examination of the patient's right eye with the ophthalmoscope held in the right hand, and the process is reversed for the patient's left eye which is viewed by the left eye with the instrument held in the left hand. It is usual to steady the patient's head with the other hand placed on the patient's forehead, which also permits the retraction of the upper lid by the thumb if there is any tendency for the patient to close the eye.

The ophthalmoscope may be used also to detect defects in the media of the eye (cornea, anterior chamber, lens and vitreous), and in fact this should precede the more detailed assessment of the fundus. The ophthalmoscope is held some distance from the patient's eye so that the fundus appears to the observer simply as a red reflex without any details of its structure, but defects of the media are revealed then as dark areas against the normal bright red background of the fundus, particularly if a fairly high convex (plus) lens is used in the head of the ophthalmoscope. Sometimes it is difficult to determine the exact situation of any such defect by this method, but this is facilitated by making use of the phenomenon of parallax so that the direction of apparent movement of an opacity in relation to a fixed point, such as the iris, is observed on movement of the patient's eye; when the eye moves upwards an opacity in front of the pupil will appear to move up but an opacity behind the pupil will appear to move down. Sometimes, of course, a defective red reflex on direct ophthalmoscopy may be the result of some fairly gross disease of the vitreous, retina or choroid.

INDIRECT OPHTHALMOSCOPY

A light from a lamp behind the patient's head is directed into the patient's eye from a concave mirror, and by placing a convex lens (of about +13 D) in the path of this light at a distance of about 7 cm from the patient's eye, an inverted image of the fundus with a magnification of about × 5 is formed between the lens and the patient's

eye. This method, which requires considerable practice, is often neg-
lected in modern times because the direct method of ophthalmoscopy
is easier to use and provides an upright image of higher magnification, but the indirect method is of great value in certain diseases
because it provides a wider field of observation, particularly in the
peripheral parts of the fundus. Its value in the examination of cases of
retinal detachment has led to the development of a specialized form
of apparatus which incorporates a bright focal beam of light so that
the use of a mirror is eliminated; it provides a binocular image of the
fundus (binocular indirect ophthalmoscope Plate VII).

The fundus may be examined also by focal illumination, using the
slit-lamp microscope, by artificially creating a flat anterior surface
of the cornea with the use of a specially designed contact lens or of a
strong concave lens (−55 D) held near the cornea. This is of particular value in evaluating subtle changes in the macular area, such as
the swelling which occurs in a central serous retinopathy and yet on
direct ophthalmoscopy may appear as a 'hole'.

2 | Estimation of the Visual Acuity

The visual acuity of each eye separately is recorded in two ways: the distant visual acuity and the near visual acuity. This distinction is sometimes of great importance, such as in a congenital idiopathic nystagmus when the near vision is usually good despite a relatively poor level of distant acuity.

DISTANT VISUAL ACUITY

This measures the form sense of the eye, which is made up of two components: first, the resolving power of the eye to discriminate between two separate but adjacent stimuli (the smallest measurement of which is the *minimum separable*), and, second, the ability of the visual cortex to appreciate the nature of a stimulus by a perceptual process (the smallest measurement of which is the *minimum cognisiable*). In general the minimum separable under conditions of normal illumination is about one minute (1') and this represents the angle which the object subtends at the nodal point of the eye (Fig. 2). This

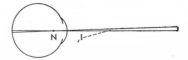

FIG. 2. *Minimum separable—angle of one minute at the nodal point of the eye*

figure is used as a basis for the construction of square-shaped serif letters or figures of Snellen's test types because the strokes which compose them and the intervals between them subtend this angle, although each letter or figure as a whole subtends 5' at this nodal point which may be regarded as an average measurement of the minimum cognisiable (Fig. 3).

Letters or figures of different sizes are constructed which subtend this angle of 5′ the nodal point when they are placed respectively at 60, 36, 24, 18, 12, 9, 6 and 5 metres from the eye and they are then placed on a card with a gradual reduction in size from above down so that the largest letter or figure is placed as a single one at the top of

FIG. 3. *Construction of a Snellen's serif test type letter*

the card and the smallest letters or figures are placed as a line at the foot of the card (Fig. 4). The distant visual acuity of each eye is recorded as an expression of the line of letters which can be discerned at a particular distance (usually 6 metres) from the eye; if, for example, only the top letter is read the acuity is recorded as 6/60, when 6 equals the distance of the chart from the eye in metres and 60 equals the distance at which the letter subtends 5′ at the nodal point of the eye. It follows, therefore, that a normal level of vision is 6/6, although under conditions of good illumination a level of 6/5 is usual. If, however, the patient is unable to read the top letter at 6 metres he is asked to approach the chart until he is able to read it; if this distance is, for example, 3 metres the vision is recorded as 3/60. It should be appreciated that, although this method of recording vision is suggestive of a 'fraction' with a numerator (the distance from the chart) and a denominator (the line of letters which is read), it is incorrect to regard it as such and, for example, a vision of 6/12 should not be considered as 'half-vision'.

If the vision is less than 2/60, a test is made for the ability to count fingers (C.F.) at different distances—2 m, 1 m, $\frac{1}{2}$ m, or, failing that, for the ability to appreciate movements of the hand (H.M.), or for the ability to have perception of light (P.L.). When this is absent the eye is blind (No P.L.).

In testing the vision of the young child who is unable to read or of the illiterate patient, a suitable method to use is the E test. This is carried out conveniently by a cube which has different-sized letter Es on each side; the cube is held by the examiner to show the different Es in different directions and at different distances from the eye and the child mimics the position of the E throughout the test with a cut-out E which he holds in his hand. It is also possible to use a Snellen's type chart with the letter Es of different sizes arranged in different directions. A further test for the young child is the Sheridan–Gardiner test, based on the Stycar charts which are composed of 9 standard Snellen letters without serifs—HLCTOXAVU—selected according to the psychological finding that a child is normally able to copy a vertical line at 2 years, a horizontal line at $2\frac{1}{2}$ years, a cross at 4 years, a square at 5 years, and a triangle at $5\frac{1}{2}$ years. Obviously, the more rapid intellectual development of certain children today determines the fact that these figures are somewhat arbitrary. In this test the child is given a card containing the Snellen letters and he points to the correct letter when the examiner presents isolated letters to him of varying sizes and at different distances.

Near Visual Acuity

This is a measure of the ability to read words composed of letters of different sizes at the normal reading distance of 33 cm ($\frac{1}{3}$ m). Jaeger's types represent a random series of different sizes of printers' types—the smallest equals J 1 and the largest equals J 20, but the modern N types are more exact because they are based on the 'point' measurement of the height of a body of letters used in printing (one point $= \frac{1}{72}$ in); the letters are of 10 different sizes—N 5 (which equals 5 points), N 6, N 8, N 10, N 12, N 14, N 18, N 24, N 36 and N 60 (Fig. 5). A modification of the Sheridan–Gardiner test using 're-duced' Snellen types may be used for assessing the near visual acuity in the young.

The Refraction of the Eye

In estimating the distant and near visual acuity, account must be taken of the spectacle requirement in order to obtain the corrected visual acuity as distinct from the unaided (uncorrected) visual acuity. This determination demands an assessment of the refraction of the eye which is dependent on two main factors: first, the influence of the refracting structures of the eye, that is, the cornea and the lens and, second, the axial length of the eyeball.

THE INFLUENCE OF THE REFRACTING STRUCTURES

Refraction takes place when rays of light travelling in one medium, for example air, fall obliquely on the surface of another medium, for

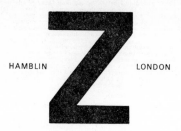

60

HAMBLIN   LONDON

36

24

18

12

9

6

5

FIG. 4. *Snellen's test types (letters)*

N.5.

The streets of London are better paved and better lighted than those of any metropolis in Europe: there are lamps on both sides of every street, in the mean proportion of one lamp to three doors. The effect produced by these double rows of lights in many streets is remarkably pleasing: of this Oxford-street and especially Bond-street, afford striking examples. We have few street robberies, and rarely indeed a midnight assassination. This last circumstance is owing to the benevolent spirit of the people; for whatever crimes the lowest orders of society are tempted to commit, those of a sanguinary nature are less frequent here than in any other country. Yet it is singular, where the police are so ably regulated, that the watchmen, our guardians of the night, are generally old decrepit men, who have scarcely strength to use the alarum which is their signal of distress in cases of emergency. It does credit, however, to the morals of the people, and to the national spirit, and evinces that the brave are always benevolent, when we reflect that, during a period when almost all kingdoms exhibited the horrors of massacre and the outrages of anarchy, when blood had contaminated the standard of liberty, and defaced the long established laws of nations, while it overwhelmed the freedom it pretended to establish, this island maintained the throne of reason, erected on the firm basis of genius, valour, and philanthropy.

cave   acorn   veneer   succour

N.8.

Water Cresses are sold in small bunches, one penny each, or three bunches for twopence. The crier of Water Cresses frequently travels seven or eight miles before the hour of breakfast to gather them fresh; but there is generally a pretty good supply of them in Covent-garden market, brought, along with other vegetables, from the gardens adjacent to the Metropolis, where they are planted and cultivated like other garden stuff. They are, however, from this circumstance, very inferior from those that grow in the natural state in a running brook, wanting that pungency of taste which makes them very wholesome; and a weed very dissimilar in quality is often imposed upon an unsuspecting purchaser.

rose   sauce   cannon   reverse

N.12.

Strawberries, brought fresh gathered to the market in the height of their season, both morning and afternoon, are sold in pottles, containing something less than a quart each. The crier adds one penny to the price of the Strawberries for the pottle, which, if returned by her customer, she abates, or will take it again at the same price on another occasion.

nuns   score   severe   careers

N.18.

Door-mats of all kinds, rush and rope, from sixpence to four shillings each, with Table Mats of various sorts, are daily cried through the streets of London.

crave   savour   concern

N.36.

The present pub-lication addresses itself, in a popular and inviting form, to foreigners who may wish to con-

FIG. 5. *Examples of N test types for near visual acuity*

example the cornea, the lens, or glass, which has a different optical density from the first medium, and the rays of light passing into the second medium become bent or refracted so that they assume a direction different from their original direction. This change occurs

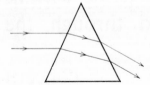

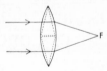

FIG. 6. *Refraction of light rays through a prism*

FIG. 7. *Convergence of parallel light rays to point of focus (F) after passing through a convex spherical lens*

because the rays of light move more rapidly in a medium of low density, for example air, than in a medium of high density, for example glass, and it is illustrated by the deviation of the light rays as they pass through a prism (Fig. 6). It follows that a convex-shaped lens, which may be considered as two prisms joined base to base, causes a convergence of parallel light rays (Fig. 7), whereas a concave-shaped lens, which may be considered as two prisms joined apex to apex, causes a divergence of parallel light rays (Fig. 8). The power of a con-

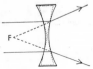

FIG. 8. *Divergence of parallel light rays apparently from a point of focus (F) after passing through concave spherical lens*

vex or concave spherical lens is determined by its focal length which is a measure of the distance from the lens to the point of focus (F) of parallel rays after passing through the lens (Figs. 7 and 8). A lens with a focal length of 1 metre is termed a 1 dioptre (I D) lens, one with a focal length of $\frac{1}{2}$ metre a 2 dioptre (2 D) lens, and one with a focal length of 2 metres a $\frac{1}{2}$ dioptre ($\frac{1}{2}$ D) lens, etc., so that the dioptric power of a lens is inversely proportional to its focal length. Convex and concave spherical lenses are distinguished from one another by the prefix plus (+) for convex lenses and minus (−) for concave lenses in front of the dioptric power.

The structures concerned in the refraction of the eye are the cornea and the lens.

The Cornea

The influence of the cornea on refraction is exerted almost entirely by its anterior surface, which is a curved convex surface producing convergence of parallel light rays entering the eye. This surface has a high refracting value and contributes significantly to the final refraction of the eye, because the corneal substance has a much greater optical density than the medium, i.e. the air, with which it is in contact. The posterior corneal surface contributes little because of the negligible difference in the optical densities of the opposing media (cornea and aqueous).

The Lens

The anterior and posterior surfaces of the lens are curved convex surfaces so that they cause increased convergence of light rays passing through the lens, although this effect is limited to some extent by the absence of any marked differences between the density of the lens and the densities of the surrounding media (aqueous and vitreous). Its effect is enhanced, however, by the fact that there is usually a slight increase in the optical density of the central part of the lens, the nucleus, as compared with the peripheral part of the lens, the cortex. It follows that a relative increase in the density of the nuclear portion increases the refracting value of the lens, and a relative increase in the density of the cortical portion decreases the dioptric value of the lens, but these differences are seldom of great significance in the normal lens.

Also, the influence of the lens is not a static one, because its refracting value may be altered by the act of accommodation. An increased effectivity of the lens during accommodation for near (positive accommodation) is produced by a contraction of the ciliary muscle (longitudinal fibres, oblique fibres and iridic fibres acting as a whole), which is innervated by the parasympathetic part of the third cranial nerve, so that there is a forward movement and thickening of the ciliary body with a consequent relaxation of the zonule, or suspensory ligament, which attaches the capsule of the lens to the ciliary body. At one time it was considered that the relaxation of the zonule allowed the lens to assume a more spherical form with an increase in the curvatures of its anterior and posterior surfaces, an increase in its antero-posterior diameter, and a decrease in its transverse diameter (theory of Helmholtz); but it is more likely that the increased curvatures are confined mainly to the regions of the anterior and posterior poles and that there is even a slight flattening of the more peripheral parts of these surfaces during accommodation (theory of Fincham) (Fig. 9), perhaps because the capsule of the lens is thicker in its more

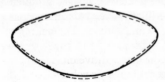

FIG. 9. *Alterations in the curvature of the lens from a resting state (solid line) to a fully accommodative state (broken line)*

peripheral parts than in its more central parts (Fig. 10). A decreased effectivity of the lens during accommodation for distance (negative accommodation) is achieved by a reversal of this process, although there is some evidence that this may involve the activity of the sympathetic nervous system, and it is certainly not a mere passive relaxation of the ciliary muscle.

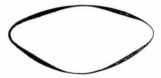

FIG. 10. *Variations in the thickness of the lens capsule*

THE INFLUENCE OF THE AXIAL LENGTH OF THE EYE

The axial length of the eyeball also determines the final refraction of the eye.

The terms used to denote the different types of refraction are:

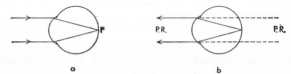

FIG. 11. *Refraction of the emmetropic eye—(a) parallel rays of light entering the eye form a focus (F) on the retina, and (b) rays of light emerging from the eye are parallel and meet at the far point (P.R.) at infinity, in front of or behind the eye*

Emmetropia

The emmetropic eye has a normal type of refraction so that parallel rays of light entering the eye come to focus on the retina (Fig. 11). It

follows that rays of light emerging from the eye are parallel and may
be considered to converge to, or to diverge from, the far point (or
punctum remotum) which lies at infinity. Emmetropia is determined
by a perfect correlation of the following factors: the axial length of the
eyeball and the dioptric power of the refracting media (curvature and
index components).

Ametropia

The ametropic eye has an abnormal type of refraction so that
parallel rays of light entering the eye do not come to a focus on the
retina. There are different forms of ametropia:

Hypermetropia. The hypermetropic eye is one in which parallel
rays of light entering the eye would come to focus (if they could be
prolonged) at a point behind the retina (Fig. 12). It follows that rays

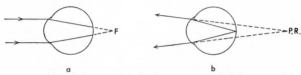

a   b

FIG. 12. *Refraction of the hypermetropic eye—(a) parallel rays of light entering
the eye, if continued, form a focus (F) behind the retina, and (b) rays of light
emerging from the eye are divergent and appear to arise from the far point (P.R.)
behind the eye*

of light emerging from the eye are divergent and appear to diverge
from the far point (or punctum remotum) which lies behind the eye.
Hypermetropia is determined by one or more of the following factors:

1. An axial failure, that is an axial length which is shorter than
normal.

2. A curvature failure, that is an insufficient degree of corneal or,
more rarely, lenticular curvature.

3. An index failure, that is a decreased density of the lens as a
whole or, more particularly, a relative decrease in density of the
nuclear part of the lens.

The hypermetropic eye is usually smaller than normal. This
affects the anterior segment so that the anterior chamber tends to
be somewhat shallow, a factor which may contribute to the development of closed-angle glaucoma (see Chap. 7). It also affects the posterior segment, and the optic disc appears ophthalmoscopically to be
unduly small; sometimes the disc margins may look blurred so that

there is a false impression of papilloedema, although this confusion is avoided by careful examination because there is no true swelling of the tissues or the disc margins and no retinal vein dilatation. Uncorrected hypermetropia may cause eyestrain because of the difficulty in maintaining an effort of accommodation in the interests of clear vision, and in young children it may precipitate the development of certain forms of convergent squint.

Myopia. The myopic eye is the eye in which parallel rays of light entering the eye come to a focus at a point in front of the retina (Fig. 13). It follows that rays of light emerging from the myopic eye

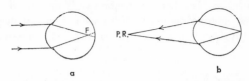

FIG. 13. *Refraction of the myopic eye—(a) parallel rays of light entering the eye form a focus in front of the retina, and (b) rays of light emerging from the eye are convergent and meet at the far point (P.R.) in front of the eye*

are convergent and converge to the far point (or punctum remotum), which lies in front of the eye. Myopia is determined by one or more of the following factors:

1. An axial failure, that is an axial length which is longer than normal.

2. A curvature failure, that is an excessive degree of corneal or, more rarely, lenticular curvature.

3. An index failure, that is an increased density of the lens as a whole, or, more particularly, a relative increase of the nuclear portion.

The myopic eye is usually larger than normal. This affects the anterior segment so that the anterior chamber tends to be deeper than normal, a factor which determines the rarity of closed-angle glaucoma in axial myopia. It also affects the posterior segment, particularly in the region of the optic disc, with the gradual development of a concentric area of choroidal atrophy, the *myopic crescent*, usually, along the temporal border of the disc but sometimes along some other border of the disc or even around the whole disc (*peripapillary atrophy*). Choroidal atrophy is also liable to occur in the submacular area with the development of degenerative changes in the overlying retina, sometimes in association with frank choroidal haemorrhage which follows a rupture of the elastic lamina (Bruch's membrane) which separates the retina from the choroid. In extreme cases a thinning of the posterior part of the sclera (including the optic disc) causes a bulging of this part of the eye backwards with the formation of a *posterior staphyloma*.

In general the occurrence of small degrees of hypermetropia or myopia is simply the result of a slight failure in correlation between the corneal refracting power and the axial length of the eyeball, but the larger degrees are produced by more elaborate failures, although an abnormality of the axial length is usually the main determining one.

Astigmatism. In the purely emmetropic, hypermetropic or myopic eye the refracting effect of the eye on parallel rays of light is identical in all meridians, but in the astigmatic eye the refracting effect is

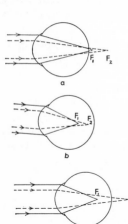

Fig. 14. *Refraction of the astigmatic eye—* (a) *hypermetropic astigmatism,* (b) *myopic astigmatism, and* (c) *mixed astigmatism.*

Note: In each diagram the rays of light in the vertical plane (solid lines) are more refracted than those in the horizontal plane (broken lines)

different according to the meridian in which these rays traverse the eye. In practically all astigmatic eyes the meridian of greatest refraction lies at right angles to the meridian of least refraction, and it is often found that one of these meridians lies in or near the vertical plane of the eyeball with the other meridian lying in or near the horizontal plane of the eyeball. Astigmatism may be associated with hypermetropia (*hypermetropic astigmatism*) (Fig. 14a), with myopia (*myopic astigmatism*) (Fig. 14b) or with hypermetropia and myopia (*mixed astigmatism*) (Fig. 14c).

Anisometropia. This is a condition in which there is an unequal degree of ametropia between the two eyes. It may be of different types; one eye may be emmetropic and the other eye hypermetropic or myopic, both eyes may be hypermetropic or myopic but to unequal degrees, or one eye may be hypermetropic and the other eye myopic (sometimes called antimetropia). It must be appreciated, of course, that small degrees of anisometropia are common and of little significance, but there is evidence that anisometropia is liable to lead to the development of a small-angle esotropia (microtropia) when it is present in early childhood.

Aniseikonia. This is a condition in which there is an unequal size of the retinal images in the two eyes. It may be produced in different ways: as a result of a significant degree of anisometropia—each 0·25 D of difference in refraction causes a 0·5 per cent size difference of the retinal images, as a result of wearing correcting lenses in the wrong positions relative to the eyes or, more rarely, as a result of some abnormality in the density of the retinal mosaic. It is possible for the visual cortex to compensate for certain degrees of aniseikonia, up to 5 per cent, by a perceptual process.

THE DETERMINATION OF REFRACTION

The refraction of the eye is measured by two main methods: first, objectively by the method of *retinoscopy*, and, second, subjectively by the effect of *correcting lenses*. These methods are discussed only briefly because detailed information about the prescription of glasses is beyond the scope of this book.

Retinoscopy

When rays of light from an electric self-illuminating retinoscope are projected into the eye they form an area of illumination on the retina. If the retinoscope is then tilted this area of illumination moves in the same direction as the tilting of the retinoscope—to the right, to the left, upwards, or downwards—and this movement of the illuminated area is independent of the type of refraction of the eye—emmetropia, hypermetropia or myopia—but the observer who is watching for such a movement through a small hole in the centre of the retinoscope is unaware of the real movement of the light on the retina because he obtains only an impression that the light originates from the punctum remotum, discussed above, which lies at infinity in emmetropia (Fig. 11), behind the eye in hypermetropia (Fig. 12), and in front of the eye in myopia (Fig. 13). It follows, therefore, that in emmetropia and in hypermetropia there is an awareness that the illuminated area moves in the same direction as the movement of the retinoscope, and in the opposite direction in myopia (Fig. 15). In emmetropia, if a convex lens of low power is placed in front of the eye, an artificial myopia is induced because parallel rays of light entering the eye come to a focus just in front of the retina, and there is then a reversal of the

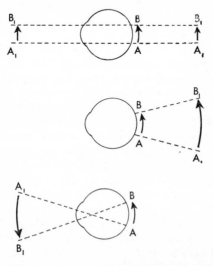

FIG. 15. *In retinoscopy the apparent movement of the illuminated retinal areas which is appreciated by the observer as coming from the punctum remotum (that is, movement from A_1 to B_1 (is in the same direction as the real movement of the illuminated retinal areas (that is, movement from A to B) in emmetropia (top) and in hypermetropia (middle), but in the opposite direction in myopia (bottom)*

apparent movement of the illuminated retinal area on moving the retinoscope. Similarly in hypermetropia a reversal is obtained by placing a sufficiently powerful convex lens in front of the eye to over-correct the hypermetropic error, and conversely in myopia a reversal of the opposite type is obtained by placing a concave lens of sufficient power in front of the eye to overcorrect the myopia. In this way the measurement of the lens, convex or concave, which is just sufficient to produce a reversal of the apparent movement of the illuminated retinal area, is a measure of the error of refraction of the eye. In theory this measurement should be recorded by the observer at an infinite distance from the eye, but in practice the observer is placed

1 metre from the eye and this introduces an error of 1 dioptre (1 D),
so that the amount of this error must be deducted from the final
measurement. Thus, the emmetropic eye is one in which a 1 D convex lens causes a reversal of the apparent movement of the illuminated
retinal areas when the observer is 1 metre from the eye. An astigmatic
error is assessed also by the method of retinoscopy by measuring
separately the refractive error which is present in the meridian of greatest refraction and in the meridian of least refraction.

Sometimes, particularly in children, it is necessary to carry out
retinoscopy after the use of a cycloplegic drug which temporarily
paralyses the accommodation of the eye, in order to permit an estimation of the correct amount of hypermetropic error (an effort of
accommodation during retinoscopy artificially decreases this measurement); such a drug also dilates the pupil (mydriasis) which facilitates
the examination of the fundus. In children, atropine 1 per cent drops
(or ointment) twice daily are effective in 3 days, and this provides
a complete cycloplegic effect, but cyclogel (Mydrilate) 1 per cent
drops are useful for rapid resting because they produce an adequate
degree of cyclopegia in 30 minutes; in adults homatropine 1 per cent
drops are effective in 30 minutes.

Subjective Test

The results of the objective method of retinoscopy are verified by a
subjective test which determines the best level of distant vision which
is obtained in each eye as measured by the Snellen's test types at
6 metres following the use of appropriate correcting lenses. These
lenses are convex (Fig. 16) in hypermetropia (although hypermetropia

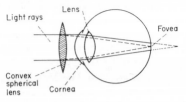

FIG. 16. *Correction of hypermetropia by a convex spherical lens*

may be corrected also by a simple act of accommodation, but the
extent of this correction will depend on the amount of accommodation available and on the degree of hypermetropia present), concave
(Fig. 17) in myopia, and cylindrical convex or concave lenses (which

have no refracting effects on rays of light which pass through them in the direction of their axes, but have the same effects as spherical lenses of equivalent dioptric power on rays of light which pass through them at 90° to their axes) in astigmatism; spherical lenses (convex or concave) are used in addition if it is necessary to correct any hypermetropic or myopic error.

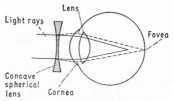

FIG. 17. *Correction of myopia by a concave spherical lens*

It is important also to determine the level of the near visual acuity of each eye after the correction of the refractive error. In the emmetropic eye there is sufficient accommodation to maintain a clear image of small print (N 5) at the normal reading range ($\frac{1}{3}$ metre) until about the age of 45 years (except in some eastern countries, for example in India, when this age is usually lower at about 38–40 years). Thereafter, however, the continued reduction in the available accommodation, due to a diminished ability of the lens to change its shape in response to a stimulus for accommodation, or perhaps to a diminished ability of the ciliary muscle to produce this change, causes blurring of small print. This is *presbyopia* and a convex spherical lens is then necessary for close reading; in emmetropia the appropriate convex lenses are used alone, but in hypermetropia, myopia or astigmatism they are used in addition to the normal correcting lenses for distant vision. In the early stages of presbyopia it is usually sufficient to prescribe + 0·50 D lenses, but this prescription is increased by + 0·50 D every few years up to a maximum of about + 2·50 D (or slightly more) by the age of 60 years. It should be noted, of course, that in uncorrected hypermetropia the onset of presbyopia will be earlier than in emmetropia because of the amount of accommodation which is expended in correcting the distant visual acuity, and that, conversely, in myopia it will be delayed; indeed in certain degrees of myopia there may be no need for the use of convex lenses for reading because the plus convex lenses for near vision would merely neutralize the minus concave lenses required for the myopia so that the correcting lenses are omitted for close reading.

CONTACT LENSES

The necessity to wear glasses for refractive errors may be avoided by the use of contact lenses which eliminate the influence of the anterior surface of the cornea as a refracting structure. There are two main types of contact lenses: first, *scleral lenses*, composed of a plastic material, which are moulded to fit accurately against the surface of the sclera and to cover the surface of the cornea without exerting any direct contact or pressure. This type of lens is designed to reduce the final refraction of the eye to a state of emmetropia, and any type of refractive error may be corrected in this way. Second, *corneal lenses* are small plastic lenses which lie on the surface of the cornea and have a similar effect to scleral lenses but with certain limitations; they are applicable only to a certain range of refractive error ($+$ 3 D to -8 D and 1·5 D of corneal astigmatism are suggested figures for this range, but there is some individual variation). They are liable to cause discomfort because of undue corneal sensitivity, although this usually becomes less after their persistent use; they are liable to cause a corneal abrasion when they are mishandled, and sometimes they are liable to be extruded during violent movements.

Of course, scleral contact lenses have a much wider application than the correction of simple refractive errors which may be corrected adequately by ordinary spectacle lenses: high degrees of myopia and astigmatism, conjunctival burns (chap. 3), keratoconus (chap. 3), corneal nebulae (chap. 3), certain serious forms of corneal ulceration (chap. 4), and ocular pemphigus (chap. 3) can all be treated therapeutically by means of these lenses. Specially designed shielded scleral lenses which limit the passage of light into the eye may be of value in albinism (chap. 6) or aniridia (chap. 6), and other lenses may be used purely for cosmetic purposes; a lens with a black centre to mask the presence of an opaque cataractous lens in a blind eye, or a lens incorporating a painted eye to wear over a useless microphthalmic eye or over a shrunken blind eye.

As a general rule scleral and corneal contact lenses are made of a fairly hard plastic material (polymethylmethacrylate), but more recently a hydrophilic acrylic soft contact lens has been devised which has advantages over a hard plastic lens because it permits some gaseous and water flow (but this advantage may be outweighed by the absence of movement of a soft lens as compared with a hard one) and also permits a rapid and permanent lid and corneal adaptation in the absence of any loss of normal corneal sensation. To some extent the soft contact lenses are still in the experimental stage and different materials are being tried; a homogeneous poly (2-hydroxyethylmethacrylate) HEMA, and a hydrophilic copolymer of the acrylate type which is a bionite material. It is possible also that silicon rubber may prove to be a suitable material, and, although not hydrophilic, this has the advantage of not being so susceptible to infection. It seems likely that further modifications of the hydrophilic contact lens will provide an improved form of lens for therapeutic purposes (such as in bullous keratopathy and in excessively dry eyes as in the Riley Day syndrome and in Sjögren's syndrome (chap. 3), quite apart from optical purposes.

Intraocular lens

It is also possible to provide an optical correction by the insertion in the eye of an acrylic lens (artificial lenticulus) which is designed to cater for the underlying refractive error; this may be placed in the anterior chamber, on the surface of the iris where it is held in place by clips, or in the position of the normal lens (that is, in the posterior chamber). As a general rule an intraocular lens is used in the correction of aphakia, but an anterior chamber implant is sometimes used in the phakic eye, as, for example, in the form of a specially shielded implant in aniridia.

Intracorneal lens

An acrylic lens inlay may be used within the cornea, but this is seldom carried out purely for refractive errors so that it is reserved largely for pathological conditions of the cornea which make a poor response to other methods of treatment (for example, bullous keratopathy chap. 4).

Keratomileusis

An attempt may be made to alter the refraction of the eye by changing the shape of the cornea. This involves removing a disc of the cornea through part of its thickness and, after freezing the tissue, the contours of the corneal disc are altered to counteract the refractive error of the eye so that when the disc is replaced (as in a lamellar keratoplasty) the refractive error of the eye is more nearly of a normal form; this operation is termed *keratomileusis*.

Colour Vision

The colour sense of the eye is its ability to distinguish different colours, and, like the form sense, it is mediated essentially by the cones. White light consists of impulses of different wave lengths so that it forms a spectrum with the following colours—red, orange, yellow, green, blue-green, blue and violet—from the longest (7000 Å) to the shortest (3800 Å) wave lengths, respectively. The true nature of colour appreciation in the retina is ill understood, but one of the most acceptable theories (the Young–Helmholtz theory) assumes the existence in the retina of three separate colour-perceiving elements and colour-transmitting mechanisms which are concerned with the three fundamental colours—red, green and blue—so that all colours are produced by varying degrees of stimulation of these elements and mechanisms and a white colour is produced by an equal stimulation of all three. In this way the person with normal colour appreciation has all three colour factors present and is termed a *trichromat* (hence its description as the *trichromatic theory*).

There are three different states of abnormal colour appreciation which are of congenital origin.

The Trichromat

The trichromat shows an anomaly (not an absence) of one factor. This may be of three types—a *protanomalous trichromat* when the red factor is weak, a *deuteranomalous trichromat* when the green factor is weak, and a *trianomalous trichromat* when the blue factor is weak. These anomalous trichromats are colour different rather than colour blind.

These forms of colour deficiency (dyschromatopsia) occur much more frequently in males than in females (8 per cent as compared with 0·4 per cent, in Western countries), and they show a well-marked hereditary pattern with a sex-linked recessive trait. Their recognition is of importance because of the use of colours in so many aspects of life; the teaching of junior mathematics at school, the labelling of electronic circuits, traffic light, etc.

The Dichromat

This person shows an absence (not an anomaly) of one factor and this may be of three types—a *protanope* when the red factor is absent, a *deuteranope* when the green factor is absent, and a *trianope* when the blue factor is absent.

The Monochromat

The monochromat shows an absence of colour appreciation so that there is a total colour blindness (*monochromatism*). This is of two types: *Cone monochromatism* (*cone dysfunction syndrome*) is a rare condition in which there is a disturbance of cone function (with a progressive loss of form and colour vision) but with no disturbance of rod function (so that peripheral vision is not lost). There are no ophthalmoscopic changes and the ERG is normal when this is of the usual scotopic type, but the photopic ERG is abnormal. In the second, *rod monochromatism*, the visual function of the eye is grossly abnormal with poor visual acuity, nystagmus and a marked intolerance of bright light.

It should be noted that the anomalous trichromat is much more common than the dichromat and that in each group the disturbance of the green factor is more common than the disturbance of the red factor and the disturbance of the blue factor is very rare. The monochromat, particularly the cone monochromat, is extremely rare.

In support of the trichromatic theory there is recent histological evidence of three types of cones in flat retinal preparations and also electrophysiological evidence of three different cone mechanisms because of the existence of three groups of modulators which are considered to subserve the function of hue discrimination in addition to dominators which are considered to subserve the function of luminosity discrimination. It is suggested also that the laminar system of the lateral geniculate body (chap. 16) is further evidence in support of the trichromatic theory, although this is largely a hypothesis. There are, however, certain objections to the theory and it is natural that other theories should have been put forward some of which are concerned with a four-colour concept with the addition of the colour yellow as well as the three other colours (red, green and blue); the introduction of this is based on psychological rather than physiological (or physical) considerations, and it is certainly important to recognize the psychological implications which are inherent in colour discrimination whereby a child is trained to appreciate the colours of different objects by name, although it is likely that such an appreciation is widely variable.

TESTS FOR COLOUR DISCRIMINATION

The Lantern Test

There are two main types of lantern: the Eldridge-Green lantern, which has a single aperture, and the Board of Trade lantern, which has two apertures. The significance of this difference is related to the phenomenon of *induction* which implies that the physiological changes which occur in the retina as the result of a stimulus are not limited to the time of the actual stimulus because of the phenomenon of *successive contrast* or *temporal induction* (the occurrence of positive and negative after-images after the primary stimulus), and also are not limited to the area of the retina stimulated by the actual stimulus because of the phenomenon of *simultaneous contrast* or *spatial induction* (the occurrence of modifications in the retina adjoining the stimulated area). The single aperture is suitable for assessing successive contrast, but the double aperture is necessary for assessing simultaneous contrast.

The Ishihara or Stilling Test

These tests are concerned with the identification of numbers on each of several plates which are formed of a series of large spots (mostly of reds or greens) against a background of large spots of other colours. The tests are more subtle than the lantern tests and are of value in identifying the anomalous trichromats (of the protanomalous or deuteranomalous types) who are often able to pass the lantern tests successfully.

There are certain diseases in which there is a change in colour appreciation, for example retrobulbar neuritis (chap. 8), toxic amblyopia (chap. 7) and chiasmal lesions (chap. 16).

Adaptation

The effect of a visual stimulus is not uniform because it depends on the state of adaptation of the retina at the time of the stimulus. In a state of light adaptation the vision is mediated largely by the cones which are concerned with the appreciation of form and colour (*photopic vision*), and in a state of dark adaptation the vision is mediated largely by the rods which are concerned essentially with the appreciation of light and movement (*scotopic vision*). This clear-cut distinction between the photopic and scotopic phases of vision is the basis of the classical *duplicity theory*. On passing from light into dark the process of dark adaptation takes place so that the retina increases markedly in sensitivity, rapidly during the first 10 minutes and then slowly up to a maximum of about 40 minutes; it follows that in dim illumination a faint stimulus is perceived which would be invisible under conditions of light adaptation. However, because the process of dark adaptation is essentially a function of the rods it does not occur uniformly throughout the retina; it occurs maximally in the peripheral parts of the retina but only minimally in the central part of the retina, so that in dim illumination the fovea and macula become virtually functionless. Conversely, on passing from dark into light the process of light adaptation occurs, a fairly rapid process, so that within a few seconds there is a marked decrease in the sensitivity of the retina; this is demonstrated by the quick acceptance of the light stimulus despite a momentary intense dazzle.

Night Blindness

This is a state in which the vision is usually fairly normal under conditions of good illumination but very defective under conditions of dim illumination; it occurs characteristically in a tapetoretinal degeneration of the retinitis pigmentosa type (chap. 7) and also in the retinal degeneration which occurs in association with keratomalacia as the result of a severe vitamin A deficiency.

Day Blindness

This is not a satisfactory term, but it is applied to a state in which there is a central scotoma (toxic amblyopia, macular degeneration, etc.) so that the eye appears to function more efficiently in dim illumination.

Depth Perception

As discussed in Chapter 13, stereopsis which is the highest form of binocular vision provides a perception of depth when there is a fusion of the retinal images of the two eyes during the bifoveal fixation of one object because of a small degree of dissimilarity of the images owing to the fact that each eye views the object from a very slightly different angle. It is evident, however, that a perception of depth is achieved by the use of one eye alone (uniocular vision) following the appreciation of various clues; the apparent sizes of different objects (the smaller the apparent size, the farther away is the object, etc.), the apparent colours of different objects (the less distinct the colour value, the farther away is the object, etc.) and the overlapping of contours of different objects (a near object may partly obliterate a distant object).

3 | Diseases of the Conjunctiva

Structure and Function

The conjunctiva is a mucous membrane which lines the under-surface of each eyelid (*palpebral conjunctiva*) and covers the surface of the eyeball (*bulbar conjunctiva*). The palpebral and bulbar conjunctivae are separated by a potential space (the conjunctival sac) which is closed above by the *superior fornix* (where the palpebral conjunctiva is reflected to form the bulbar conjunctiva), below by the *inferior fornix*, medially at the *medial canthus* (where there is a junction of the medial ends of the upper and lower lids) and laterally at the *lateral canthus*. The conjunctival sac is open externally between the upper and lower lid margins (*palpebral fissure*). The bulbar conjunctiva ends at the corneal margin (*limbus*) although its epithelium is continuous there with the corneal epithelium. The bulbar conjunctiva is separated from the underlying Tenon's capsule by a space (the sub-conjunctival space) and this capsule is separated from the underlying sclera by another space (the episcleral space) which contains the episcleral tissues.

The conjunctiva is richly supplied by arteries and veins, but under normal conditions most of these vessels are contracted so that they are scarcely visible. Two other structures lie in the conjunctival sac.

1. The *plica semilunaris* which is a crescentic shaped fold of conjunctiva arising from the region of the medial canthus immediately lateral to the caruncle with a free border directed towards the cornea. It corresponds to the third eyelid of certain animals (the nictitating membrane).

2. The *caruncle* which is a small red fleshy body lying on the medial side of the plica at the medial canthus. It represents a part of the margin of the lower lid which becomes isolated during early development.

28

The conjunctiva forms a protective coat over the underlying sclera and provides moisture to the eye by means of two types of gland:

Mucous glands. Mucus is secreted by goblet cells which are widespread in the conjunctival epithelium.

Serous glands. Lacrimal fluid is secreted by accessory lacrimal glands which are present in various parts of the conjunctiva, although the chief source of tears is from the main lacrimal gland (chap. 12).

Injuries

Haemorrhage. Any direct injury of the conjunctiva may cause a subconjunctival haemorrhage which is often widespread owing to the free nature of the subconjunctival space, although the haemorrhage shades off posteriorly and seldom spreads as far as the tissues of the orbit. This is in contrast to a haemorrhage which reaches the subconjunctival space from the orbit (for example after a fracture of orbit), which is intense posteriorly without any limiting edge.

Note: Subconjunctival haemorrhages may occur quite spontaneously in normal healthy people because of the exposed situation of the relatively fragile conjunctival vessels, although they are more likely in arteriosclerotic persons particularly after bouts of coughing. The haermorrhage usually persists for a week or so and remains red during this time because of free oxygenation of the blood through the thin conjunctival covering.

Laceration. Any direct injury of the conjunctiva is liable to cause its laceration. This heals readily, but when extensive it should be sutured with silk or catgut.

Foreign Body. Foreign bodies commonly enter the conjunctival sac from the atmosphere—particles of dirt, cigarette ash, steel from a grinding machine, husks of bird seed, etc. They are readily identified on the bulbar conjunctiva by opening the lids and on the palpebral conjunctiva of the lower lid or in the inferior fornix by pulling down the lower lid, but their identification on the palpebral conjunctiva of the upper lid demands eversion of the lid. This is achieved by standing behind the patient and, with the patient looking down and relaxing his lids by keeping them open, pulling the upper lid margin upwards with the forefinger and thumb of one hand whilst pressing on the upper border of the tarsal plate with the forefinger of the other

hand or with a glass rod. When it is necessary to expose the full extent
of the superior fornix, the fold of conjunctiva which projects from the
everted lid is everted also (double eversion of the upper eyelid) by the
use of a Desmarres eyelid retractor.

Chemical Burn. Chemical burns usually involve the lower part of
the bulbar conjunctiva because the reflex closure of the lids, which
follows the awareness of an approaching foreign substance, is preceded by an upturning of the eyeball (Bell's phenomenon). Ideally an
acid substance should be washed out by a weak alkali solution, such as
sodium bicarbonate, and an alkali substance by a weak acid solution,
such as boracic acid, but these are not always available and the
essential measure is to dilute and then to eliminate the chemical substance by rapid irrigation with water, often achieved effectively by
plunging the head with the eyes open into a basin of water. Thereafter
any secondary infection is avoided by giving local antibiotics supplemented by atropine 1 per cent drops if there is any associated corneal
damage.

Certain chemical agents, especially *lime*, may cause serious injury
because of their severe burning effects which tend to persist owing to
a collection of particles which are not readily removed by simple irrigation. Damage to the bulbar and palpebral conjunctivae may lead to
adhesions with obliteration of parts of the conjunctival sac (symblepharon). The cornea is also liable to be affected by direct damage, by
an encroachment of the affected conjunctiva on to the cornea, or by
excessive exposure when a symblepharon interferes with normal lid
closure; adhesions may be avoided by passing a glass rod across the
fornices each day until healing is complete. However in severe cases
an immediate amniotic membrane graft or the insertion of a large
specially moulded flush-fitting contact lens may sometimes be
necessary. If extensive adhesions develop they should be divided once
the condition becomes static (usually several months after the injury),
and an attempt made to retain the conjunctival space by the immediate fitting of a contact lens or to re-form the sac by the use of a
mucous membrane graft from the inner surface of the lower lip.

Conjunctivitis

Conjunctivitis, an inflammatory condition of the conjunctiva, is
usually of an infective nature, bacterial or viral, and may be acute,
subacute or chronic. Some cases, however, are of an allergic nature
and others are related to certain skin disorders.

INFECTIVE CONJUNCTIVITIS: ACUTE OR SUBACUTE CONJUNCTIVITIS

This almost invariably affects both eyes simulanteously, or within a short period of each other. It is the result of a variety of organisms (bacterial or viral), usually exogenous; it is therefore essentially a contagious disease fostered by crowded conditions and poor standards of cleanliness, although rarely the cause is endogenous. It commences as a feeling of discomfort of the eyes which often becomes intense with a sensation of grittiness but without any deep-seated pain except sometimes on exposure to bright light (photophobia). Characteristically there is a profuse discharge from the eyes which may be watery, mucous, mucopurulent or purulent according to the severity of the condition and according to the nature of the organism, and this accounts for the stickiness of the eyelids, particularly after sleep, and for the excoriation of the lid margins in the later stages. Sometimes the discharge may cause the appearance of rainbow effects as it passes across the cornea, but these, unlike the rainbows which occur in closed-angle glaucoma, disappear on blinking.

The degree of redness of the eyes also varies according to the severity and nature of the infection. It affects the bulbar and palpebral conjunctivae and is of a vivid type. Its superficial situation in the bulbar conjunctiva may be demonstrated by the movement of the reddened area on rubbing the margin of the lower lid against the bulbar conjunctiva (in contrast to the darker and deeper immovable type of redness which characterizes an episcleritis). The redness is less intense in the circumcorneal region (in contrast to the marked *circumcorneal* or *ciliary injection* which characterizes an iritis or closed-angle glaucoma). In severe cases the inflamed conjunctiva may be so congested that it becomes swollen (chemosis). Rarely the cornea becomes involved secondarily in a conjunctivitis, although there are certain inflammatory conditions in which the conjunctiva and cornea are involved together (*keratoconjunctivitis*).

Conjunctival Injection. This term refers to the redness which occurs in a conjunctivitis and also in other noninflammatory conditions, such as allergic disorders or as reactions to many irritants, e.g. foreign bodies, chemical agents, tobacco smoke and smog.

There are special features which characterize different forms of infective conjunctivitis according to the nature of the organism:

Bacterial Conditions

Morax-Axenfeld Diplobacillus. This causes a mild but fairly persistent catarrhal or occasionally mucopurulent conjunctivitis which is the result of the macerating effect of an enzyme secreted by the organism. The effect is usually limited to the regions of the lateral and medial canthi (hence the name *angular conjunctivitis*) because the action of the organism is inhibited to some extent by the lysozyme of the tears in the main part of the conjunctival sac. There is often a collection of froth-like secretion on the lid margins which produces a red and eczematous condition of the lids with a sensation of intense irritation and itchiness of the eyes.

Staphylococcus aureus (*Coagulase Positive*). This produces a conjunctivitis which is usually of the acute catarrhal type, but occasionally of a chronic nature with a marginal keratitis in which small white infiltrates (subepithelial keratitis) occur at the limbus with a tendency to spread circumferentially; this keratitis may be a sensitivity reaction to the staphyloccus (or to some other antigen).

Note : Staphylococcus aureus (*coagulase negative*) and *Staphylococcus albus* are not pathogenic in the conjunctiva.

Koch-Weeks Bacillus (*Haemophilus influenzae*). This is responsible for the large epidemics of mucopurulent conjunctivitis (*pink eye*) which are particularly common in closely confined communities.

Pneumococcus. This commonly follows an infection of the tear sac (dacryocystitis) and is prone to be associated with subconjunctival haemorrhage.

Gonococcus (*Micrococcus gonorrhoeae* or *Neisseria gonorrhoeae*). This organism is usually harboured by the abundant leucocytes within the secretion. The infection may occur in the newborn causing a severe bilateral conjunctivitis (ophthalmia neonatorum) within a few days of birth following a direct infection from the infected vaginal passage. Large amounts of purulent secretion accumulate under tension behind tightly closed swollen and red eyelids, necessitating great care during examination because of the tendency for pus to spurt into the examiner's eyes when attempts are made to prise the lids open. In severe cases there is rapid involvement of the cornea with ulcer formation which may lead to corneal perforation, loss of the anterior chamber and, frequently, damage to the anterior part of the lens (*anterior polar cataract*). Sometimes the perforation heals with a restoration of the anterior chamber although a fairly dense corneal scar persists, but at other times the underlying iris becomes adherent to the cornea with the formation of a *leucoma adherens*. In severe cases the infection may spread rapidly to involve the whole eye (*endophthalmitis* or *panophthalmitis*) with a subsequent shrinkage of the eye (*phthisis bulbi*), which becomes blind. At one time it was customary to try and prevent ophthalmia neonatorum by the routine use of silver nitrate 1 or 2 per cent drops (Credé's method) or sulphacetamide 10 per cent drops in the eyes of the newborn after the careful washing of the outer surfaces of the eyelids with simple lotion, but this prophylactic treatment has largely fallen into abeyance because it is not sufficient to prevent a severe infection like a gonococcal one and indeed it may mask the immediate effects of the infection so that its diagnosis (and, therefore, its treatment) are delayed. The only adequate prophylactic treatment for the child is to recognize and treat any infection of the mother during the pregnancy.

Ophthalmia neonatorum may also occur as a result of infection in the newborn infant by other organisms—*Koch-Weeks bacillus, pneumococcus, staphylococcus, Bacterium coli,* the *virus of trachoma or inclusion conjunctivitis* (TRIC agent), etc.—but these cause a much less severe condition, often with only slight mucopurulent discharge from the eyes, except for the TRIC agent (see chap. 3) which may be as lethal as the gonococcus. There is sometimes an associated failure of canalization of the nasolacrimal duct (chap. 12).

All cases of ophthalmia neonatorum—defined as 'a purulent discharge from the eyes of an infant commencing within 21 days from the date of its birth'—must be notified by the medical practitioner in attendance under the Public Health Regulations of 1926.

Gonococcal or TRIC agent conjunctivitis may occur also in other age groups, particularly in the adult following the direct introduction of the infective agent into the eye from a source of infection, for example a gonococcal urethritis of the patient or some other individual. It usually remains confined to one eye provided the spread of infection is avoided; a useful method is to enclose the affected eye in a special rubber shield (Buller's shield). The conjunctivitis develops after an incubation period of 2 to 5 days and is very acute with abundant creamy purulent discharge, massive chemosis and swelling of the lids. In contrast to most other forms of conjunctivitis the cornea is prone to develop ulceration of a severe type so that a perforation of the cornea and other complications (chap. 4) are likely.

Corynebacterium diphtheriae. This is liable to cause a severe conjunctivitis with the formation of a true membrane involving the mucosal and even the submucosal parts of the conjunctiva with an occasional spread of the membrane on to the skin of the lid. Removal of the membrane is usually followed by haemorrhage. Later it may be replaced by scar tissue with obliteration of parts of the fornix (symblepharon) or with some deformity of the eyelid such as an entropion.

Diphtheroid bacilli (for example, *Corynebacterium xerosis*) are not pathogenic in the conjunctiva. Other organisms, such as *Streptococcus haemolyticus, pneumococcus, meningococcus, Koch-Weeks bacillus*, may be associated rarely with membrane formation as part of a severe conjunctivitis, but in these conditions the membrane is a false one because it is not incorporated in the underlying tissues.

Pseudomonas pyocyanea (*Pseudomonas aeruginosa*). This rarely causes a primary conjunctivitis although a conjunctivitis may occur following inflammatory changes of the cornea (chap. 4).

Micrococcus catarrhalis. This causes a mild form of conjunctivitis.

Treatment of Bacterial Conjunctivitis

Discomfort is relieved by the removal of crusts and excessive secretions by simple irrigation with bland saline or boracic lotion, but too frequent irrigations are undesirable because they dilute the lysozyme of the tears which is an effective antibacterial substance. The eyes should not be bandaged. Dark glasses may be necessary if there is photophobia.

Antibacterial Treatment. There are many chemotherapeutic or antibiotic drugs which may be used locally in the eye in the form of drops during the day and in the form of ointment at night to prevent the adherence of the lids to one another. Penicillin in concentrations of 5000 units per ml or even higher is of great value against most Gram-positive cocci (except sometimes the staphylococcus), but it may be contraindicated in some cases because of an allergy or resistance to the drug. In gonococcal ophthalmia neonatorum the treatment must be intense—penicillin (10,000 units per ml) drops every minute for 30 minutes, every 5 minutes for 30 minutes and then every 30 minutes until the condition is controlled; systemic sulpha drugs are necessary when there is corneal involvement. Other drugs, such as chloramphenicol 0·5 per cent drops or 1 per cent ointment, neomycin 1 per cent drops or ointment, and bacitracin 1 per cent drops or ointment, have a fairly wide spectra of action. Polymyxin ointment 10,000 units per g is effective against the *Pseudomonas pyocyanea* and many other bacteria. Zinc sulphate drops 0·5 per cent or 1 per cent, often combined with adrenaline (1 in 1000) because of its vasoconstrictive effect, are specific against the effects of the enzyme of the Morax-Axenfeld bacillus. Silver preparations, for example in the form of Argyrol drops, are seldom used nowadays and so argyrosis—black-staining of the bulbar and palpebral conjunctiva particularly in the region of the inferior fornix—which follows their prolonged use is rarely seen.

Note: There is a tendency to omit the examination of the conjunctival secretion for the pathogenic organism as a routine procedure in cases of conjunctivitis because of the wide range of effectiveness of many of the modern drugs, but a culture of the organism and its sensitivity to various drugs should be carried out whenever possible and certainly in all cases which fail to show a quick response to treatment.

Viral Conditions

Conjunctivitis caused by a virus is usually associated with the formation of follicles, hence the term *follicular conjunctivitis*; but follicles occur in other conditions such as allergic ones so that it should not be considered as indicative only of a viral condition. The follicles represent proliferations of the normal lymphoid tissue, which is present in the submucosal (adenoid) layer of the conjunctiva, and appear as pale slightly raised patches of relatively small size, which are arranged in regular rows within the palpebral conjunctivae, particularly of the lower lids. More rarely a virus infection is associated with ulcerative or granulomatous changes.

There are several different forms of viral conjunctivitis:

1. *Inclusion conjunctivitis.* This is produced by one of the TRIC viruses (Chlamydia oculogenitale). It develops after an incubation period of 5 to 9 days. The virus may be isolated in the cervix or male urethra. It is confirmed by the presence in conjunctival scrapings of characteristic basophilic cytoplasmic inclusion bodies within the epithelial cells. It is usually self-limiting but sometimes resolution may be accelerated by the use of topical antibiotics. Rarely this virus may be responsible for a form of ophthalmia neonatorum (chap. 5) Sometimes an inclusion conjunctivitis is associated with limbal lesions (pannus) or with a punctate keratitis.

2. *Trachoma.* This is an endemic condition in certain parts of the world, for example in the Middle East and in parts of Eastern Europe, but it is rare in this country although sporadic cases have appeared since it was introduced first in the early part of the nineteenth century under the name of *Egyptian ophthalmia*. It is a highly contagious condition caused by one of the TRIC viruses (Chlamydia trachomatis). It is characterized by the formation of Halberstaedter

Prowazek inclusions (elementary bodies) within the affected conjunctival and corneal cells, but many of the later and severe complications are largely from a secondary invasion of the affected tissues by bacteria; this explains the prevalence of such complications in crowded and unhygienic surroundings, although these conditions also favour the spread of the causative virus. The disease presents, after an incubation period of about one week, as an acute bilateral conjunctivitis with intense discomfort, photophobia and redness of the eyes. There is an associated marked thickening of the palpebral conjunctiva resulting from *papillary hypertrophy*, with a gradual thickening and engorgement of the surface layers so that the conjunctiva assumes a rich velvety red appearance which obscures the underlying conjunctival vessels and tarsal glands. *Follicular formations*, which are localized accumulations of lymphocytes, plasma cells and epithelioid cells in the subconjunctival tissues, project through the surface of the conjunctiva to form round translucent prominences suggestive of sago grains or frog spawn. These follicles occur to some extent over the whole conjunctiva but are most obvious on the palpebral conjunctiva, particularly of the upper lid, and are responsible for the granular appearance which provides the name *trachoma* (from Greek 'roughness'). The cornea is also involved, not simply because of the rubbing on the cornea of the granular undersurfaces of the upper lids, but as the result of a primary involvement which causes punctate epithelial erosions, punctate epithelial keratitis, and punctate subepithelial keratitis with the production of distinctive yellowish coloured subepithelial opacities. These changes occur particularly in the upper part of the cornea and are accompanied by a superficial vascularization of the affected area with the formation of scarring (*superficial pannus*) which causes a disturbance of vision when it extends into the central parts of the cornea.

The infective stage of trachoma tends to be self-limiting after a period of months or even years, but changes continue in the tissues of the lids because of the proliferation of scar tissue which occurs in the previously hypertrophied subepithelial tissues and within the tarsal plate so that the palpebral conjunctiva, although becoming relatively white and smooth, develops radiating lines of scarring which are important diagnostic features of the disease. This scarring is liable also to lead to adhesions between the bulbar and palpebral conjunctivae, particularly of the upper lid, with partial obliteration of the fornices (symblepharon), and to entropion of the eyelids, particularly the upper one, so that the eyelashes turn in and rub on the cornea.

Trichiasis may occur also by the development of aberrant lashes. Ptsosis of the upper lid may follow an increased bulk of the lid or an involvement of the levator muscle (or its associated smooth muscle). The corneal pannus may become less marked in time, but some permanent scarring is inevitable and the development of small irregular faceted scars, which are often difficult to detect, is liable to affect the vision markedly.

The diagnosis of trachoma is often easy because of the many distinctive clinical features, but it is confirmed in the laboratory by an identification of the specific inclusion bodies within damaged epithelial cells in conjunctival scrapings, by the isolation of the virus, and by the presence of polymorphonuclear leucocytes and mononuclear cells, in the absence of eosinophils, in conjunctival scrapings. This typical cytology is a feature of TRIC infection.

The treatment of trachoma is aimed at the control of the causal agent and of the secondary infection. Local antibiotics or chemotherapeutic agents are instilled (frequent chloramphenicol 0·5 per cent drops or Albucid 30 per cent drops, or less frequent long-acting sulpha drugs such as tetracycline ointment), and chemotherapeutic drugs given systemically (sulphadiazine $\frac{1}{2}$ g tablets: adults 4 tablets initially, 2 tablets four times daily for one week, 1 tablet three times daily for a further week; the dose is appropriately reduced for children). Rarely if excessive conjunctival hypertrophy persists the follicles may be expressed by specially designed pressure forceps (*Graddy's forceps*) or roller forceps (*Knapp's forceps*), or the general bulk of the conjunctiva may be reduced simply by repeated local cauterizations with copper sulphate (the classical 'blue-stone stick') or with silver nitrate 1 per cent solution. In the later stages surgical treatment may be necessary to correct the deformities of the lids (removal of the thickened tarsal plate, correction of the entropion, transplantation of the lashes, etc.) or keratoplasty for severe corneal scarring (a contact lens may provide a useful level of vision without recourse to keratoplasty, the results of which may be prejudiced by the unhealthy state of the cornea and by the vascularization).

3. Conjunctivitis in *lymphogranuloma venereum*.

4. Conjunctivitis in *Reiter's Disease* in which a mild catarrhal conjunctivitis is associated with urethritis, polyarthritis and pyrexia.

5. Conjunctivitis in virus conditions of the skin: (*a*) *Molluscum contagiosum*, (*b*) *Vaccinia* and *Variola*.

6. Conjunctivitis in virus conditions of the cornea: (*a*) epidemic

keratoconjunctivitis, (*b*) herpes simplex, and (*c*) herpes zoster (chap. 4).

7. Conjunctivitis in systemic virus conditions such as measles and mumps which may be exogenous or endogenous.

The two other forms of infective conjunctivitis are:

Granulomatous Conjunctivitis. This is characterized by the formation of granulomatous masses together with a generalized conjunctivitis of the affected eye, a regional adenitis particularly the preauricular lymph nodes, and sometimes a pyrexia—a symptom complex known as *Parinaud's oculoglandular syndrome.* It may be exogenous or endogenous in association with certain diseases: syphilis in the form of a large painful ulcer (*primary chancre*) or of a localized inflammatory mass (*gumma*) of the underlying episcleral tissues or tarsal plate; tuberculosis in the form of a raised mass of the bulbar conjunctiva which may form indolent ulceration; viruses such as *lymphogranuloma venereum*; leprosy in the form of nodules in the palpebral conjunctiva particularly near the lid margins or in the bulbar conjunctiva usually near the limbus with subsequent involvement of the cornea (unlike other forms of granulomatous conjunctivitis it may be bilateral); and *glanders, tularaemia* and *fungus conditions* such as *rhinosporidiosis.* The treatment is aimed at the general disease with local treatment to combat any secondary infection, although sometimes it is necessary to excise the nodular lesions (which should of course be examined histologically).

Endogenous Conjunctivitis. This occurs in certain systemic disorders, e.g. measles, influenza, glandular fever, leptospirosis, and gonorrhoea (in its later stages), as a result of an endogenous infection, although the exogenous type of conjunctivitis is more common.

CHRONIC CONJUNCTIVITIS

This is induced in various ways: as the aftermath of a severe attack (or repeated attacks) of acute or subacute conjunctivitis sometimes in association with an excessive or prolonged use of topical drugs; as the result of undue exposure of the bulbar conjunctiva in exophthalmos, proptosis, facial paralysis or ectropion; or as the result of defective tear drainage through the lacrimal passages which is usually associated with some recurrent infection from the tear sac. The symptoms are similar to those of 'eyestrain'—a tiredness and heaviness of the eyes particularly after prolonged use, a sensation of grittiness and a feeling of excessive heat of the eyes. The affected conjunctiva is hyperaemic, and there is a persistent discharge, sometimes of an infective nature but usually merely an excess of the normal mucous secretions of the conjunctiva and often also of the sebaceous discharges from the tarsal (Meibomian) glands of the eyelids; these account for the redness of the lid margins which is a common feature.

Treatment is aimed at removing the cause of the condition, the control of any infection, the discontinuance of harmful drugs, the relief of any nasolacrimal obstruction and the correction of any deformity of the eyelids. Sometimes the local application of an astringent, such as silver nitrate 1 per cent, to the palpebral surfaces, or more simply the use of saline or boracic lotion may relieve the symptoms.

Allergic Conjunctivitis and Keratitis

Vernal Conjunctivitis and Keratitis (*Spring Catarrh*). This allergic condition follows exposure to certain external agents, such as pollens, and occurs usually but not invariably during the summer (the term *spring catarrh* is a misnomer) in children and young adults. The conjunctivitis is a constant feature with the development of a slightly milky-white translucence of the bulbar conjunctivae of both eyes and with the formation of flattened papillae ('cobblestones') of the palpebral conjunctivae particularly of the upper lids. Similar conjunctival thickenings may occur at the limbus. The predominant symptoms are discomfort and intense itching during the active stages. The *keratitis* occurs in certain cases following an extension of the limbal conjunctival lesions with the formation of a vascularized pannus which resembles the pannus of trachoma, except that it is not invariably at the upper part of the cornea, or sometimes as a separate entity in the form of a punctate keratitis with minute dull grey spots particularly in the upper part of the cornea but not at the extreme periphery. Rarely the keratitis may be of the ulcerative type with the formation of a transversely oval ulcer involving the anterior part of the stroma, causing a permanent scar. The keratitis of spring catarrh is aggravated by the roughened undersurfaces of the upper lids and by the deposits of any therapeutic agent which forms suspensions. Scrapings of the conjunctiva show an inflammatory exudate which contains lymphocytes, plasma cells, usually abundant eosinophils, and often damaged epithelial cells.

Treatment. The local condition may be relieved by steroid solutions, but these should be limited to soluble preparations, for example prednisolone drops. Sometimes systemic steroid therapy may be advisable. Care should be exercised, however, in the long-term use of steroids because of the complications which may occur, particularly a form of glaucoma in the susceptible individually by topical steroids and cataract by systemic steroids. The cobblestones may be excised when excessively large with or without a replacement mucosal graft (for example, from the buccal mucosa). Atropine and antibiotic drops are necessary when there is active keratitis. In severe and unresponsive cases small doses of beta irradiation may suppress the condition. It should be noted that it is usually a self-limiting disease which seldom persists into adult life.

Phlyctenular Keratoconjunctivitis. This is an allergic condition, almost certainly of an endogenous nature, which occurs as a response to tuberculoprotein or perhaps to a toxic agent in association with a septic focus. The basic lesion (*the phlycten*) represents a responsive reaction of tissues which have been sensitized to the allergen following infection by the specific agent. It occurs almost exclusively in young children, particularly in conditions of poor hygiene and defective nutrition. The phlyctens appear as discrete raised pink spots on the bulbar conjunctiva or on the cornea particularly near the limbus, and are associated with leashes of superficial vessels. They represent subepithelial aggregations of polymorphonuclear leucocytes and usually form ulcerated areas as a result of a loss of their overlying epithelial covering, although without any involvement of the deeper tissues unless there is a marked associated secondary infection. These areas cause severe pain, intense photophobia, lacrimation and tight closure of the reddened lids (blepharospasm). There is usually a positive skin sensitivity to tuberculoprotein. The condition is prone to recurrences.

Treatment. This is sometimes ineffective, but corticosteroid drops are often of value in relieving the symptoms. Any secondary infection should be treated by local antibiotic drops, and any frank corneal ulceration should be treated by the usual methods taking care to avoid cortisone during the active stage.

Other Forms of Allergic Conjunctivitis. These occur on contact with many substances in patients who develop a sensitivity to their use. Certain drugs such as atropine and penicillin are liable to produce an allergic reaction, although usually only after prolonged use. Similarly pollens may induce an allergic conjunctivitis in association with profuse watery discharge from the nose (hay fever), and cosmetics, particularly those which are applied near the eye such as mascara or which are introduced into the eye by rubbing with the fingers such as nail varnish, may cause an allergic conjunctivitis. The condition is characterized by a profuse watery discharge from both eyes with a marked hyperaemia of the conjunctiva, an eczematous and swollen condition of the lids, and by a tendency for follicles to occur in the palpebral conjunctiva, particularly of the lower lids.

Treatment. Antistin-Privine drops may relieve some of the irritation and redness but corticosteroid drops are usually more effective. Systemic antihistamine therapy may also be necessary. It is important to identify the allergic agent; sometimes this is determined by sensitization skin tests, but in the case of cosmetics it is usually sufficient to omit all cosmetics for a period and then to reintroduce them one by one until a reaction becomes apparent. It is then possible to avoid the allergen or to desensitize the patient by graduated injections.

CONJUNCTIVITIS AND KERATITIS IN ASSOCIATION WITH SKIN DISEASES

Acne Rosacea

This condition is probably a metabolic disorder with perhaps also some hormonal disorder because it is most common in females after the onset of the menopause; it is interesting, however, that particularly severe cases may occur in men. Characteristic changes occur in the skin of the face with a 'butterfly-wing' distribution over the cheeks and nose associated with ocular changes, which may be more or less severe than the skin changes. There is usually a fairly marked chronic blepharoconjunctivitis, but the characteristic lesions occur on the cornea as a marginal keratitis particularly of the lower (and more exposed) region with the formation of fairly large, tongue-shaped, greyish-white, superficial infiltrations spreading from the limbus towards the more central part of the cornea with leashes of superficial vessels from the limbal circulation. Sometimes fine or coarse forms of epithelial keratitis also occur with the later occurrence of subepithelial opacities of a slightly yellow colour. The condition generally pursues a relatively mild but chronic course with periods of recession and recrudescence, but sometimes it is severe with widespread involvement of the cornea and a consequent disturbance of vision and even an associated deep keratitis. A generalized feeling of discomfort of the eye and eyelids is associated with photophobia when there are active corneal lesions.

Treatment. Most cases respond initially to topical corticosteroids

and to antibiotics which control any secondary infection, but
recurrences are common. In severe cases small doses of beta irradiation are of value. It is important to treat any associated skin lesions
and gastric dysfunction (sometimes from an achlorhydria, but more
often from dietary indiscretions) by appropriate measures.

Pemphigus

Generalized Pemphigus. In the acute form the conjunctiva and
cornea may be associated in the generalized changes of the skin
and mucous membranes, but they are overshadowed by the acute-
ness of the other manifestations often in association with signs of
marked toxaemia.

Localized Pemphigus. The surface tissues of the eye may be
involved in a condition which resembles pemphigus, and often
without any obvious changes in the skin. The lesions occur in the
conjunctiva with a secondary fibrosis of the subconjunctival tissues; in
the early state lines of tension form between the bulbar and palpebral
conjunctiva and later develop into a symblepharon with partial
obliteration of the conjunctival sac. There are subsequent degenerative changes in the cornea because of exposure due to faulty closure
of the eyelids and to loss of the normal moisture of the eye. This latter
follows destruction by fibrosis of the conjunctival mucous glands and
obliteration of the lacrimal ducts which discharge the lacrimal fluid
(tears) into the conjunctival sac from the main and accessory lacrimal
glands. Suppuration of the degenerate cornea is a likely terminal
event leading to an endophthalmitis and subsequent phthisisis
bulbi.

Treatment. An attempt is made to retain the integrity of the conjunctival sac by a division of any adhesions and by the immediate
insertion at operation of a haptic contact shell which is maintained
indefinitely. Unfortunately this shell may be extruded by further
scarring, but this method of treatment probably offers a better chance
than an attempt to line the re-formed sac by a mucous membrane
graft.

Erythema Exudativum Multiforme (Stevens-Johnson Syndrome).
This occurs in young people and causes a widespread exudative
erythema of the skin, particularly the hands, forearms and neck,
and of the mucous membranes of the conjunctiva, mouth and genital
passages. Its affect on the eye is similar to ocular pemphigus—symblepharon formation and a marked tendency to severe corneal ulceration.
The treatment also is similar.

Keratoconjunctivitis sicca

This follows a grossly diminished tear formation in association with a diminution of the secretions of the salivary, sweat and mucous glands so that the dryness of the eyes is accompanied by a dryness of the mouth, skin, and other mucous surfaces. There may be an associated rheumatoid arthritis, Raynaud's phenomenon, or lupus erythematosis, a symptom-complex which is termed *Sjögren's syndrome*. It is also sometimes associated with *Felty's syndrome* (leucopenia, splenomegaly, and rheumatoid arthritis). The condition probably has some hormonal background because it occurs predominantly in women after the onset of the menopause. It may also follow a destructive autoimmune process of the glandular tissues which leads ultimately to atrophy. Interestingly there is a close resemblance between the histology of the lacrimal gland in this disease and the histology of the thyroid gland in Hashimoto's disease (which follows an autoimmune process), particularly as the lacrimal and thyroid glands are immunologically related tissues.

Scattered foci of desiccation occur in epithelium of the conjunctiva and cornea; this is demonstrated by a vital dye like Rose Bengal. Sometimes the epithelium of the desiccated cornea is not shed and remains attached at one end with the formation of small filaments which may have a mucous covering—*filamentary keratitis* (this also occurs in viral keratitis).

Treatment. The dryness is relieved by artificial tears (for example, methyl cellulose 1 per cent drops, which have the merit of a more persistent action than a lotion such as saline, because of their slightly oily nature). Sometimes sealing of the lacrimal puncta by cauterization may help to conserve any available moisture of the eye, but this is reserved for cases without any hope of spontaneous recovery.

Degenerations

Concretions

These occur in the crypts of the palpebral conjunctiva following a gradual accumulation of inflammatory or degenerative products. They usually remain as small white spots, of little or no significance, but sometimes they become calcareous and project beyond the surface level causing irritation. They may be removed easily by a sharp-pointed instrument such as a capsulotomy needle using a surface anaesthetic (cocaine 4 per cent drops).

Pingueculae

These are yellow-coloured oval slightly raised masses which form on the bulbar conjunctiva on either or both sides of the cornea in the interpalpebral area; the slightly broader part of the lesion is directed towards the cornea. They occur almost universally, particularly after middle age, and represent hyaline degenerative changes in an area exposed to dust and wind. Treatment is by simple excision, although this is seldom indicated because the resultant scar tissue is likely to be as obvious as the pinguecula. Sometimes, however, a pinguecula extends to form a pterygium.

Pterygium

This degenerative condition of the conjunctiva is associated with similar changes in the cornea. It presents as a wing-shaped vascular thickening of the bulbar conjunctiva which begins on either or both sides of the cornea, more commonly on the nasal side, often following enlargement of a pinguecula. It only merits the name *pterygium* when the part adjacent to the cornea (its head) encroaches on to the cornea and insinuates itself between the epithelium and Bowman's membrane. This encroachment occurs when there are superficial degenerative changes in the cornea of a primary nature, which are shown by the grey edge in the superficial corneal tissues distal to the spreading head of the pterygium. The main part (the body) of the pterygium also extends in the opposite direction so that its terminal part (the tail) reaches the region of the medial (or lateral) canthus. It occurs essentially following persistent exposure to wind and dust so that it is common in parts of the world like the Middle East and Australia, but it may occur in any country.

Treatment. If a pterygium is threatening to involve the central part of the cornea or if it is cosmetically unsightly it should be removed. It is usual to shave the head of the pterygium from the cornea, and to remove the bulk of the pterygium by a subconjunctival approach; a fairly large portion of the conjunctiva near the limbus is also removed so that a bare area of sclera remains after the operation which should prevent a further encroachment of the conjunctival tissues on to the affected part of the cornea before healing is complete. Postoperative beta irradiation is useful in recurrent cases or sometimes following the first operation when the pterygium is fleshy and 'active' looking. The affected part of the cornea remains permanently scarred even after a successful operation so that it is essential to operate before the central part of the cornea is involved, although in advanced cases this complication may be overcome by combining the removal of the pterygium with a lamellar keratoplasty.

Note: Pseudopterygium. When a fold of conjunctiva becomes adherent to a limbal corneal lesion like an ulcer the appearance is similar to a true pterygium, but it is distinguished by demonstrating the bridge-like nature of the encroachment in a pseudopterygium so that a probe is readily passed under it.

Cysts

Lymphatic Cysts

These appear as small worm-like dilatations of clear thin-walled vessels. They may be removed by simple excision (although care should be taken to localize them by a suture before opening the conjunctiva otherwise they may be obscured by haemorrhage); simple incision is liable to be followed by recurrence.

Implantation Cysts

These occur in the subconjunctival tissues following the implantation of a fragment of conjunctiva after injury or operation. If they become large they are readily excised.

TUMOURS

Various tumours may arise in the conjunctiva, particularly at the limbus, but they are rare.

Papilloma

This is a benign epithelial tumour which appears as a small raised vascular mass with an irregular surface.

Epithelioma

This may follow malignant change in a papilloma, but it also occurs spontaneously or in a previously inflamed or injured area. It forms a raised vascular mass which is often only locally invasive, but sometimes it may spread to the regional lymph nodes (preauricular and cervical) or it may even form distant metastases. The histological appearances are variable; it is usually a *squamous cell carcinoma* but may be a *basal cell carcinoma* or an intraepithelial epithelioma (*Bowen's disease*) in which the lesions appear as slightly elevated diffuse patches of highly vascular gelatinous tissue of a yellowish-grey colour, characteristically in elderly men.

Melanoma

This term is applied to a group of tumours composed of pigment-producing (melanocytic) cells which clinically and histologically may be subdivided into different groups:

Simple Melanoma and Malignant Melanoma. A simple melanoma is a congenitally determined tumour and usually presents as a small red spot which only becomes obviously pigmented some years later, often around puberty. Commonly it lies in apposition to the basal epidermal layers (*junctional naevus*) but sometimes it involves the underlying tissues (*deep* or *intradermal naevus*). It is uncertain whether it has a neurogenic or epidermal mode of origin. Rarely it may become malignant (*malignant melanoma*) with the formation of a raised pigmented spreading mass and with inflammatory changes in the surrounding tissues.

Precancerous Melanosis and Cancerous Melanosis (Malignant Melanoma). Precancerous melanosis is an acquired disease which occurs particularly in the middle-aged, more commonly in women. One or more flat pigmented areas, each of which may show evidence of progression of regression at various stages, form within the basal layers of the epithelium (*intraepithelial melanoma*). The condition may remain benign for an indefinite period, but sometimes malignancy develops after a period of 5 to 10 years with the formation of a typical *malignant melanoma (cancerous melanosis).*

Blue Naevus and Malignant Blue Naevus. These are exceedingly rare tumours of the conjunctiva.

Granuloma

This is liable to follow operative trauma if Tenon's capsule is incorporated in the conjunctival wound or if there is a reaction to suture material (usually catgut, as in a squint operation). It may also occur in the palpebral conjunctiva as an extension of a Meibomian cyst (chalazion).

Various Tumours of Vascular Origin

These, which include *lymphoma, lymphosarcoma, angioma, lymphangioma,* and *endothelioma (perithelioma)*, occur rarely.

Dermoid and Dermolipoma

These are benign growths which are congenitally determined.

Treatment of Conjunctival Tumours. In general benign tumours may be treated by simple excision and malignant tumours by excision and postoperative irradiation.

4 | Diseases of the Cornea

Structure and Function

The cornea forms the anterior one-sixth of the outer coat of the eyeball (the sclera forming the remaining five-sixths), and is composed of the following five layers (Fig. 18).

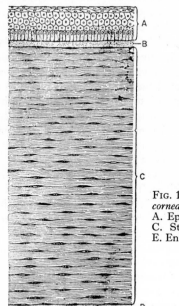

FIG. 18. *The histological appearances of the cornea*
A. Epithelium; B. Bowman's membrane; C. Stroma; D. Descemet's membrane; E. Endothelium.

The Epithelium. The delicate squamous surface epithelium is continuous with the conjunctival epithelium at the limbus. It is analogous to skin epithelium except that there is no keratinization of the surface cells (and it is therefore transparent) and there is no close union with the underlying tissue (Bowman's membrane). The epithelium is maintained in position by a suction pressure exerted by the under-lying stromal tissues. The epithelium permits the passage of water into the cornea but restricts the passage of salts so that there is a very limited entry of tears into the intact cornea. The integrity of the epithelium is dependent on a free supply of oxygen, hence the oede-matous changes which follow ill-fitting contact lenses. Defects of the epithelium heal readily by a rapid sliding process of the surrounding epithelial cells.

Bowman's Membrane. A thin lamina of condensed stromal tissue which is fairly resistant to injury or disease, but once perforated it does not regenerate and is replaced by scar tissue.

The Stroma. This represents 90 per cent of the thickness of the cornea and is continuous with the sclera. It is composed of many lamellae which lie parallel to one another with little or no inter-lacing. Each lamella contains uniform collagen fibrils which extend across the cornea in parallel sheets. The stroma is avascular, and the fibrils are separated from one another by a ground substance or tissue fluid, probably of a mucinous nature, which creates a suction mech-anism so that certain constituents of the aqueous humour, and to a slight extent of the tears, are drawn into the cornea to maintain its nourishment; some nourishment also reaches the stroma from the limbal circulation. The rigid layering of the lamellae is of surgical importance because it facilitates the removal of a uniformly thick disc of corneal tissue (lamellar graft) along a precise plane of cleavage; it also permits a fairly marked swelling of the stromal tissues by fluid under certain pathological conditions. To a large extent the precise arrangement of the collagen fibrils in the stroma determines its transparency. If this arrangement is disturbed by mechanical stress following injury, by a sudden rise of pressure within the eye, as in the acute phase of a closed-angle glaucoma, or by an oedema of the ground substance, as in deep keratitis, there is a scattering of the light rays by interference with a loss of transparency. The avascularity of the stroma also determines its transparency so that the entry of vessels into the stroma, often as a result of an increase in the spaces between the fibrils permitting the entry of capillary vessels in certain diseased conditions, results in some loss of transparency.

Descemet's Membrane. This is a thin lamina which separates the stroma from the underlying endothelium. It is fairly resistant to injury and disease.

The Endothelium. This is a thin single layer of cells on the inner surface of the cornea in continuity with the endothelial covering of the trabecular tissues in the filtration angle and with the surface endothelial layer of the iris. It has a protective function in controlling the access of the intraocular fluid (*aqueous humour*) into the stroma, and it plays an active part in pumping fluid out of the cornea so that a loss of the endothelium may result in a 'water-logging' of the corneal stroma. It follows that changes in the endothelium as a result of injury, for example during an intraocular operation such as cataract extraction, or as a result of degenerative changes, may indirectly result in oedematous changes in the epithelium and stroma (*bullous keratopathy*). The diameter of the normal cornea is about 11·7 mm horizontally and 10·6 mm vertically.

The Corneal Reflexes

Light from a window or electric light source is mirrored on the anterior surface of the cornea as a bright reflex—this is one of the Purkinje-Samson images (the other images being formed by the posterior surface of the cornea and by the anterior and posterior surfaces of the lens)—and the clarity and uniformity of this corneal reflection are dependent on the normal transparency and curvature of this corneal surface.

The two drugs which are of diagnostic value in corneal lesions are:

Fluorescein (2 per cent drops). This dye stains immature epithelial cells (exposed by the removal of the surface cells following injury or disease) a very bright shade of green, and areas of defective epithelium) a less bright shade of green. Fluorescein will also stain the fluid layer which is normally present on the cornea (this precorneal fluid is composed of tears from the lacrimal gland, mucus from the conjunctival glands and sebaceous material from the Meibomian or tarsal glands of the lids). If excess dye is removed by an irrigation with saline before examining the eye, fluorescein staining of epithelium will not be confused with fluorescein in the precorneal fluid.

Rose Bengal (1 per cent drops). This is a dye which stains diseased epithelial cells, for example as a result of intense viral invasion or as the result of desiccation.

Corneal Sensitivity

The normal corneal epithelium is very sensitive to touch; the sensation which is mediated is essentially one of pain and serves a protective function. Any prolonged infective condition of the epithelium impairs this sensation thus rendering the cornea more liable to subsequent disease; this is noted particularly after recurrent bouts of viral keratitis, the so-called *keratitis metaherpetica.*

Congenital Anomalies

Microcornea

A small cornea occurs in a small eye (*microphthalmos*) which follows a developmental failure of the whole eye, but it occurs also in an otherwise normal eye. It produces a hypermetropic refractive error and its association with a narrow filtration angle may predispose to a closed-angle glaucoma.

Megalocornea

A large cornea occurs in an otherwise normal eye of males only and may predispose to a dislocation of the lens or to a cataract. It causes myopia and is distinguished from the enlarged cornea which occurs in high axial myopia by the absence of changes in the posterior segment of the eye (chap. 2), and from the enlarged cornea which occurs in buphthalmos by the absence of the other defects which develop in the cornea (chap. 15).

Injuries

Abrasion

The cornea is highly susceptible to superficial injury because of the delicate state of its epithelium. It is usually the lower part of the cornea which is affected because the eye turns up during the instinctive closure of the eyelids as a protective response to an approaching object. An abrasion causes immediate and often severe pain, redness of the conjunctiva, particularly in the circumcorneal region, and intense lacrimation. The abrasion usually heals rapidly within 12 to 24 hours unless a secondary infection of the abraded area causes a corneal ulcer with all its subsequent complications.

Treatment. This consists of the prevention of secondary infection by antibiotic drops, and of pupillary spasm by atropine drops, of the relief of pain by covering the eye, and of the avoidance of any adhesions between the abraded area of the cornea and the under-surface of the upper lid by a lubricating agent such as liquid paroleine or an antibiotic ointment.

Recurrent Erosion

Any form of corneal abrasion (classically the scratch from a baby's fingernail) may break down repeatedly, even months after an injury. It usually occurs on opening the eye in the early morning when an adhesion between the undersurface of the upper lid and the epithelial cells of the healed cornea area which formed during sleep is broken, stripping cells from the cornea (it can also occur at other times). It seems likely that some acquired defect renders these cells more 'tacky' than usual.

Treatment. Each recurrence is treated as an abrasion, and an attempt is made to avoid recurrences by the prolonged use of a lubricating agent (for example, paroleine drops) at night until the injured area is completely healed. Cauterization of the affected corneal area in a recurrent erosion is sometimes advocated but this is a procedure of doubtful validity because it may not avoid further recurrences and it may cause certain complications. The development of scarring of the region of Bowman's membrane creates an irregular surface which prevents the epithelium of the surrounding cornea from covering it adequately, and the development of an oedematous reaction within the corneal stroma may be followed by the production of a disciform keratitis with permanent scarring and vacularization. Recalcitrant cases may benefit by superficial beta irradiation.

Superficial Foreign Bodies

The cornea is a frequent target for foreign bodies which are wind-swept into the eyes or directed into the eyes in occupations which utilize grinding machines. The foreign body usually lodges in the lower part of the cornea because of the reflex turning up of the eye as the eyelids close forcibly on the awareness of an approaching object (Bell's phenomenon). The impact of the foreign body causes immediate pain, redness and lacrimation and a gritty sensation on movement of the eyelids over the affected area. The foreign body is readily visible on focal illumination against the background of the iris, but sometimes it comes into view only on looking at the cornea in a particular direction or by the use of a slit-lamp microscope.

Treatment. It is sometimes possible for the patient to dislodge the foreign body by rapid and forcible movements of the lids over the corneal surface, a process aided by the intense lacrimation associated with the injury; but this ability is short-lived because a rapid swelling of the corneal cells causes the foreign body to become firmly lodged, particularly when there is destruction of the epithelium. The foreign body is removed under a local anaesthetic (cocaine drops 2 to 4 per cent) by a variety of techniques:

1. A capsulotomy needle is the ideal instrument because it permits removal of the foreign body with minimum damage to the surrounding cornea together with removal of any underlying rust-staining or retained particles. It is, however, a method which has obvious dangers in unskilled hands.

2. A blunt instrument like a 'spud' can be used to remove a foreign body without risk of perforating the cornea, but it has the disadvantage of causing considerable damage to the surrounding unaffected epithelium and thus leads to delayed healing.

3. A cotton-wool swab, usually impregnated with liquid paraffin, is of value only in removing very superficial foreign bodies. However, this is dangerous as it can remove large parts of the surrounding corneal epithelium, particularly if the cornea is unduly dry, so that it is not a valid method for the unskilled person.

After removal of the foreign body the cornea is treated in the same way as a corneal abrasion (see above). An effective way of reducing subsequent infection is the routine use of sulphacetamide drops (10, 20, or 30 per cent), or other similar antibacterial agent.

Deep Foreign Bodies

The cornea is fairly resistant to perforation by a foreign body because of the layering of its lamellae and because of the presence of Descemet's membrane, so that even a small sharp foreign body which enters the cornea at considerable speed may become lodged within the stroma without entering the eye. Sometimes a foreign body may be present in the stroma without causing any immediate discomfort because the surface wound is so small that it heals rapidly. Such a foreign body may be removed, but this demands the skill of an experienced surgeon, and in certain cases the surgeon may elect to avoid any interference because of the damage to the surrounding cornea which might follow.

Perforating Wounds

This subject is covered in Chapter 17.

Ultraviolet Light

Ultraviolet light may affect the eyes during its therapeutic administration, following a flash from a welder's arc, or following intense exposure to the glare of the sun (so-called *snowblindness*). There is a severe reaction in the conjunctiva and cornea, usually of both eyes, although only after an interval of a few hours because the reaction represents a photochemical response. There is marked hyperaemia of the conjunctiva, diffuse superficial oedema of the corneal epithelium (which stains vividly with fluorescein drops), intense photophobia, lacrimation, blepharospasm and pain. The condition responds fairly rapidly to the immediate instillation of cocaine 2 per cent drops to relieve the pain (this is one of the few occasions in which cocaine is justified therapeutically), and adrenaline drops to relieve the congestion. The condition should be prevented by wearing protective tinted goggles during any likely exposure to ultraviolet light, but the associated reduction in clarity sometimes engenders a casual attitude to their use in certain industrial procedures.

Keratitis

Keratitis is the name applied to inflammatory conditions of the cornea which are mostly exogenous (of bacterial, viral or mycotic origin) or sometimes endogenous.

BACTERIAL KERATITIS

This can be caused by many bacterial organisms which have been discussed in Chapter 3, for example, pneumococcus, staphylococcus, streptococcus, gonococcus, *Pseudomonas pyocyanea, B. proteus, Bact. coli*, and it is usually associated with some degree of conjunctivitis.

The characteristic lesion of a superficial bacterial keratitis is a *corneal ulcer* which may be single or multiple, and because of its infective nature it is sometimes termed a *catarrhal ulcer*. This appears as a grey circular area on the surface of the cornea, often initially without any loss of corneal substance but invariably with oedema of the surrounding corneal epithelium (*corneal bedewing*) which dulls the normal brightness of the cornea within and around the affected area and distorts the normal corneal reflex. The defective area may be determined by using fluorescein drops. The eye becomes red in the circumcorneal region (*circumcorneal injection*) and the deep vessels here may be involved also (*ciliary injection*), but a generalized redness occurs when there is an associated conjunctivitis. The ulcer causes severe pain, lacrimation, photophobia, spasm of the eyelids (*blepharospasm*), and sometimes spasm of the pupil (*miosis*) as a result of stimulation of the abundant sensory nerve endings within the corneal epithelium. Most catarrhal corneal ulcers have a marginal distribution, but infection with the pneumococcus, or more rarely with the *Pseudomonas pyocyanea*, tends to cause the formation of a more centrally placed ulcer which often shows irregularly spreading edges (hence the term *acute serpiginous ulcer*). Rarely the ulcer is confined to the epithelium so that it heals without leaving any significant scar, but usually there is involvement of the corneal stroma which leads subsequently to fibrosis and to permanent scarring. The scar may be small (a *nebula*) or large (a *leucoma*), and sometimes it may be marked only by a slight depression (a *facet*). In the later stages, particularly when the ulcer is near the limbus, vessels from the conjunctival circulation (*superficial vascularization*) pass over the limbus to the affected area and these tend to persist for a prolonged time. Sometimes the ulcer fails to heal, particularly when it is in the central part of the cornea. It then extends through the stroma to the level of Descemet's membrane, which may protrude through the ulcerated area as a thin vesicle (*descemetocele*) because of the pressure of the intraocular fluid even when the pressure is normal. Later this vesicle may rupture (*corneal perforation*), although as a rule Descemet's membrane is remarkably resistant to perforation. This type of severe deep ulcer usually occurs when there is considerable sepsis, and an associated collection of purulent inflammatory cells in the anterior chamber may form a mass in the lower part of the anterior chamber (*hypopyon keratitis*).

In a corneal perforation aqueous humour is expressed from the anterior chamber through the corneal opening at the moment of perforation and the patient is often aware of warm fluid running down the cheek. Sometimes this is followed by healing of the perforated area—an occurrence which prompted the use of a wide surgical incision (*Saemisch section*) through the whole thickness of the cornea including the affected area, but this drastic method of treatment is now discarded because of modern methods of therapy to control infection. It is rare for a corneal perforation to heal with normal restoration of the anterior chamber so that it is often followed by serious complications. Part of the iris may be expressed through the perforation (*iris prolapse*) leading eventually to an extensively thickened and scarred cornea containing iris tissue (*corneal staphyloma*). Parts of the iris may remain in contact with the inner aspect of the perforation without actually prolapsing (*anterior synechia*), and in such cases there is often an extensively scarred area of cornea (*leucoma adherens*). A corneal perforation is also liable to result in the lens coming into contact with the cornea so that an *anterior capsular cataract* occurs. Occasionally in elderly people there may be an extensive choroidal haemorrhage following the sudden lowering of the intraocular pressure (*expulsive choroidal haemorrhage*) and this is fostered by an abnormality of the choroidal vessels or of the elastic lamina of Bruch's membrane. It is also possible for adhesions to form between the peripheral part of the iris and the filtration angle (*peripheral anterior synechiae*) so that there may be the development of *secondary glaucoma*. Sometimes a corneal ulcer may lead to an *anterior uveitis* and even to an inflammation of the whole eye (*panophthalmitis*) so that there may be a subsequent shrinkage of the eye which becomes blind and degenerate (*phthisis bulbi*).

Prevention and Treatment. The soluble sulphonamides (sulphacetamide 10, 20 or 30 per cent drops or 2·5 per cent ointment) and more recently various antibiotic preparations have reduced the incidence of bacterial keratitis because of their widespread use in the treatment of superficial injuries and infections of the eyes in factory first-aid departments, hospital casualty departments and in general practice. In established cases the infection is treated by appropriate antibiotics, and the nature of the infection and its sensitivity to particular drugs should be ascertained unless there is an immediate response to treatment. In severe cases antibiotics, such as Soframycin or neomycin, may be injected subconjunctivally to provide a high concentration of the drug. The use of atropine (1 per cent drops or ointment) reduces pain and accelerates the process of healing because the mydriasis eliminates the spasm of the sphincter muscle of the iris (although it causes an increased photophobia so that it may be necessary to keep the eye covered by a pad or to wear tinted glasses). Topical steroids are contraindicated because, although they may accelerate the resolution of the inflammatory process, they delay healing and favour a perforation if the ulcer is deep; furthermore they are dangerous if there is any associated viral or fungal condition. Sometimes in a descemetocele a scleral contact lens may be of value in preventing perforation, but a corneal graft operation is often necessary.

The application of heat to the affected eye is of value in relieving pain and accelerating the healing processes; it may be applied in the form of hot spoon-bathings (chap. 11), as an electrically heated eye-pad or as short-wave diathermy.

In bacterial keratitis cauterization of the ulcerated area with phenol or even with the actual cautery was a common method of treatment in indolent cases before the advent of modern drugs, but it is seldom, if ever, required now and the method is prone to cause permanent scarring.

When the vision is affected by severe scarring, a corneal graft operation may be performed when the condition is no longer active; sometimes a contact lens may be of value in improving the vision, particularly when the residual scar causes corneal distortion.

VIRAL KERATITIS

This is becoming an increasingly common condition. The term *superficial punctate keratitis* is sometimes regarded as synonymous with viral keratitis, but this is a misconception because the former includes many different forms of viral keratitis and also several other conditions of a bacterial nature (for example, the keratitis which may be associated with staphylococcal blepharoconjunctivitis), of a non-infective nature (for example, *keratitis sicca* which occurs in excessive dryness of the eye, *rosacea keratitis* which occurs in association with acne rosacea, or *neurotropic keratitis* which follows lesions of the ophthalmic division of the trigeminal nerve), or of a traumatic nature (for example, the *neuroparalytic keratitis—exposure keratitis*—which follows paralysis of the facial nerve, the keratitis which follows exposure to ultraviolet light, and the keratitis which follows persistent trichiasis). These varied conditions are more aptly termed *punctate epithelial erosions* and represent fine very slightly depressed areas on the surface of the corneal epithelium which stain with fluorescein because of a loss of the surface epithelial cells.

The five more common forms of viral keratitis are: (*a*) epidemic keratoconjunctivitis; (*b*) herpes simplex; (*c*) herpes zoster; (*d*) trachoma; and (*e*) vaccinia and variola (for a detailed discussion of (*d*) and (*e*), see chap. 3).

Epidemic Keratoconjunctivitis

This is due to an adenovirus and occurs usually in epidemics, although sometimes only sporadically. It is characterized by relatively circumscribed areas of infiltration in the superficial parts of the corneal stroma (*subepithelial keratitis*) which are sufficiently large to be readily visible, although it is often preceded by a mild transient epithelial keratitis. The epithelial lesions usually clear quickly without leaving any scars and the deeper lesions also clear to a large extent over a period of weeks. In the early stages there is invariably an intense conjunctivitis and enlargement of the preauricular lymph glands. Scrapings of the conjunctiva show an abundance of mononuclear cells, few eosinophils, few polymorphonuclear leucocytes and an absence of inclusion bodies.

Herpes Simplex

This is associated with multiple small vesicular formations in the epithelial cells (*fine punctate keratitis*) which stain vividly with Rose Bengal; they also stain with fluorescein although only after they rupture to form minute superficial areas of ulceration. More rarely the punctate areas may be coarse, stellate, areolar or even filamentary in nature. These early punctate epithelial lesions become associated with subepithelial lesions of a greyish-white colour which tend to be permanent. Sometimes there are associated herpetic vesicles of the skin of the face, particularly on the eyelids or the side of the nose. These lesions are prone to recur especially during some other infection, for example of a respiratory nature, presumably following a lowering of the natural immunity to the virus.

A distinctive form of herpes keratitis is the *dendritic ulcer* in which vesicles coalesce to form an irregular line of superficial ulceration with many small extensions from the main stem each of which ends in a 'bud-like' formation. There is a tendency for this to lead to a deep stromal type of keratitis (*disciform keratitis*) which begins as an oedema of the stroma particularly centrally with haziness and impaired vision; these features may be permanent although they usually become less marked after a prolonged time. The inflammatory process favours the entry of deep vessels from the episcleral plexus into the cornea thus leading to further scarring; their deep nature is indicated by their disappearance beyond the limbus in contrast to more superficial vessels which may spread to the cornea from the conjunctival vessels (Fig. 19). Deep vessels usually persist indefinitely within the cornea although after many months or even years there may be an absence of any circulating blood; these 'ghost vessels' appear as thin white lines which are distinguished from prominent corneal nerves by their sites of entry at the limbus and by their fairly regular course within a particular layer of the stroma. There may be an accompanying iritis. These changes in the stroma may represent an immunological response due to the meeting of the virus with an antibody which enters the cornea from the limbal circulation. The more superficial epithelial changes may persist during the active period of the deep keratitis, and it is likely that the abnormal condition of the stroma prevents the overlying epithelium from healing so that it remains defective despite an absence of any active disease within its cells.

Treatment. It is imperative to destroy the virus at a stage when it is confined to the epithelial cells, and this may be achieved by cauterizing the affected areas lightly with iodine, phenol, or alcohol.

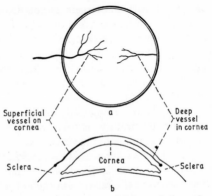

FIG. 19. *Corneal vascularization—superficial vessels from the conjunctival circulation and deep vessels from the ciliary plexus—as shown on surface view and on vertical section of the cornea*

In certain cases this may result in some damage to the underlying stroma which becomes oedematous, thus favouring the development of a deep keratitis, so it is better to remove the diseased areas carefully with a sharp knife. Secondary infection is avoided by the use of local antibiotic drugs. There is evidence that IDU (5 iodo-2-deoxyuridine), a substance which affects the cellular and viral synthesis of DNA (deoxyribonucleic acid), acts as a viral antibiotic so that its use may eliminate the need to apply cauterizing agents. It is essential to use the IDU drops at frequent intervals (hourly during the day and 2 hourly at night) for 24 hours each day for several days in order to ensure eradication of the virus, and even after this intensive treatment recurrences are not uncommon; when IDU ointment is available it is used 2 hourly and 4 hourly.

In unresponsive cases a tarsorrhaphy (closure of the lids by uniting the lid margins) may be of value, but sometimes this is unwise because it masks the case which is deteriorating, and a therapeutic lamellar keratoplasty to replace the diseased area of cornea with donor material may be more satisfactory.

In a developing disciform keratitis the use of steroids, topically or sometimes by subconjunctival injection, may decrease the extent of the stromal changes, but their use is contraindicated if there are any active surface lesions because they favour the spread of such lesions, although sometimes this adverse effect may be avoided by the use also of IDU. In cases suitable for topical steroids it is essential to continue their use for many weeks or even months with a gradual reduction in amount, otherwise a recrudescence is likely. In the later stages permanent scarring may necessitate a keratoplasty to restore the vision of the eye, sometimes preceded or followed by beta irradiation to diminish the vascularization.

Herpes Zoster

This is usually the result of infection by a virus which is related to the virus of herpes simplex, and to that of chicken pox. In herpes zoster ophthalmicus the virus affects the ophthalmic division of the trigeminal nerve or sometimes the Gasserian ganglion. Rarely the condition may be of a noninfective nature as the result of an involvement of these structures by some traumatic, toxic or neoplastic process.

The rapid development of severe neuralgic pain over part or the whole of the area of distribution of the ophthalmic division of the trigeminal nerve (the scalp, the forehead, the upper lid and the side and tip of the nose) is usually the first manifestation. It persists for several hours, or even days, before redness and swelling of the affected area with the formation of characteristic vesicles develop. The condition affects one side of the head only and this is presumably a measure of the rapid immunity which develops in the condition. There is usually well-marked conjunctival injection sometimes with a frank conjunctivitis, and the cornea often shows epithelial oedema which may be followed by corneal vesicles and subepithelial opacities which may persist indefinitely with a consequent disturbance of vision. Sometimes there is a severe iritis which may be followed by a secondary glaucoma, or an episcleritis. Ophthalmoplegia (external or internal) occurs rarely. Involvement of the eyeball is more likely when the tip of the nose is involved by vesicles (Hutchinson's sign), and this is scarcely surprising in view of the fact that the nerve supply of this region (the external nasal nerve) is the terminal branch of the sensory nerve of the eyeball (the nasociliary branch of the ophthalmic division of the trigeminal nerve).

Some cases are complicated later by a *neurotrophic keratitis*, a degenerative condition which is presumably the result of permanent damage to the sensory nerves of the cornea. A similar condition may follow other forms of severe long-standing keratitis, or after section or alcohol injection of the Gasserian ganglion for persistent trigeminal neuralgia.

Treatment. The treatment is as described for conjunctivitis, keratitis, iritis, secondary glaucoma, and external ophthalmoplegia. Pain of the affected area is difficult to control because of its intense nature and its persistence long after the active stage of the disease. Analgesics are often only of limited value. A neurotrophic keratitis usually demands a liberal tarsorrhaphy, particularly of the central parts of the lids, which must be maintained for several months or even years.

MYCOTIC KERATITIS

This results from infection by a fungus such as *Aspergillus* or *Streptothrix*. It is a rare condition but in recent years an increased incidence has followed the topical use of antibiotics and corticosteroids which favour an accumulation of fungi within ulcerated areas following a bacterial or viral keratitis, or within areas of simple abrasion. There is an apparent healing, followed by relapse, of the original lesion; a yellow-white infiltration of the affected area develops with surrounding concentric zones of faint opacification—a serious complication because it may lead to a hypopyon ulceration. The fungus is identified in scrapings from the lesion.

Treatment. The topical use of copper sulphate ⅓ per cent combined with potassium iodide by mouth, or one of the newer fungistatic agents, such as amphotericin B.

OTHER FORMS OF KERATITIS

Interstitial Keratitis

This deep keratitis presents as a white cloudiness of the stroma following an oedematous process, often localized initially but becoming more generalized. Severe loss of vision may be the only symptom for several days or even weeks, although usually there is also severe pain, photophobia and blepharospasm because of an intense iritis.

The oedema of the stroma favours the ingrowth of vessels into the cornea from the deep episcleral plexus of vessels at the limbus (these vessels cannot be traced beyond the level of the limbus because of their deep origin) which cause a patchy pink appearance (the 'salmon patches'). The iritis is associated with the production of keratic precipitates ('KP') and often also of posterior synechiae although these may be masked by the gross disturbance of corneal transparency. The oedematous and vascularized state of the corneal stroma causes the formation of dense scar tissue; this is permanent to some extent although it gradually becomes less diffuse so that small 'windows' of partial clearing may permit a reasonable return of vision particularly for close reading, a factor of great importance from an educative point of view when the condition occurs in a child. The corneal vessels also become less obvious in time and eventually are free of circulating blood ('ghost vessels'). Sometimes, however, the condition may recur, or in later life degenerative changes may occur in the cornea. In this way the vision in interstitial keratitis may show three phases: extremely poor in the early and acute stage; considerable improvement some years later; and a gradual deterioration in advancing years.

In the more localized forms of interstitial keratitis the disease occurs characteristically near the limbus, although it may spread later to the more central parts of the cornea when it tends to be more persistent. Sometimes the changes are limited to several large punctate foci in the posterior third of the corneal stroma.

Most cases of interstitial keratitis are associated with congenital syphilis with or without the other stigmata of the disease (such as Hutchinson's teeth and saddle-shaped depression of the nose); they occur usually between the ages of 5 and 18 years. Only one eye is involved initially but the other is almost inevitably attacked some weeks or months later. It may also occur in acquired syphilis, tuberculosis, leprosy, Leishmaniasis, trypanosomiasis, onchocerciasis and lupus erythematosus; it is commonly confined to one eye. It is essentially an endogenous condition.

There are other forms of interstitial keratitis—*disciform keratitis* which follows herpes of the cornea (discussed above) and *keratitis profunda* which is associated with an anterior unveitis (chap. 6).

Treatment. Topical steroids reduce the ravages of the disease, particularly when they are applied early. The pupil is dilated with atropine to prevent the formation of posterior synechiae. Treatment is directed also to the cause of the condition—for example, systemic penicillin in massive doses in syphilis. When the degree of permanent scarring is sufficient to cause marked impairment of vision a keratoplasty may restore useful vision, despite the presence of vessels within the diseased cornea provided perfect apposition is achieved between the donor and host cornea with a satisfactory method of suturing.

Mooren's Ulcer

This is a chronic indolent but often painful type of ulceration which occurs without any obvious infective element in an elderly person. It is usually unilateral initially, but there is a tendency for the other eye to be involved later. The lesion begins as a concentric depression of a wide area of the cornea at the limbus with a characteristic undermining of the edge of the depression away from the limbus so that there is an overhanging thickened portion of cornea which spreads gradually (hence the term *chronic serpiginous ulcer*) across the whole cornea leaving behind a somewhat attenuated but densely scattered and vascularized cornea.

Treatment. This is often fairly hopeless; keratoplasty is of limited value because the donor cornea is liable to become scarred and vascularized by a spread of the disease from the affected host cornea, and such an operation is often not feasible in an elderly and debilitated patient. The main aim is to limit the spread of the disease early before the central cornea is affected; the protection of the cornea by a conjunctival flap over the affected area may be of value, and sometimes beta-irradiation is an effective procedure.

Neuroparalytic Keratitis

This is a degenerative condition which follows exposure of the eyeball in conditions such as facial paralysis. The lower part of the cornea is more commonly affected because the upper part is protected by the fact that the eye turns up when an attempt is made to close the partially paralysed lids (Bell's phenomenon).

Treatment. The main aim is to protect the eye by an adequate tarsorrhaphy. A lateral tarsorrhaphy is effective in limiting the exposure of the cornea and has the merit of not interfering with the vision, but a central tarsorrhaphy is necessary in severe cases.

Mustard Gas Keratitis

Mild exposure to mustard gas causes an immediate and intense conjunctival irritation which usually subsides within a few days or weeks, but in more severe exposures there is an associated corneal involvement with the development of superficial ulcerated areas which become scarred and vascularized and may even lead to perforation. Other characteristic changes in the cornea become evident many (as long as 30) years later with the formation of multiple ulcers in association with areas of stromal collapse, and with the entry of vessels in the superficial parts of the cornea which show varicosities and have a tendency to cause haemorrhages. This is essentially a degenerative condition as a result of the changes which occur in the cornea following contamination with this radiomimetic substance. The vision is affected by the scarring and by the corneal irregularities and distortions which tend to cause repeated alterations in the refractive error.

Treatment. The keratoconjunctivitis is treated along the usual lines (pp. 34 and 55), but a more specific form of treatment is the use of a flush-fitting contact lens; this lessens the discomfort of the eye, protects it from repeated attacks and improves the visual acuity by eliminating the effect of the continually changing corneal irregularities.

The remaining forms of keratitis are: *phlyctenular keratitis; keratitis in spring catarrh; filamentary keratitis; keratitis secondary to membranous conjunctivitis; keratitis in acne rosacea* (all discussed in chap. 3); and *sclerosing keratitis* (see chap. 5).

OPHTHALMIA NODOSA

This is essentially a foreign-body reaction to the presence of fine hairs which may be animal (e.g. from a caterpillar) or vegetable (e.g. from a cactus) in origin. These hairs tend to migrate in the tissues so that they may produce flat-topped yellow nodules in different ocular tissues—the conjunctiva, the cornea and the iris—with accompanying inflammatory changes. The lungs may be affected similarly.

KERATOPLASTY (CORNEAL GRAFTING)

This operation consists of the replacement of a diseased area of cornea (the host cornea) by part of the cornea from another human eye (the donor cornea) which is usually obtained from the cadaver (a homograft). The Human Tissue Act of 1953 allows an individual to bequeath his eyes for such a purpose, but it is essential for the eyes to be enucleated within a few hours of death otherwise the cornea is unsuitable for transference when use is made of natural tissue, but the cornea may be preserved for considerable periods by a freeze-drying process. It is essential for the donor cornea to be transparent and to be free from disease. Sometimes the donor cornea is obtained from an eye removed because of a disorder not involving the integrity of the cornea and not liable to be transmitted to the host eye as in certain infective conditions such as syphilis or in malignant disease within the anterior segment of the eye. The cornea, unlike other parts of the body, accepts this transference of corneal tissue because the absence of vascularization prevents the occurrence of the immunological reactions which cause the discarding of other transplanted tissues; this unique property of the cornea is lost to some extent when the host cornea is vascularized as a result of disease. The donor cornea may be provided by the patient himself (an autograft) in the rare event of a person having one potentially sighted eye with a diseased cornea and another irrevocably blind eye with an intact cornea.

There are two main forms of keratoplasty: lamellar keratoplasty which involves the transplantation of the anterior half or two-thirds of the cornea (usually about 0·4 mm) so that the anterior chamber remains intact during the operation, or penetrating keratoplasty which involves the transplantation of the whole thickness of the cornea. A keratoplasty is usually performed to restore vision when the cornea is scarred, but sometimes it is also performed for therapeutic reasons; for example, to prevent the spread of a Mooren's ulcer, to restore the integrity of the anterior chamber after the rupture of a descemetocele, to accelerate the healing of the cornea after severe chemical burns, or to remove a diseased portion of cornea which has suffered repeated attacks of dendritic ulceration. A lamellar keratoplasty is only valid as an optical procedure when the diseased condition of the cornea is confined to the anterior part, but it is of particular value as an emergency procedure to maintain the integrity of a diseased cornea; in such a case a penetrating keratoplasty may be performed subsequently for optical purposes.

Keratoprostheses

In an extensively diseased cornea when a keratoplasty is unsuccessful an attempt may be made to substitute the central part of the scarred and vascularized cornea with various forms of acrylic keratoprostheses. An ingenious example is the *osteo-odontoprosthesis*, which represents a narrow disc prepared from one of the canine teeth of the patient together with bone from the socket of the tooth so that the outer ring of bone becomes adherent to the edge of the diseased cornea and the acrylic lens is placed within the inner ring of dentine.

The use of dentine is based on the unique properties of a tooth which shows a ready acceptance of foreign material (dental fillings).

Keratomalacia

Keratomalacia results from a lack of vitamin A and occurs only in infants suffering from severe malnutrition; it is an extremely rare condition in Western countries. The surface epithelium of the cornea becomes dry and insensitive so that it loses its normal lustre, and this is followed by a rapid opacification of the whole cornea which may slough and perforate without any obvious inflammatory changes. Other changes in the eye are dryness of the conjunctiva (*xerophthalmia*) with the formation of *Bitôt's spots* (small triangular foam-like white areas near the limbus) and night blindness (chap. 27).

Treatment. Massive doses of vitamin A are effective and must be provided with great urgency.

Note : It has been suggested that vitamin B deficiency (*ariboflavinosis*) causes a superficial vasculization of the cornea near the limbus, but this occurs only when there is an associated element of trauma.

Pigmentary Disturbances

Blood-staining. This occurs after a leakage of blood in a keratitis which is associated with intracorneal vascularization. It also occurs when a haemorrhage in the anterior chamber (*hyphaema*) develops in association with a secondary glaucoma (chap. 15).

The *Kayser-Fleischer ring*, a green-brown ring in the region of Descemet's membrane in the peripheral part of the cornea near the limbus, which develops at an early stage of *Kinnear Wilson's disease* (*hepatolenticular degeneration*) is probably of haematogenous origin, although it may be the result of deposits of copper or silver perhaps following an atrophic state of the liver.

Melanin. A thin brown horizontal line—the so-called *Stahli-Hudson line*—may develop in the lower central part of the cornea after middle age, particularly in an area of scarring; this is usually an infiltration of melanin but sometimes it may be derived from blood (*haemosiderin*). Melanin pigment on the posterior surface of the cornea, sometimes in the form of a *Krukenberg's spindle*, is described in Chapter 6.

Silver Pigment. Small black particles are deposited in the region of Descemet's membrane in *argyrosis* (chap. 3).

Iron Pigment. Small brown particles are deposited in the corneal stroma when an iron foreign body is retained within the eye (*siderosis*) (chap. 17).

Copper Pigment. Small brown particles are deposited in the corneal stroma, particularly in the peripheral parts, when a copper foreign body is retained within the eye (chap. 17) or after the prolonged use of a copper stick in trachoma (*chalcosis*).

Toxic and Metabolic Disturbances

Lignac-Fanconi's Syndrome

This is an inherited defect of amino acid metabolism; it is characterized by dwarfism and renal rickets. Deposits in the cornea, possibly cystine in nature, cause photophobia, and are apparent on slit-lamp microscopy as shiny rod or needle-shaped crystals in the superficial stroma. Deposits may also occur in other ocular tissues; conjunctiva, sclera, uvea and rarely the retina. Cystine-storage disease (cystinosis) is a related disorder.

Synthetic Antimalarial Drugs

Drugs such as mepacrine and chloroquine are liable to cause the deposition of whitish-grey particles in the corneal epithelium and in the most superficial layers of the stroma; these may cause a subjective awareness of coloured halos (a symptom which is generally indicative of closed-angle glaucoma). Chloroquine, which is used in the treatment of certain skin disorders such as lupus erythematosus) and also in malaria, is liable to cause a pigmentary disturbance in the retina (chap. 7). It is rare for these effects to occur when the drug is used in small doses (for example, as a prophylactic measure) except in unduly susceptible individuals. The corneal changes are reversible when the drug is discontinued.

Tumours

Tumours are discussed in Chapter 3, those of particular note are the limbal dermoid, Bowen's disease, and the melanomata.

Degenerations

Fatty Degeneration

This occurs most commonly in the ageing eye. There are circumscribed circular deposits of lipoid material in the peripheral part of the corneal stroma, the so-called *arcus senilis* (*gerontoxon*) which is separated from the limbus by a narrow zone of unaffected cornea; in contrast in the similar but rare condition which occurs in infants, *arcus juvenalis* (*embryotoxon*), the deposits extend to the limbus. An arcus senilis develops gradually during adult life, usually starting in the lower part of the cornea and then the upper part before extending round the sides to form a complete ring; it never affects the transparency of the central cornea. It is almost invariably present in the elderly, but its presence before the age of 40 years may indicate a hyperlipoidaemia with sometimes a predisposition to coronary heart disease, and this may apply also between the ages of 40 and 60 years when it may be an indication of significantly raised serum cholesterol and phospholipid values.

Fatty degeneration may develop in an old corneal scar (following previous infection or injury) or it may occur in a more generalized form in an extensively diseased eye. Sometimes active ulceration may develop in a fatty area, the so-called *atheromatous ulcer*, and a marked secondary infection may lead to a severe hypopyon keratitis, often a terminal event because of the poor response of such a diseased eye to treatment.

Extensive infiltration of the cornea by mucopolysaccharides and perhaps also by lipoids is a feature of *gargoylism* (*Hurler's disease; dysostosis multiplex*); this condition occurs in early infancy and produces characteristic general changes in the skull (widely spaced orbits and frontal bossing), in the abdomen (swelling due to involvement of the liver and spleen) and in the skeleton (dwarfism). The corneal change may be very extensive and lead to gross loss of vision.

Sometimes small aggregations of lipoid material containing calcium form fine white rings in the anterior part of the corneal stroma (*Coats' white rings*) usually at the site of a previous minor injury.

Calcareous Degeneration

This occurs in eyes which are seriously damaged by long-standing disease such as keratitis, iridocyclitis, and glaucoma; it is a characteristic feature of the uveitis which occurs in early childhood, particularly in the presence of a rheumatic diathesis as in Still's disease. It develops in a superficial vascularized granulation tissue which forms between the epithelium and Bowman's membrane and later destroys this membrane with subsequent involvement of the anterior corneal lamellae (*pannus degenerativus*). The calcareous changes occur particularly across the lower part of the cornea which is exposed when the lids are open, hence the term *band-shaped degeneration*, but it is more usually termed *band keratopathy*. It may occur also in association with hyperparathyroidism, extensive vitamin D intake, tuberose sclerosis and Fanconi's syndrome, and rarely as an isolated event (idiopathic type) in the elderly.

Treatment. The calcareous area in the central part of the cornea may be scraped away with a sharp knife and the operated area heals with or without the use of a lamellar corneal graft; obviously, however, such an operation is of no value when the rest of the eye is grossly diseased. The calcareous area may also be removed by a chelating agent such as disodium versenate.

Dellen

These represent shallow saucer-like excavations (dimples, facets) of the surface layers (epithelium and to some extent Bowman's membrane) of the cornea near the limbus, each with a well-defined edge and with faint opacification of the floor. They are sometimes of a transient nature persisting for only a few days or changing in extent within a few days. It is possible that they occur as the result of a compression of the limbal capillaries such as by a patch of episcleritis or tumour formation adjacent to the limbus or as the result of an obliteration of the limbal capillaries after trauma (injury or operation) or in the elderly in association with vasosclerosis, but they may occur simply as the result of the dehydration of the peripheral cornea which follows a limbal lesion.

Dystrophies Affecting the Cornea

Hereditary Dystrophies

These usually become evident in the early years of life, before or at puberty, particularly in males. There are different forms: the *granular* or *nodular form* (the so-called *Groenouw's dystrophy*), the *lattice form*, and the *macular form*. The granular and lattice forms are inherited as dominant and the macular form as recessive conditions.

The opacified areas gradually extend from the central to the peripheral parts of both corneas with a gradual impairment in the vision; the granular form usually shows the slowest progress, and reasonable vision may be retained until middle age.

Treatment. A lamellar corneal graft is the only effective form of treatment, but it should be delayed until the vision is severely affected because, although the absence of vascularity favours a corneal transplant, there is a tendency for dystrophic changes to develop later in the donor cornea, particularly in the macular form.

Fuchs' Dystrophy

This was originally described as an epithelial dystrophy, but the earliest changes occur in the endothelium which develops a bronzed appearance interspersed with black vacuoles representing localized thickenings of Descemet's membrane; the later epithelial changes are accompanied by opacities in the stroma which follow an oedema because of an impairment of the endothelial barrier. The condition, which seldom occurs before late middle age, is bilateral and progresses slowly, but ultimately the vision is impaired considerably; unfortunately it progresses more rapidly after any form of intraocular operation, particularly a cataract extraction, even when any corneal endothelial damage is minimal (chap. 9).

Salzmann's Dystrophy

This is a nodular type of dystrophy which is usually confined to one eye only, unlike the other forms of corneal dystrophy; it is likely, however, that it occurs essentially in an area of previous inflammatory change, such as a phylcten, so that it is not primarily a dystrophy.

Keratoconus (Conical Cornea)

This is a form of corneal dystrophy affecting the central part of the cornea which gradually becomes attenuated, bowed forwards and insensitive. It is a bilateral condition which usually starts around puberty and, unlike other forms of hereditary corneal dystrophy, affects females particularly. Its progress is unpredictable, but the vision becomes impaired by the development of a form of myopic astigmatism which is not susceptible, except in the early stages, to correction by ordinary spectacle lenses because of its irregular nature. The condition is detected to some extent by retinoscopy because of the distortion of the normal reflex from the fundus, but it is confirmed by demonstrating the distortion of the corneal reflection by means of Placido's disc (Fig. 20) or more precisely by careful examination of the cornea with the slit-lamp microscope. The vision deteriorates markedly when ruptures develop in Descemet's membrane in the affected area so that the aqueous passes freely into the corneal stroma with consequent permanent scarring.

Treatment. Provided opacification has not occurred, many cases respond well to the use of contact lenses which restore the vision to a

normal level by eliminating the effect of the abnormal curvature of
the anterior corneal surface. Contact lenses also prevent, to some
extent, a further increase in the corneal protrusion, although this
applies mainly to the use of haptic (flushfitting) contact lenses rather

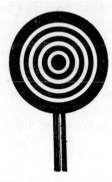

FIG. 20. *Placido's disc*

than microcorneal lenses. A perforating keratoplasty is also an effective method of treatment because of the avascularity of the diseased
cornea, but this should be attempted only after contact lenses have
been tried and the nature of the corneal changes necessitates a fairly
large graft of 7 mm, or even more, in diameter.

5 | Diseases of the Sclera

Structure and Function

The *sclera* forms five-sixths of the protective outer coat of the eye and its dense fibrous tissue is continuous anteriorly with the stromal part of the cornea (which forms the remaining one-sixth). Its outer surface is covered by a loose vascular tissue (the *episcleral tissue*) which is separated from the overlying conjunctiva by a thin layer of more dense fibrous tissue (Tenon's capsule).

Injuries

The sclera is fairly resistant to injury but perforation may occur directly, for example by metallic fragments which strike at high speed or by injury with a sharp instrument, or indirectly, as a rupture of the sclera following a severe concussion of the globe.

Episcleritis and Scleritis

An episcleritis is an inflammatory condition of the episclera which is characterized by a localized area of redness of the eye; this differs from the redness of a conjunctivitis by being more intense and deep-seated and not moving on displacing the conjunctiva. The affected area may be swollen. The condition is sometimes confined to one eye only, there is a sensation of pain, not irritation, with tenderness on palpation through the closed lids, and there is no discharge. Sometimes the patch of episcleritis is short-lived ('*episcleritis fugax*'). The condition is prone to recurrence in the same or in another area.

Scleritis is an inflammatory condition of the sclera which tends to be associated with an episcleritis, a uveitis or a keratitis (*sclerosing keratitis*).

71

Episcleritis and scleritis are essentially collagen diseases, so they may be associated with rheumatic or arthritic conditions. They may occur also in Wegener's granulomatosis.

Scleromalacia Perforans. Sometimes an area of scleritis is so intense that the whole thickness of the sclera is involved, with a tendency for the affected area to become attenuated and even to perforate.

Wegener's Granulomatosis

Wegener's granulomatosis is a necrotizing granulomatous scleritis or sclerouveitis which causes localized areas of thinning of the sclera; unlike scleromalacia perforans it seldom progresses sufficiently to cause perforation. Similar pathological conditions may occur in the cornea (the ulceration resembles a Mooren's ulcer), in the nasal sinuses, in the lungs (abscess formation), and in the kidneys (focal glomerulo-nephritis).

Treatment. Episcleritis and scleritis usually respond well to local steroids, although these are dangerous if there is any tendency to the development of a scleromalacia perforans because they may hasten the perforation; systemic steroids are less dangerous in such cases. The local effects of Wegener's granulomatosis may respond to irradiation.

Blue Sclerotics

A blue discoloration of the sclera may occur as a pathological entity in *fragilitas ossium*, an hereditary condition associated sometimes with deafness and a marked tendency, particularly in childhood, to develop fractures after relatively trivial injury. It should be noted, however, that under normal conditions a slight bluish tint of the sclera may be caused by a shining of the choroidal pigment through an unduly transparent sclera, a phenomenon often seen during operation when the sclera becomes translucent following dehydration.

STAPHYLOMA OF THE SCLERA

This is an area of thinned sclera which bulges outwards with the underlying uveal tissue. Different parts of the sclera may be involved: an *intercalary staphyloma* occurs immediately in front of the ciliary body and is lined by the root of the iris, a *ciliary staphyloma* is lined by the ciliary body, and an *equatorial staphyloma* is lined by the equatorial part of the choroid; the equatorial region of the sclera is weak because it marks the exit from the choroid of the four large vortex veins. These staphylomata usually follow prolonged periods of glaucoma and therefore often occur in blind eyes.

Posterior staphyloma is a feature of high axial myopia and is associated with extensive choroido-retinal changes around the optic disc and in the macular area (chap. 2).

6 | Diseases of the Uveal Tract

Structure and Function

The uvea forms the middle coat of the eyeball. It has three different parts—iris, ciliary body and choroid—in anatomical continuity.

THE IRIS

This forms a forwards projection from the ciliary body in front of the lens and its more or less circular and central opening forms the pupil. The *anterior chamber* lies between its outer surface and the inner surface of the cornea, and the shallow *posterior chamber* between its inner surface and the outer surface of the lens.

The pupils average about 4 mm in diameter but, because of the balancing influences of the opposing parasympathetic and sympathetic impulses, they vary considerably in size under normal conditions, quite apart from the variations which occur during changes of illumination. In the infant they are relatively small, increase in size during childhood and adolescence, and in later life again tend to become small. In hypermetropia they are usually smaller than in myopia. In emotional states they tend to become large following increased sympathetic tone. In sleep they are small. In heavily pigmented (brown) eyes they are smaller than in lightly pigmented (blue) eyes. Normally the pupils of the two eyes are more or less equal in size and an obvious difference in size (*anisocoria*) is usually of pathological significance.

The iris is composed of an endothelial layer, a stromal layer, and two layers of pigment epithelium (Fig. 21).

The thin *endothelial layer* on its outer surface is continuous with the corneal endothelium and with the endothelial lining of the trabecular spaces in the filtration angle of the anterior chamber. It is absent over the iris crypts which are irregular areas in which the superficial part of the stromal layer is defective.

The thick *stromal layer* is continuous with the stroma of the choroid and contains blood vessels running radially except at the collarette—the junction between its thicker portion (the ciliary part) and its thinner portion (the pupillary part)—where they run circumferentially (the minor arterial circle of the iris). It contains two muscles in

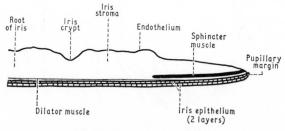

FIG. 21. *The structures of the iris*

its deeper part: the sphincter muscle which runs circumferentially in the pupillary part and causes a constriction of the pupil, and the dilator muscle which runs radially in its ciliary, and to some extent pupillary, parts and dilates the pupil. In infancy there is no pigment within the stroma so that the iris appears blue; this may persist indefinitely, but usually after a few years pigment is deposited so that it assumes varied patterns of colour—green, yellow and brown—which may be uniform or mottled.

Heterochromia iridis is an iris which has one sector different in colour from the rest.

Heterochromia iridum is a difference in colour between the two irides, for example one blue and the other brown. It may occur normally or pathologically (heterochromic cyclitis, p. 94).

Of the two layers of *pigment epithelium*, the outer one is continuous with the outer pigment epithelial layer of the ciliary body and is concerned with the formation of the sphincter and dilator muscles, and the inner one is continuous with the inner nonpigmented epithelial layer of the ciliary body.

The Pupillary Reflexes (Fig. 22)

The sphincter muscle is innervated by the parasympathetic fibres of the oculomotor nerve (cranial nerve III) which arise in the parasympathetic parts of the oculomotor nucleus (nuclei of Edinger-Westphal and Perlia) in the midbrain. These fibres separate into two groups in the orbit; one is relayed in the ciliary ganglion and subserves the constriction of the pupil to light, the other is relayed in an

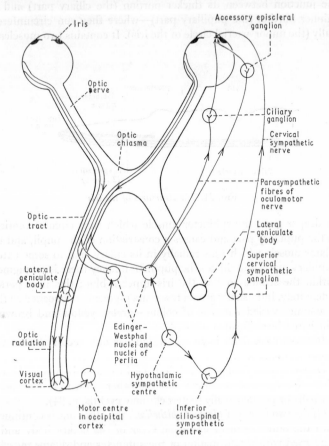

FIG. 22. *The nerve pathways of the pupillary light and accommodation reflexes*

accessory episcleral ganglion and subserves the constriction of the pupil to a near stimulus. The parasympathetic parts of both oculomotor nuclei are stimulated by light stimuli from each retina because the afferent pupillary (visual) fibres from each eye pass to both sides of the midbrain, so that a light stimulus to one eye produces a constriction of the pupil of the stimulated eye (*direct reaction to light*) and of the pupil of the other eye (*consensual reaction to light*). The parasympathetic parts of the nucleus are also concerned with the constriction of the pupil during accommodation (the accommodation pupil reflex) and during convergence (the convergence pupil reflex); these are initiated by a centre in the occipital cortex which is controlled by the visual cortex (part of the psychooptical reflex, chap 13). The dilator muscle is innervated by the sympathetic fibres; these travel in the cervical sympathetic nerve from the ciliospinal centre (in the upper part of the spinal cord), are relayed in the superior cervical ganglion and pass to the eye by the sympathetic plexus around the internal carotid artery, and by the nasociliary branch of the ophthalmic division of the trigeminal nerve. The ciliospinal centre is controlled by a sympathetic centre in the hypothalamus which also produces a dilatation of the pupil by sending inhibitory impulses directly to the parasympathetic nuclei so that dilatation follows relaxation of the sphincter; this is the type of dilatation which follows psychical stimuli.

THE CILIARY BODY

The stroma contains the ciliary muscle (longitudinal, oblique and iridic fibres) which on contraction causes a forward movement and thickening of the ciliary body, thus producing an accommodative change in the lens by a relaxation of the suspensory ligament (see chap. 2).

The Accommodation Reflex (Fig. 23)

The ciliary muscle is innervated by the parasympathetic fibres of the oculomotor nerve (cranial nerve III) which arise in the parasympathetic parts of the oculomotor nucleus and are relayed to the eye in the ciliary ganglion. The accommodation reflex is initiated from a centre in the occipital cortex which is controlled by the visual cortex (part of the psychooptical reflex) and produces a contraction of the ciliary muscle. The relaxation of the muscle may be the result simply of an inhibition of the parasympathetic, but it is likely that the sympathetic nerves, which pass to the ciliary muscle by a route similar to those which supply the dilator muscle of the pupil (Fig. 22), are responsible also for this. The anterior part of the stroma contains the major arterial circle of the iris. The inner surface, which shows many ciliary processes containing highly vascularized tissue, is lined by two layers of epithelium: an outer layer of pigmented epithelium which is continuous with the pigment layer of the retina, and an inner layer of ciliary epithelium which is continuous with the terminal part of the rest of the retina at the ora serrata. The ciliary epithelium is concerned in the formation of aqueous humour by processes of dialysis and secretion.

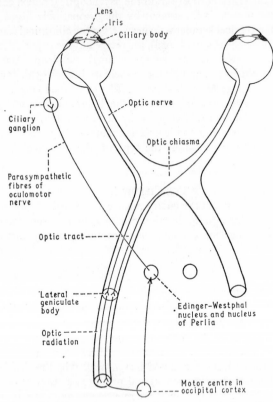

FIG. 23. *The nerve pathways of the accommodation reflex*

THE CHOROID

This is a vascular coat composed of arteries and veins with a layer of capillaries (the *choriocapillaris*) on its inner surface which is separated from the underlying retina by Bruch's membrane; these capillaries nourish the oute half of the retina. The outer surface of

the choroid is separated from the overlying sclera by a potential space
(the suprachoroidal space).

Congenital Anomalies

Persistent Pupillary Membrane
  Late in fetal life the pupil is formed by a complete disappearance
in a central circular area of the vascularized mesodermal tissue which
covers the anterior surface of the lens. There is also a partial disappearance of this tissue over the pupillary part of the iris as far as the
collarette (see above), but sometimes small strands remain (*persistent
pupillary membrane*) which pass across the pupil; sometimes one end

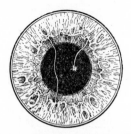

FIG. 24. *Strands of persistent pupillary membrane and an epicapsular star on the
anterior lens capsule*

of the strand lies free in the anterior chamber or is attached to the
anterior lens capsule with the formation of small golden pigment
deposits (the so-called *episcapsular stars*) (Fig. 24). None of these
changes interferes significantly with vision.

Aniridia
  In this familial condition the iris fails to develop except for small
rudimentary stumps in the region of the filtration angle. It is usually
bilateral but seldom to the same degree in each eye. There is marked
photophobia because of the unrestricted entry of light, and usually a
pendular (ocular) type of nystagmus (chap. 13); there is also a likelihood of glaucoma in early adult life (or even in childhood) because of
the abnormality of the filtration angle. The photophobia is relieved
by dark glasses or goggles; sometimes a specially shielded contact
lens may be of value. The treatment of the glaucoma is discussed in
Chapter 15.

Coloboma of the Uvea

In this familial condition a failure in closure of the fetal cleft causes a coloboma in the lower part of the eye. This may involve the iris, ciliary body and choroid together or alone, and the extent of the choroidal coloboma is variable; it may affect the peripheral part only or a whole sector so that it approaches the lower border of the optic disc with a white appearance of the affected area because of the exposed sclera; the retina is also involved in the coloboma except for a few retinal vessels which pass across the coloboma. Sometimes there is also a coloboma of the optic disc. The condition is usually bilateral although each eye may be involved in different ways and to different extents.

Choroideremia

This is a rare inherited condition in which there is a progressive atrophy of the choroid and of the retinal pigment epithelium starting in the periphery and spreading to the whole fundus (except the macula) by middle age, so that the fundus appears white although the overlying retinal vessels persist and the macula and optic disc are normal in colour. There is a progressive loss of peripheral vision with a marked night blindness, but there may be retention of central vision. The established disease is confined to males, but affected females may show modified 'pepper-and-salt' degenerative changes in the periphery of the fundus. Rarely an apparent choroideremia results from a confluence of areas of gyrate atrophy (p. 97).

Albinism

This is a hereditary condition with a Mendelian type recessive inheritance showing a marked deficiency in the pigment of the whole body (white hair, white eyelashes, pink skin, etc.). The eye appears pink because of the absence of pigment in the uveal tract and in the retina which also causes a scattering of light so that there is photophobia and almost invariably a pendular nystagmus. The fundus appears unduly pale with a prominence of the retinal and choroidal vessels against the white background of the sclera. The eyes invariably become myopic. The photophobia may be relieved by dark glasses or goggles. A flush-fitting shielded contact lens, which prevents light from entering the eye except by a small central aperture, is also of value. It is possible that the fitting of such lenses shortly after birth before the development of nystagmus may prevent its occurrence, although the photophobia and nystagmus do not prohibit a reasonable level of corrected vision, particularly for close reading, so that a normal education is possible.

Ocular Albinism

Sometimes the albinotic changes may be confined to the tissues of the eyes (ocular albinism), and this may be overlooked because of the absence of the general features of albinism and also because some pallor of the fundus is a normal finding in childhood. An undue translucency of the iris, particularly near its root, is a characteristic feature.

Injuries

IRIS

Hyphaema

Haemorrhage into the anterior chamber from the iris may follow blunt or perforating injury (chap. 17). The haemorrhage is often completely absorbed within a few days; but sometimes, particularly if the haemorrhage is extensive, the filtration angle becomes clogged causing a secondary glaucoma which may lead to a blood-stained cornea (chap. 4). It should be noted that a small traumatic hyphaema may be followed some hours, or even days, later by further haemorrhages, so that such cases should be admitted for observation. If necessary the hyphaema should be evacuated through a small *paracentesis* opening near the limbus in the lower outer quadrant of the eye; this may be reopened on subsequent days by depressing the outer lip of the incision to release further haemorrhage. If the haemorrhage is clotted it is removed by irrigation of the anterior chamber through a keratome incision in the upper part of the cornea near the limbus; fibrinolysin in the irrigating fluid helps to liquefy the clots.

Traumatic Mydriasis

A paralysis of the sphincter may follow blunt trauma so that the pupil becomes dilated and shows no response to light or near stimuli. There is usually a gradual recovery within a few weeks or months, but this is often only partial.

Iridodialysis

This represents a tear in the iris, usually at its junction with the ciliary body. It is seldom advisable to attempt to repair this defect because of its proximity to the filtration angle.

Iridoschisis

In this condition there is a generalized disruption of the iris stroma so that free ends of strands of iris tissue pass into the anterior chamber following forcible entry of aqueous into the iris as the result of blunt trauma of the eye. A similar condition in elderly people is simply the result of degenerative changes in the absence of trauma (p. 97).

CILIARY BODY

The ciliary body is seldom affected by injury except a perforating one (chap. 17), but sometimes severe contusion of the globe causes a temporary reduction in the intraocular pressure (*hypotonia*) following a diminished production of aqueous from the ciliary body.

CHOROID

Severe blunt trauma may cause a *rupture of the choroid*. In the early stages this is usually masked by choroidal haemorrhage which appears dark red in colour because it lies deep to the retina, although some haemorrhage may also pass into the retina. Later it appears as a narrow crescentic white area which often runs concentrically with the optic disc because of an exposure of the underlying sclera; any retinal vessel passing over it appears normal.

Uveitis

An inflammation of the whole uveal tract is termed *panuveitis* (*endophthalmitis*). When it is confined mainly to the anterior segment it is termed *anterior uveitis* or *iridocyclitis* (sometimes separated into *iritis*—an inflammation of the iris, and *cyclitis*—an inflammation of the ciliary body); in the posterior segment it is termed *posterior uveitis* or *choroiditis*. Uveitis is usually a primary disorder, but it may follow some other infection (e.g. interstitial keratitis, chap. 4; scleritis, chap. 5).

ANTERIOR UVEITIS (IRITIS, CYCLITIS OR IRIDOCYCLITIS)

This condition usually starts fairly acutely with severe pain (often likened to the pain of toothache), intense dislike of light (photophobia), and a mild to severe degree of blurred vision. The condition is frequently confined to one eye. There are many clinical features:

1. *Redness.* There is some general conjunctival injection as in a conjunctivitis, but there is also intense redness in the circumcorneal region with involvement of the deep episcleral vessels (*ciliary injection*); similar redness also occurs in closed-angle glaucoma (chap. 15).

2. *Lacrimation.* This is usually profuse, particularly on exposure to light, but unlike a conjunctivitis it is not mucopurulent.

3. *Tenderness.* The eyeball is very sensitive on palpation.

4. *Exudation.* Exudate containing inflammatory cells enters the anterior chamber so that the aqueous becomes visible (*aqueous flare*) instead of being optically 'empty' as in the normal eye. Cells may also be visible in the retrolental space which lies between the posterior surface of the lens and the anterior face of the vitreous. The exudation in the anterior chamber causes the *keratic precipitates* (*K.P.*) to form on the posterior surface of the cornea as the result of an oedema of the corneal endothelium. This oedema is apparent early in the iridocyclitis because of the continuity of the endothelium of the cornea with the endothelium of the iris and causes a tackiness of this surface. The cells in the anterior chamber circulate because of movement of the aqueous upwards over the surface of the iris and downwards behind the inner surface of the cornea which is induced by the thermal currents (Fig. 25) caused by the temperature of the anterior

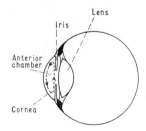

FIG. 25. *The convection currents of the aqueous humour in the anterior chamber*

chamber being higher than the air outside the eye, so that the K.P. usually assume an axial distribution in the lower part of the cornea (Fig. 26). The K.P. are often variable in size and colour. The large nonpigmented K.P. (the 'mutton-fat' K.P.) are characteristic of the granulomatous forms of uveitis found in tuberculosis or sarcoid. Sometimes, however, they may be small with a widespread distribution over the cornea even in its upper part (Fig. 27), as in heterochromic cyclitis or in the Posner-Schlossman syndrome. K.P. tend to become pigmented after an interval so that these are usually indicative of long-standing disease, although in a few cases they may be pigmented from the outset. Old K.P. tend to become crenated and they persist long after the active stage of infection.

Note: Fine particles of iris pigment may be deposited on the posterior surface of the cornea in any form of iris atrophy (for

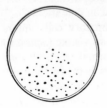

Fig. 26. *An axial distribution of keratic precipitates (K.P.)*

example in old age or after prolonged glaucoma) even in the absence of uveitis; they sometimes have a spindle-shaped vertical distribution (*Krukenberg's spindle*).

The exudation also produces other effects. It may form a purulent deposit in the lower part of the anterior chamber (*hypopyon*), and in severe cases there may also be some haemorrhage (*hyphaema*). It readily causes adhesions between the posterior surface of the iris and the anterior surface of the lens (*posterior synechiae*), particularly when

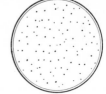

Fig. 27. *A widespread distribution of keratic precipitates (K.P.)*

the pupil is allowed to remain constricted. When the whole pupillary area is involved there is a *seclusion of the pupil* which is liable to be followed by a bulging forwards of the main part of the iris (*iris bombé*) because the aqueous cannot pass into the anterior chamber from the posterior chamber, a condition of pupil block which leads to *secondary glaucoma*. It may cause adhesions between the anterior surface of the iris and the posterior surface of the corneoscleral junction in the filtration angle (*peripheral anterior synechiae*) which leads to a *secondary glaucoma* when a sufficiently large area of the filtration angle is occluded by the synechiae. It may form an organized exudate on the anterior surface of the lens in the pupillary area (*occlusion of the pupil*), a condition which may also lead to a *secondary glaucoma*. It may orm an organized exudate from the ciliary body into the anterior part of the vitreous (*cyclitic membrane*) which may be associated with a retinal detachment.

5. *The intraocular pressure.* The intraocular pressure of the eye is seldom affected in the early stages, although sometimes the pressure may be slightly lower than normal. In the later stages, particularly after repeated attacks, a secondary glaucoma may ensue in various ways as discussed above.

6. *Nodule formations.* These are characteristic of the granulomatous forms of the disease (see below).

7. *Cataract.* Prolonged uveitis predisposes to cataract.

8. *Atrophic changes.* It is not uncommon for an eye to recover more or less completely from an attack of iridocyclitis, particularly after the use of modern therapeutic methods, but repeated severe attacks ultimately lead to atrophic changes of the iris with a decrease of pigmentation and sometimes with more generalized atrophic changes (*atrophia bulbi*)—scarring and vascularization of the subepithelial parts of the cornea (*pannus degenerativus*), chronic inflammatory changes in the uveal tract leading ultimately to calcareous and even osseous changes, cataract and shrinkage of the globe. A shrinkage may also follow a severe septic inflammation of the whole eye (*panophthalmitis*); this is termed *phthisis bulbi*.

POSTERIOR UVEITIS (CHOROIDITIS)

This seldom produces symptoms other than blurring of vision which may vary from a very slight lack of definition to a well-marked diffuse haze. In the active stage there is an outpouring of inflammatory cells (exudation) into the vitreous, which causes the blurring of vision; these cells may be visible also in the retrolental space, but they are seldom present to any significant extent in the anterior chamber. The vitreous exudate is liable to form persistent opacities. In the acute stage the affected area of the choroid is swollen and fluffy white due to intense inflammatory changes, although this may be difficult to observe if the vitreous haze is intense or if the area lies in the periphery. In the method of fluorescein angiography (chap. 7) there is a diffuse leakage of the dye so that there is a pronounced fuzziness around the edges of the lesion when the focus of choroiditis is active. There is also some leakage of dye into the overlying oedematous retina which is particularly evident when there is an

involvement of the macular area. The underlying retina is involved
and produces a scotoma in the visual field due to destruction of the
deeply placed visual receptor cells (rods and cones). Later the scotoma
is associated with a sector-shaped field defect extending from the
region of the scotoma to the periphery of the field due to a destruction of the superficially placed retinal nerve fibres which pass
through the affected area from the sector of the retina peripheral to
the lesion. The surrounding retina is oedematous to varying degrees.
After several weeks the acute stage subsides and one or more atrophic
areas of the choroid and retina develop, so that the sclera is visible as
a white, often fairly circular focus, surrounded usually by varying
amounts of pigmentary disturbance.

The area of involvement may be localized (*focal choroiditis*), widespread (*diffuse choroiditis*), or multiple (*disseminated choroiditis*); and
it may occur in the macular region (*central choroiditis*), adjacent to
the optic disc (*juxtapapillary choroiditis*), or in the peripheral region
(*anterior choroiditis*).

The final visual result depends on the area of the retina involved;
direct implication of the macular area usually destroys the central
vision, but even indirect implication by oedema, as in a juxtapapillary
choroiditis, tends to be followed by fine pigmentary disturbances at
the macula which affect the central vision to some extent. Involvement of a peripheral retinal area may leave little or no subjective
awareness of the defect.

Pars Planitis (*Chronic Posterior Cyclitis*)

In a form of uveitis which involves the peripheral part of the uvea
(the pars plana of the ciliary body) there are certain distinctive
features: scanty inflammatory changes in the anterior chamber,
exudative inflammatory changes of the pars plana which may lend to
a detachment of the peripheral retina and choroid, marked inflammatory disturbance of the anterior part of the vitreous with dust-like
opacities which may eventually form confluent exudates ('snowball'
opacities) on the surface of the peripheral retina, and an oedema of
the macular region which may cause a cystoid degenerative change
(chap. 7).

PAN-UVEITIS (ENDOPHTHALMITIS)

A generalized uveitis occurs classically in sympathetic ophthalmitis
(p. 95), almost invariably in the uveitis of Still's disease (p. 92), and in
other nonspecific forms. It presents with blurring of vision and some-

times in the early stages the apparently mild state of the anterior uveitis (fine K.P., slight flare and relatively few cells in the aqueous humour) is in contrast to the marked oedema of the retina, particularly surrounding the optic disc, due to a widespread posterior uveitis which is revealed in the later stages by the development of scattered areas of choroido-retinal atrophy. The papilloedema may be followed by a secondary optic atrophy, presumably as a result of damage to the capillary circulation of the disc during the active stage; the ultimate visual prognosis is poor. Sometimes, particularly in infants, the retina becomes detached as a result of proliferation of the inflammatory products in the underlying choroid: this disorganized mass of retinal and uveal tissue may be termed a *pseudoglioma* and it must be distinguished from a retinoblastoma (chap. 7).

Treatment. In addition to the usual treatment for anterior uveitis (p. 96), systemic steroids or adrenocorticotrophic hormone (ACTH) are essential to lessen the severity of the inflammatory process in the posterior part of the uvea.

Aetiology of Uveitis

The condition may be primary (endogenous or exogenous) or secondary.

Endogeneous Uveitis. There are two main forms, granulomatous and nongranulomatous uveitis, and frequently cases show features of both forms.

Granulomatous uveitis follows a direct involvement of the uveal tract by infective organisms—tuberculosis, syphilis, sarcoidosis, toxoplasmosis, histoplasmosis, brucellosis, certain virus conditions etc.—and may occur without any acute episode. Focal lesions produce visible nodules in the iris with associated large K.P., or in the choroid with associated marked vitreous haze. The inflammatory response varies according to the nature of the organism and according to the response of the tissues. Immunity as a result of a previous infection or of some innate characteristic provides a resistance to the spread of the disease, but a hypersensitivity resulting from a previous infection provokes an exuberant and rapidly progressing response; this is seen in the temporary flare-up (*Jarisch-Herxheimer reaction*) which may occur early in the treatment of a syphilitic uveitis.

Nongranulomatous uveitis follows an indirect involvement of the uveal tract, so that the response is an allergic one to bacteria such as the streptococcus, gonococcus and tubercle bacillus which are present in an active state within some remote focus of the body (for example, the sinuses, teeth, prostate, gall bladder, or lung). It usually presents acutely. It is characterized by small K.P., few posterior synechiae, only slight vitreous haze, an absence of any focal lesions, and often a widespread retinal oedema. These features, however, are seldom maintained in subsequent attacks and 'granulomatous' appearances become evident.

Exogenous Uveitis. This follows the direct introduction of infection into the uveal tract following a perforation of the globe (injury, operation, perforated corneal ulcer, etc.). A special form is sympathethic ophthalmitis.

General aspects of the systemic conditions which are sometimes associated with uveitis are discussed below and methods of treatment of uveitis itself on page 96.

TOXOPLASMOSIS

This follows an infestation by the Toxoplasma, a protozoal organism which has long been recognized in many animals, particularly rodents and birds, but more recently in man. Infection may be acquired at any age as well as congenitally by transmission from the mother (who may never have shown any signs of the disease) to the fetus. Infection may be widespread in the infant.

Central Nervous System. In the early stages there is a meningo-encephalitis of varying intensity leading in some cases to convulsions and even to death. Later there may be hydrocephalus, epilepsy, spasticity, comatous attacks or mental retardation. Foci from previous cerebral involvement are often visible on radiographical examination of the skull because they become calcified.

Digestive System. Involvement of the liver may be associated with jaundice.

Lymphatic System. Involvement of the spleen may cause spleno-megaly.

Eye. Isolated patches of acute choroido-retinitis are prone to occur with a predilection for the central part of the fundus, so that the macula may be implicated directly or indirectly by a spread of oedema from an adjacent focus. Later the focus appears as a white atrophic area with usually dense surrounding pigmentation. There is a tendency to recurrence after a prolonged interval, and a frank choroido-retinitis in the older child or adult may be the result of a previously undetected congenital lesion. It follows that aetiologically there are two types of lesion: one which is the direct result of the organism in the absence of any immunity and the other which

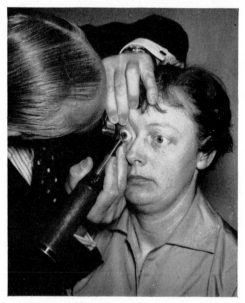

PLATE I Examination of the right eye with an ophthalmic loupe and focal
illumination

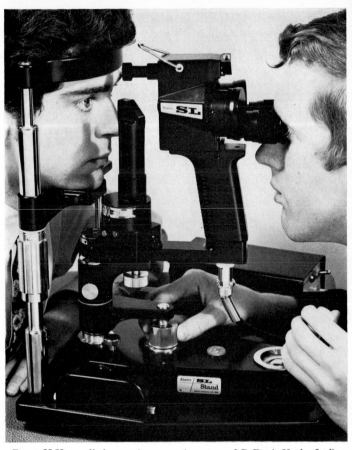

PLATE II Kowa slit-lamp microscope (courtesy of C. Davis Keeler Ltd)

is hypersensitive reaction in the presence of immunity. The effects of the posterior uveitis are so marked that toxoplasmosis is discussed in the chapter dealing with diseases of the uveal tract, but the marked predilection of the organism for nervous tissues determines the likelihood that it is primarily an infection of the retina with a secondary involvement of the underlying choroid.

Other ocular defects such as cataract, nystagmus, microphthalmos and ophthalmoplegia are more rare.

Serological Diagnosis

The antibody titre in the blood may be determined by a methylene blue test: the dye stains the toxoplasma deeply when it is incubated with normal serum, but less deeply when there are antibodies in the serum. A high titre (for example 1 in 64,000 or 1 in 32,000) may persist for several years after an infection. A low titre (for example 1 in 32) is not diagnostic unless repeated tests show a rising titre with an active choroiditis. The complement fixation test is of less value.

Treatment. In lesions which show a poor response to systemic steroids (and this appears to apply particularly to the more peripheral ones), Daraprim (pyrimethamine), an antimalarial drug, is effective in some cases (25 mg twice daily, reducing to once daily), but as it may cause a macrocytic type of anaemia and leucopenia a blood examination should be carried out at weekly intervals. Yeast tablets may diminish the adverse effects of Daraprim.

HISTOPLASMOSIS

This is a fungal condition which occurs particularly in parts of the United States. It causes small disseminated peripheral foci of choroiditis, and sometimes isolated spherical yellow-white nodules in the choroid usually without any obvious pigmentary disturbance. The vitreous remains clear and an anterior uveitis is rare. There is often also a disciform type of choroidal haemorrhage in the submacular or peripapillary area. Foci of disease may occur in the lungs. A skin test using fresh antigen provides a positive result in the majority of cases.

TUBERCULOSIS

Tuberculous uveitis may occur by a direct (primary) or indirect (secondary) involvement.

Primary infection

Direct ocular involvement by *Myobacterium tuberculosis* produces an extensive lesion in the anterior uvea, particularly in the region of the root of the iris with involvement of the ciliary body, or in the posterior uvea. This is serious because the inflammatory and caseous changes may cause perforation of the globe before the onset of the usual reparative processes of fibrosis. Fortunately it is rare and there is no specific treatment.

Secondary Infection

Indirect ocular involvement by tuberculous toxin from some remote source is more common, and the uveitis may be anterior (with the formation of characteristically large 'mutton fat' K.P.) or posterior. Its intensity is variable because it depends on the tissue immunity, which is lowered in states of malnutrition or in the presence of active disease, and on the tissue hypersensitivity.

Diagnosis. The *Mantoux skin test* measures the sensitivity to intracutaneous injections of dilute tuberculin, but this test is becoming of less value because of the widespread use of B.C.G. vaccination. A positive reaction indicates a tuberculous focus, but this is only significant in the child because a positive reaction is common in the adult due to an old and quite inactive lesion. It should be noted also that it is a measure of *skin* and not necessarily *uveal* sensitivity. A *radiographic examination* may show an active or inactive focus of the disease in the chest.

Treatment. A general sanatorium regimen of rest, good diet and sunshine may be combined with systemic treatment (streptomycin 1 g daily and para amino-salicyclic acid (PAS) 12–15 g daily for several weeks) in severe cases. Desensitization with repeated injections of tuberculin, initially in low dilutions but thereafter in gradually increasing concentrations, although not sufficient to cause acute exacerbations, is largely an outmoded therapeutic procedure.

SARCOIDOSIS (BESNIER-BOECK DISEASE)

This disease is characterized by the production of nodules in different sites of the body: in the lymph nodes (*benign lympho-granulomatosis*) commonly in the hilar glands (apparent on radiographic examination) or underlying the skin (the diagnosis is confirmed by biopsy excision), in the salivary glands (*Heerfordt's disease* or *uveoparotid fever* when the uveitis is associated with an involvement of the parotid gland so that there may also be a facial paralysis; *Mikulicz's syndrome* when the uveitis is associated with involvement of the lacrimal gland in addition to the salivary glands), rarely in the bones with the production of areas of rarefaction, and in the lungs with the development of fibrosis. Certain cases appear to be induced in response to carcinomatous or traumatic influences. A granulomatous type of uveitis with the formation of profuse large white K.P. is common and may be the only obvious manifestation; sometimes there are large nodules in the iris which subside spontaneously but recur in a subsequent attack. The Mantoux reaction is negative.

SYPHILIS

Congenital Syphilis

An anterior uveitis occurs with an interstitial keratitis (chap. 4), but also as a separate entity particularly in the very young. More rarely a posterior uveitis, affecting the peripheral parts of the choroid, occurs with or without an anterior uveitis. Both eyes are usually involved and it is apparent in the first year of life as a diffuse pigmentary change in both fundi, the so-called 'pepper and salt' appearances. The management of congenital syphilis is discussed in Chapter 4.

Acquired Syphilis

An anterior uveitis may occur in the secondary or tertiary stages of the disease and, without effective systemic treatment, is prone to recurrence; occasionally the affected iris shows patches of dilated capillary blood vessels, the so-called *roseolae*. Posterior uveitis may also occur in the secondary or tertiary stages. In the serological diagnosis of syphilitic conditions of the eye it is evident that reliance can no longer be placed solely on the *Wassermann Reaction (W.R.)* or the *Kahn Test*. There are two main aims in such serological tests: first, the detection of antibodies against the Treponema pallidum using living or dead suspensions and these include the *Treponemal Immobilization (TPI)*, the *Reiter Protein Complement Fixation Test (RPCFT)*, the *Fluorescent Treponemal Antibody Test (FTA–200)*, and the *Fluorescent Treponemal Antibody Test (FTA–ABS)*; and second, the detection of antibody-like substances (*'reagins'*) and these include the *Complement Fixation Tests (Wassermann Reaction (W.R.)* and *Cardiolipin W. R.)* and *Flocculation Tests (Khan Test, Price's Protein Reaction (PPR)*, and the *Venereal Diseases Reference Laboratory Slide Test (VDRL)*. It is recommended that the *Cardiophilin W. R.*, the *VDRL Slide Test* and the *RPCFT* should be used as routine tests with the inclusion of other tests such as *TPI* and *FTA–ABS* only when these three tests prove to be inconclusive. The treatment is usually massive doses of penicillin (one million units per day for at least 10 days).

GONORRHOEA

A nongranulomatous anterior uveitis may occur in the late stages in association with a chronic prostatitis or vesiculitis; there is often also an arthritis. The uveitis is usually intense with severe pain, and a gelatinous exudate rapidly develops in the anterior chamber, sometimes with obvious haemorrhage. The diagnosis is confirmed by a prostatic or cervical smear for the causative organism; the *Gonococcal Fixation Test (GCFT)* is largely discarded because it is positive, result is obtained in only about 30 per cent of the cases, a false positivity is common, and it remains positive many years after a cure of the disease.

BEHÇET'S DISEASE

A severe relapsing uveitis occurs with episodes of recurrent oral and genital ulceration, and more rarely thrombophlebitis, polyarthritis or carditis. The uveitis appears as an iritis but the severity of this often masks more widespread inflammatory changes in the eye: choroiditis, retinal vasculitis and optic neuritis. The disease tends to affect people between 20 and 40 years of age and is usually bilateral. The response to treatment is poor, but systemic streptomycin may be of value. The influence of steroids is unpredictable.

STILL'S DISEASE

In this condition of childhood a rheumatoid form of arthritis, affecting particularly the lower extremities, is associated with a persistent bilateral uveitis initially of the nongranulomatous type but later with granulomatous features. The brunt of the inflammatory changes appears to be in the anterior segment but almost invariably there is involvement of the posterior uvea with an associated low-grade oedema of the overlying retina. Sometimes an identical form of uveitis develops in the absence of any arthritic changes, although these may develop later. Cataract is prone to develop even relatively early in the disease and its removal is of limited value because of the poor state of the eye. Optic atrophy may follow a secondary glaucoma or sometimes simply as a result of the uveitis. Band-shaped degeneration of the cornea is a characteristic feature. The aetiology is unknown;

a sensitivity reaction to some antigen, perhaps bacterial in origin or perhaps a denatured gamma globulin, is suggested, but it may be of virus origin. The uveitis seldom responds to local measures. Prolonged systemic steroids probably provide the best chance of saving some sight, but these may induce adverse side-effects such as an increase in girth but a stunting of growth; ACTH is less prone to side-effects, and sometimes subconjunctival injections of a long-acting steroid every few weeks may be of value.

VOGT-KOYANAGI SYNDROME

This usually occurs in childhood with a granulomatous anterior uveitis, alopecia, vitiligo, dysacousis and poliosis (whitening of the hair or eyelashes). There may be an underlying hypothalamic disturbance, but the aetiology of the condition, which is perhaps induced by some virus or sensitivity factor, is unknown.

HARADA'S DISEASE

An anterior uveitis may occur, although the retinal involvement is the main feature (see chap. 7).

HERPES ZOSTER

This is associated with a granulomatous anterior uveitis (p. 87).

LYMPHOGRANULOMA VENEREUM

This virus condition is associated with a granulomatous anterior uveitis.

DIABETES

Roseolae may occur in the iris, but it is doubtful if there is a form of uveitis which is unique to diabetes.

LEPROSY

An anterior uveitis with the formation of nodules may occur in leprosy.

SPECIFIC INTESTINAL CONDITIONS

Conditions such as *typhoid, paratyphoid*, and *dysentery* may be associated with uveitis.

ACUTE SPECIFIC FEVERS

A uveitis, often mild and transient, may occur in certain virus conditions, such as *measles, rubella, mumps, varicella* and *variola*, or in certain bacterial conditions, such as *meningogoccal meningitis*.

BRUCELLOSIS (MALTA FEVER OR UNDULANT FEVER)

A granulomatous anterior uveitis, sometimes recurrent, or a posterior uveitis with disseminated nodular foci of exudative choroiditis, may be features of brucellosis.

ANKYLOSING SPONDYLITIS

This is associated with a recurrent anterior uveitis and rheumatoid changes within the spine which lead eventually to extreme rigidity so that the body becomes flexed at the hips.

GOUT

An anterior uveitis sometimes occurs in gout, which is characterized by acute episodes of arthritis affecting particularly the feet and by periods of remission before becoming chronic; it may follow a disturbance of purine metabolism.

There are also certain special forms of uveitis which are not associated with any systemic disorder.

Heterochromic Cyclitis

Heterochromic cyclitis is a distinctive uveitis which occurs most commonly in young adults, usually in one eye only, with a mild but persistent course. There is a gradual depigmentation and atrophy of the iris stroma so that the alteration in the colour of the iris of the affected eye is a characteristic feature of the condition. It is interesting that there is a complete absence of any posterior synechiae despite the persistent nature of the uveitis. The K.P. are small, white and somewhat crenated, with a widespread distribution over the entire posterior corneal surface (as in the *Posner-Schlossman syndrome—see below*). A few cells occur sporadically in the anterior chamber and in the retrolental space with the formation sometimes of fine opacities in the anterior part of the vitreous, but the vision is relatively unaffected until, after a interval of several years, a posterior cortical cataract ensues with eventually widespread cataractous changes; the removal of the cataractous lens is usually a satisfactory procedure. Sometimes glaucoma occurs in the affected eye with pathological cupping of the optic disc and consequent visual field loss, probably because of deposits of inflammatory material in the filtration angle.

Posner-Schlossman Syndrome (Glaucomatocyclitic Crisis)

The Posner-Schlossman syndrome is a distinctive form of anterior uveitis in which an apparently mild form of iritis, characterized by small, white, somewhat crenated K.P. which are widespread over the entire posterior corneal surface (as in heterochromic cyclitis), is associated with a high intraocular pressure, although, unlike congestive glaucoma, mistiness of vision and the appearance of haloes are seldom marked and the condition remains confined almost invariably to one eye.

Sympathetic Ophthalmitis

Sympathetic ophthalmitis occurs only after a perforating injury of the eye particularly involving the ciliary body. Its nature is unknown; it may be of a viral origin (there is certainly no consistent evidence of any bacterial agent) with an associated allergic response in the injured eye, the *exciting eye*, and in the uninjured eye, the *sympathizing eye*. The uveitis of the sympathizing eye which becomes intense after a mild start occurs some weeks, months, or even years after the injury in association with an intense uveitis of the exciting eye. Thus an injured eye which remains inflamed some weeks after a perforating injury is potentially dangerous unless it is removed before the onset of inflammation in the uninjured eye, and its removal *after* this is of no value in arresting the uveitis of the sympathizing eye; indeed its removal then is most unwise because it may retain finally more vision than the sympathizing eye, although the vision of both eyes is likely to be poor unless there is a rapid and sustained response to intensive treatment with steroids. It follows that it is most unwise to retain a severely injured eye which shows persistent inflammatory changes some weeks after the injury when the long-term visual prognosis is poor.

Phacoanaphylactic Uveitis (Lens-induced Uveitis)

Phacoanaphylactic uveitis occurs as an allergic response to lens material liberated during an extracapsular cataract extraction, following a rupture of the lens capsule, or following seepage through the abnormally permeable lens capsule in a hypermature cataract; the allergic response is usually induced by previous exposure to lens material, for example, after an extracapsular extraction in the other eye. The uveitis is intense, and, when lens material is present, it is usually necessary to remove it.

TREATMENT OF UVEITIS

1. The maintenance of full pupillary dilatation during the active stage to prevent the formation of posterior synechiae which leads to complications (chap. 15). This may be achieved by mydriatics—atropine 1 per cent drops or ointment, hyoscine 0·25 per cent to 0·5 per cent drops, cyclopentolate 1 per cent drops, or phenylephrine 10 per cent drops—and their effects are enhanced by heat (hot spoon-bathings or short-wave diathermy), but sometimes it is necessary to inject mydricaine (a solution of atropine, procaine, and adrenaline, which has a most powerful mydriatic effect, into the subconjunctival tissues after adequate surface anaesthesia with cocaine 4 per cent drops because it causes fairly severe pain.

2. The restriction of the inflammatory response by topical steroids, for example, predsol drops hourly or two-hourly in anterior uveitis, and of systemic steroids, for example, prednisolone 15 to 25 mg daily in posterior uveitis. Their use has eliminated the need for protein shock therapy, the effect of which is largely to mobilize the cortisone reserves of the patient. During prolonged systemic steroid therapy care should be taken to recognize any marked increase in fluid retention or any significant rise in the blood pressure; undue changes in the blood chemistry may be avoided by the use of potassium chloride, 2 G daily.

3. The relief of pain and photophobia by the application of heat, the prevention of pupillary movement by maintaining full mydriasis, the use of dark glasses (or even an eye pad), and various analgesics.

4. The control of any septic element by the use of chemotherapeutic agents or antibiotics topically, subconjunctivally or systemically, in hypopyon iritis.

5. The eradication of the cause of the uveitis if known, for example, treatment of any systemic condition, such as syphilis, gonorrhoea, or of any form of focal infection, such as septic tonsils, or an apical dental abscess.

6. Certain forms of at one time well-established therapy: prolonged periods of rest in persistent uveitis, if necessary by in-patient treatment with a sanatorium type of regimen; the use of a vaccine in nongranulomatous uveitis, for example, the streptococcal form; the use of tuberculin in uveitis due to tuberculosis and also in other cases to produce a nonspecific protein reaction, are of doubtful value and have fallen largely into abeyance since the advent of steroid therapy.

The treatment of complications are discussed elsewhere; for example, secondary glaucoma (chap. 15), cataract (chap. 9).

RUBEOSIS IRIDIS

In rubeosis iridis networks of new vessel formations develop on the anterior surface of the iris, particularly in certain retinal diseases, for example, diabetic retinopathy, thrombosis of the central retinal vein, retrolental fibroplasia, old-standing retinal detachment (all discussed in chap. 8). It is possible that the new vessels are a response to a 'vaso-formative factor' from the diseased peripheral retina, and this 'stimulus' may be diminished by destroying the retina beyond the equator by diathermy. Rubeosis iridis is liable to cause an obliteration of the filtration angle by the formation of peripheral anterior syne-chiae with the production of an intractable secondary glaucoma.

DEGENERATIONS

Iris

Iris atrophy is usually secondary to prolonged anterior uveitis or glaucoma, but rarely it occurs as a primary entity—*essential atrophy of the iris*—in which irregular areas of atrophy lead to distortions of the pupil and ultimately to hole formations. A secondary glaucoma may follow involvement of the filtration angle. Another form of iris atrophy —*iridoschisis*—is usually traumatic in origin (p. 82).

Choroid

Gyrate Atrophy. In this familial condition circular, or irregular, areas of choroidal atrophy occur in the central parts of both fundi with atrophic changes in the overlying retina; the affected areas appear white because of the exposed underlying sclera. Later these areas become confluent and it is suggested that ultimately there may be a *choroideremia* (complete absence of the choroid), but it is more likely that this occurs only as a congenital anomaly (p. 80).

Central Areolar Choroidal Sclerosis. In this familial condition irregular areas of choroidal atrophy occur in the central parts of both fundi but, unlike gyrate atrophy, the degenerative changes are confined to the choriocapillaris; the exposed choroidal vessels appear ophthalmoscopically to be sclerosed, hence the term *sclerosis*, but there are seldom sclerotic changes histologically.

Disciform Degeneration. This follows a massive haemorrhage which forms under the retina usually in the submacular area. It has

been considered that the haemorrhage follows a degeneration of the
choroidal vessels, particularly the capillary layer (the choriocapillaris),
but it is more likely that the primary lesion is a disruption of the
elastic lamina of Bruch's membrane, as the result of an ageing
process, so that the haemorrhage follows a failure of the normal
supporting role of the choroidal capillaries by the elastic lamina. Sometimes the subretinal extravasation is more exudative than haemorrhagic. In fluorescein angiography there is a central pooling of
fluorescence which represents the dye which has leaked from the
choriocapillaris into the area of detached retinal pigment epithelium
with a surrounding dark nonfluorescent area which represents the
haemorrhage. Inevitably there is a disruption of the function of the
overlying retina. Ophthalmoscopically the lesion appears as a dark
swelling without any obvious haemorrhage unless this tracks into the
overlying retina. Eventually the deep haemorrhage usually absorbs
with atrophic changes in the retina and choroid, but it may become
organized with the formation of a raised, often pigmented, mass of
tissue (Fuch's black spot). Sometimes the deep haemorrhage is surrounded by white patches (macrophages) arranged in a concentric or
annular manner—the so-called *circinate retinopathy*.

Anterior Segment Necrosis (*Ischaemic Ocular Inflammation*)

A peculiar form of anterior uveitis may result from a disturbance
with the blood supply to the anterior segment of the eye (*ischaemic
ocular inflammation*), particularly when there is an undue interference
with the recti muscles which contain the anterior ciliary arteries; this
may occur in extensive retinal detachment surgery or in certain
muscle transplant procedures. It may occur also simply as the result
of long-standing ocular disease. There are other features: diffuse
episcleral redness, corneal oedema with a wrinkling of Descemet's
membrane, neovascularization of the iris, atrophy of the iris with an
irregular semidilatation of the pupil which responds poorly to light
and drugs, cataract, and a greyness of the peripheral part of the retina
with haemorrhages. There is a poor response to anti-inflammatory
measures, and blindness usually ensues.

Tumours

Melanoma

This humour probably has a neuroectodermal origin in the uveal
tract and may be simple (benign melanoma, pigmented mole, naevus), often present in early life, or malignant (malignant melanoma).

Iris

A simple melanoma presents as a localized pigmented mass on the surface of the iris or within the stroma, and it is composed largely of spindle cells; it is different from an *iris freckle* which is simply a proliferation of normal stromal melanocytes. A change to malignancy is indicated by an increase in its size so that it may project into the anterior chamber, sometimes with an area of corneal contact, or into the posterior chamber where it lies against the lens. It may also extend to the tissues of the filtration angle and the anterior part of the ciliary body. A ^{32}P test is sometimes of value in establishing its maliganant nature. When malignancy is suspected the tumour should be excised completely together with a strip of normal iris (*iridectomy*) and also with a portion of the ciliary body (*iridocyclectomy*) when necessary. Early and adequate local excision carries a good prognosis and avoids the removal of the eye.

Choroid

A simple melanoma appears as a bluish-grey mass under the retina, and its benign nature is favoured by certain features; no obvious increase in size over a prolonged period, no marked elevation of the retina over the affected area, the retention of visual function in this area of retina (because the benign tumour does not involve the choriocapillaris which supplies the outer part of the retina), and the absence of any surrounding serous retinal detachment. In fluorescein angiography there is an area of nonfluorescence corresponding to the area of the tumour because this screens the background fluorescence of the choroid. In a change to malignancy, which seldom occurs before middle age, these features are lost, and of particular importance is the development of an area of retinal detachment, quite apart from the retina overlying the tumour, because of fluid in the subretinal space; the formation of this fluid confirms the active nature of the choroidal lesion, and the free nature of the subretinal space determines the fact that, although the serous detachment usually is adjacent to the tumour, it may be remote from it because the fluid from the tumour gravitates to the lower part of the subretinal space. There is a disturbance of retinal function over the tumour and in the area of the serous detachment, but sometimes this is not noticed by the patient until the central vision becomes affected. A few haemorrhages may occur in the retina in the area of the tumour.

A ^{32}P test is of value in certain cases; the radioactive phosphorus is taken by mouth and its concentration over the surface of the affected and unaffected eyes is determined with a Geiger counter 24 hours later. An excessively high uptake over the affected area is of diagnostic importance, but the results are sometimes inconclusive particularly as it depends largely on a comparison of values between corresponding parts of the affected and unaffected eyes. It follows that the result of any one test should not sway unduly clinical judgement. Transillumination of the globe by shining a bright light into the eye through the sclera may reveal a shadow over the affected area, but this test is not always reliable. In fluorescein angiography there is a filling of the vessels of the tumour with the dye and throughout the substance of the tumour there is an abnormal pooling of fluorescein with a finely flecked fluorescence at the border of the tumour as the result of a leakage of the dye. The main lesions which may be confused with a malignant melanoma are an extensive choroidal haemorrhage (p. 97), a simple retinal detachment (chap. 7), and a metastatic carcinoma (see below). A malignant melanoma usually remains confined to the eye for a considerable period before involving the extraocular tissues by direct spread through the sclera or before forming more distant metastases (classically in the liver, but sometimes in the skin or in other regions) as a result of blood spread. Indeed the tumour in the eye may become so large that it causes a secondary glaucoma (caused sometimes by obliteration of the filtration angle by new vessel formations on the surface of the iris), so that the eye becomes blind and painful; it follows that sometimes an 'unknown' blind eye should be removed if it is not possible to examine the fundus ophthalmoscopically in case it harbours a malignant melanoma.

Treatment. Enucleation of the eye is the treatment of choice, and, provided there is no evidence of extraocular extension at operation or on histological examination of the eye and provided there are no metastases within a few years, there is a good prognosis. Sometimes if the other eye has poor vision (or has been lost by injury or disease) it may be justified to try to control the tumour by irradiation (for example, the application of a cobalt disc) or by photocoagulation of the affected area.

Haemangioma (*Angioma*)

A haemangioma may occur in any part of the uveal tract—very rarely in the iris and ciliary body but less rarely in the choroid. A *haemangioma of the iris* because of its vascular nature accounts for the development of periodic bleeding (hyphaema). A *haemangioma of the choroid* may not become evident until adult life despite its congenital nature. It is usually situated near the optic disc. It grows slowly with the formation of a raised mass and eventually with the development of a remote serous retinal detachment in the lower part of the eye. In fluorescein angiography the tumour shows a brilliant fluorescence because of its vascular nature with a coarsely flecked fluorescence at the border of the tumour because of a leakage of the dye; both these features are usually more prominent than in a malignant melanoma of the choroid.

Quite frequently a haemangioma of the uveal tract is associated with a naevus flammeus, port-wine stain, affecting the skin of the face in the distribution of the ipsilateral trigeminal nerve (cranial nerve V), with similar abnormal vessels in the episcleral region near the limbus so that glaucoma may ensue following obliteration of the filtration angle, and with similar lesions in the ipsilateral cerebral cortex causing hemiplegia, epilepsy, mental deficiency (the *Sturge-Weber syndrome*, one of the phakomatoses (chap. 7)).

Neurofibroma

This tumour occurs rarely in the choroid usually as a manifestation of Von Recklinghausen's disease, one of the phakomatoses.

Metastatic Carcinoma

The choroid is a common site for carcinomatous metastatic deposits from a primary focus in the lungs or breast, and it is usually an indication of widespread dissemination. The lesion responds readily to irradiation and, unless the patient is moribund, this should be carried out because it permits the retention of some vision and prevents the complications which may follow a later total retinal detachment such as a secondary glaucoma. Removal of the eye is seldom justified unless it becomes blind and painful.

Cysts

A *spontaneous cyst* of the iris as a result of a separation of the two pigmented layers following an accumulation of fluid, sometimes of an inflammatory nature, is extremely rare, but an *implantation cyst* on the surface of the iris is slightly more common and may follow a proliferation of epithelial tissue which is introduced into the eye from a corneal wound at the time of a perforating injury or operation; sometimes this cyst becomes sufficiently large to necessitate its removal, otherwise glaucoma may ensue.

Anomalies of the Pupillary Reflexes

These follow lesions of the afferent or efferent parts of their nervous pathways.

A Lesion of the Afferent Pupillary (Visual) Pathway in the Retina or Optic Nerve

Stimulation of the affected eye by light causes a defect in the pupillary constriction of the affected eye (direct light reflex) and of the unaffected eye (consensual light reflex) because the afferent pupillary fibres from each eye are transmitted to the parasympathetic parts of the oculomotor nuclei on both sides of the brainstem. The defects are complete if the lesions are complete and partial if the lesions are partial. In contrast, the consensual light response of the affected eye and the direct light response of the unaffected eye are normal. The constriction of the pupil of the affected eye which occurs in the consensual response is followed by a dilatation of the pupil when the light stimulus of the unaffected eye is discontinued and the dilatation continues even when the affected eye is stimulated by light (*Marcus Gunn pupillary phenomenon*).

A Lesion of the Afferent Pupillary (Visual) Pathway in the Optic Chiasma or Optic Tract

This causes defects similar to those described above, but only when the affected part of the pathway is stimulated because of the partial decussation of the afferent pupillary (and visual) fibres in the optic chiasma (chap. 16); this 'hemianopic' pupil response is difficult to determine clinically because of the scattering of light on illuminating any part of the retina.

A lesion of the afferent visual pathway caudal to the exit of the afferent pupillary fibres from the optic tract does not interfere with the pupillary light reflexes; it follows that total blindness caused by lesions of both cortical visual areas is compatible with unimpaired pupillary light reflexes.

A Lesion of the Efferent Parasympathetic Pupillary Pathway

This causes a defect in the pupillary constriction of the eye on the side of the lesion to a light stimulus of the ipsilateral eye (direct light reflex) and to a light stimulus of the contralateral eye (consensual light reflex), but there is no defect in the light responses of the other eye. There is also a defect in the pupillary constriction of the eye on the side of the lesion to a near stimulus (accommodation and convergence pupillary reflexes). This represents an internal ophthalmoplegia.

A Lesion of the Efferent Peripheral Sympathetic Pupillary Pathway
This causes little interference in the pupillary reaction to light because the main effect of the hypothalamic sympathetic centre is an indirect one on the parasympathetic nucleus so that pupillary dilatation follows an inhibition of the nucleus rather than a peripheral sympathetic stimulation. However, it causes other characteristic features (*Horner's syndrome*)—a somewhat constricted pupil (miosis) resulting from the unopposed action of the sphincter muscle of the pupil, a narrowing of the palpebral fissure from a failure of the superior (and inferior) palpebral smooth muscles, a decreased sweating of the ipsilateral forehead, and (occasionally) a decreased pigmentation of the affected iris. The enophthalmos which is sometimes described is more apparent (following the narrowing of the palpebral fissure) than real, because there is no effective smooth muscle in the orbit which alters significantly the position of the eye. Conversely, an irritative lesion of the sympathetic pathway (for example, the early stages of a neoplasm in the upper part of the chest) produces the opposite effects; a somewhat dilated pupil (mydriasis), a widening of the palpebral fissure, and an increased sweating of the ipsilateral forehead.

The other pupillary anomalies are:
Myotonic Pupil (Adie's Pupil). This is more common in females and occurs usually in early adult life, almost invariably confined to one eye. The pupil is somewhat dilated with an apparent absence of any response to light, directly or consensually, except for slight worm-like heavings of the pupil margin. The pupil constricts to a near stimulus, but this is slow, becoming effective only after a considerable time. There is also a slowness of the pupil to revert to its usual size after removing the near stimulus; this retention of some form of near response distinguishes the myotonic pupil from the dilated pupil which follows a mydriatic like atropin, and the myotonic pupil, unlike the atropinized pupil, constricts after the instillation of mecholyl 2·5 per cent drops. Sometimes the tendon reflexes (particularly the knee

and ankle jerks) are defective, but there are no other neurologic complications and the site of the lesion is unknown.

Argyll Robertson Pupil. This is characterized by a persistent but somewhat irregular miosis with an absence of (or, in the early stages, with an impaired) response to light, directly and consensually, and with a brisk response to near stimulus. It is almost invariably bilateral although the degree of miosis may be unequal. It occurs in lesions affecting the pretectal region of the mid-brain (hence its bilateral nature) in a wide variety of cerebral disorders (encephalitis, vascular abnormalities, traumatic lesions) but characteristically it occurs in neurosyphilis (tabes dorsalis and general paralysis of the insane); in the juvenile form of neurosyphilis the pupils may be involved in a similar way except for an absence of miosis. A unilateral Argyll Robertson pupil rarely follows a cerebral disorder but may follow a lesion of the ciliary ganglion in the orbit with involvement of the efferent pathway subserving the constriction to light (the pathway subserving constriction to a near stimulus is not mediated by the ciliary ganglion so that the near response is retained).

Hippus. This term applies to a state of pupillary unrest with constant slight fluctuations without any change in illumination. It has been described in some cases of disseminated sclerosis and chorea.

Anomalies of Accommodation

Paralysis. This occurs in lesions of the part of the oculomotor nucleus or nerve subserving the intrinsic ocular muscles of the ciliary body, but it is rare.

Insufficiency. This occurs commonly at any age and is usually precipitated by some emotional factor, such as overwork, worry, or by some debilitating disease which causes a functional (not an organic) disorder. The blurred reading vision is associated with symptoms of eyestrain, such as aching and redness of the eyes, headaches, and there may also be weakness of convergence. These may be relieved partly by the correction of any refractive error, but it is essential to treat the underlying cause. It occurs, of course, naturally with age (*presbyopia*, chap. 2).

Spasm. This may also occur at any age because of emotional factors. The persistent excess of accommodation causes a blurring of vision in the distance, an inability to read small print unless held close to the eyes, and the symptoms of eyestrain. There may be an associated spasm of convergence which results in a latent or even manifest convergent squint, and an associated spasm of the sphincter of the pupils. The treatment is directed at the underlying cause.

Influence of Drugs on the Pupils and the Ciliary Body

The mydriatic and cycloplegic effects of drugs such as atropine and hyoscine, and the miotic and cyclospastic effects of drugs, such as eserine and pilocarpine, are discussed elsewhere (chaps. 2 and 15).

7 | Diseases of the Retina

Structure and Function (Fig. 28)

The retina forms the inner coat of the eye and is concerned with the reception of the images of the fixation object (central vision) and of the other objects in the visual panorama (peripheral vision). It has two main parts—the pigment epithelium (the outer layer) and the optical part (the inner layers)—a distinction of importance because the two parts lie in apposition without any form of union, except around the optic disc and in the extreme periphery at the ora serrata so that there is a potential space (this is the site of the subretinal fluid in a retinal detachment). This peculiarity of 'apposition without adherence' is the result of the development of the retina in the embryo by an invagination of the primary optic vesicle to form the secondary optic vesicle, whereby the invaginated portion forms the optical part of the retina and the uninvaginated portion forms the pigment epithelium. An abnormal closure of the cleft of the secondary optic vesicle determines the formation of a uveal coloboma (chap. 6).

The optical part is complex but it functions as three main layers:

1. An *outer layer of rods and cones* which lies immediately beneath the pigment epithelium; their nuclei form the *outer nuclear layer*.

The *rods* are concerned under conditions of bright illumination with an appreciation of light and movement, but under conditions of dim illumination their function is enhanced because the visual purple (rhodopsin) which is a constituent of the rods and is bleached on exposure to light, becomes re-formed as a photochemical response which is dependent on an adequate supply of vitamin A and on an adequate contact of the rods with a normally functioning pigment epithelium. The rods are responsible for *scotopic vision*. They are present throughout the retina, particularly in the more peripheral parts, but are absent in the fovea.

The *cones* are concerned with an appreciation of form and colour under conditions of bright illumination (*photopic vision*). They are present throughout the retina but particularly in the fovea, where there are no rods, and in the parafovea or macula, where there are few rods.

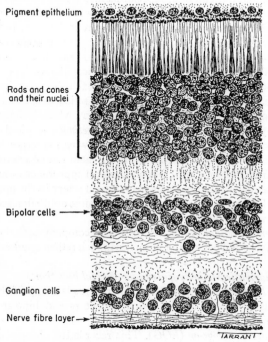

Pigment epithelium

Rods and cones and their nuclei

Bipolar cells

Ganglion cells

Nerve fibre layer

FIG. 28. *The minute structure of the retina (after Duke-Elder)*

2. *A middle layer of bipolar cells* which provide the connecting link between the rods and cones and the ganglion cells. It forms the *inner nuclear layer*.

3. *An inner layer of ganglion cells* which give rise to the nerve fibres which pass along the innermost part of the retina (*nerve fibre* later) to the optic nerve-head, optic nerve, optic chiasma and optic tract to reach the lateral geniculate body. This layer is absent directly over the fovea which is, therefore, less thick than the rest of the retina.

BLOOD SUPPLY (Fig. 30)

The central retinal artery, which is a branch of the ophthalmic artery (a branch of the internal carotid artery), enters the eye through the optic nerve-head within the optic cup and divides into four main branches which supply each retinal quadrant—the superior temporal, inferior temporal, superior nasal and inferior nasal arteries. Each of these arteries (or their branches) acts as an end artery so that its occlusion causes a loss of function in a retinal sector, but it supplies only the inner half of the retina (as far as the bipolar cells)—the outer half, containing the rods and cones, is supplied indirectly by the capillaries of the choroid (the choriocapillaris). The fovea is devoid of retinal vessels and is nourished exclusively by the choriocapillaris. Rarely a small artery passes to the retina, usually its macular part, from the circle of Zinn within the sclera which is derived from the ciliary circulation. This is termed a *cilioretinal* artery and ophthalmoscopically it appears as a small artery which emerges from the border of the optic disc (in contrast to the main retinal arteries which emerge from the optic cup), but an identical appearance occurs when a small retinal artery leaves the main retinal artery in the optic nerve behind the lamina cribrosa, which is not visible ophthalmoscopically, to pass independently to the retina.

The central retinal vein leaves the eye in company with the central retinal artery and has similar branches in each retinal quadrant.

Electrodiagnostic Methods of Assessing Retinal Function

The Electroretinogram (ERG). This records the sum of the action potentials generated by the retinal receptors and bipolar cells in response to a flash of light.

The Electrooculogram (EOG). This records the changes of ocular potential caused by metabolic activity, mainly in the retinal pigment epithelium.

These electrodiagnostic methods provide evidence of abnormal responses in lesions involving the circulation of the choroid or involving the pigment epithelium, receptor cells or bipolar cells of the retina. They are of particular value when it is not possible to view the fundus because of a dense opacity of the media such as a cataract, or in certain abiotrophic, degenerative or vascular lesions of the retina at a stage when there are no obvious ophthalmoscopic changes. However, the ERG provides a mass response so that half the retina must be involved before the result is abnormal.

Fluorescein Angiography

In recent years the method of fluorescein angiography has assumed an important role in the assessment of certain retinal and choroidal disorders. Fluorescein (5 ml of 10 per cent solution) is injected intravenously (the antecubital vein of the right arm), and the appearance of the dye in the fundus and its final disappearance are recorded by a camera containing high-speed film which photographs the fundus at regular intervals (about every second) and incorporating a blue filter (with maximum transmission between 4800 and 5000 Å units). In the normal eye the following sequence of events is recorded; a *choroidal flush* which lasts for less than a second, an *early retinal arteriolar phase* which spreads outwards from the optic disc, a *late retinal arteriolar phase* in which the whole arteriolar tree is brightly fluorescent, a *retinal capillary phase* which appears first as a reticular pattern in the late retinal arteriolar phase and persists beyond that phase, an *early retinal venous phase* which appears in the late retinal arteriolar phase as a layering or streaming along the venous walls, and a *late retinal venous phase* at a stage when the retinal arterioles lose their fluorescence; finally the brightness of the venous fluorescence fades, but persists to some extent because of a recirculation of the dye particularly within the optic disc and the outline of the choroidal vessels is visible against the background of scleral fluorescence.

Congenital Anomalies

Opaque Nerve Fibres

The optic nerve fibres in the retina are normally nonmyelinated so that they are not visible ophthalmoscopically—the myelinating process which spreads along the optic nerve from the central nervous system in the fetus, and even for a short time after birth, terminates at the lamina cribrosa in the deeper part of the optic nerve-head. Rarely the myelination extends into part of the retina so that the nerve fibres in the affected area become visible as an opaque white slightly striated patch with 'feathery' edges which characteristically tends to obscure partially the retinal vessels in the affected region because of the superficial position of the optic nerve fibres; this is in direct contrast to other white patches such as exudates, colloid material or choroidal atrophy which lie deep to the retinal vessels. Opaque nerve fibres are usually contiguous with the optic disc, but rarely an isolated patch may occur in another part of the retina. There is some depression of visual function in the affected area.

Abnormal Pigmentation

The uniform 'redness' of the normal fundus on ophthalmoscopic examination is caused by the blood within the underlying choroidal circulation and the pattern of the choroidal vessels is obscured by the dense pigmentation of the retinal pigment epithelium; but if this pigmentation is less dense than usual, these vessels become visible to some extent so that the fundus has a tigroid appearance (the so-called 'tigroid' fundus). A marked deficiency or even a complete absence of pigmentation, as in albinism, gives the fundus a pale pink appearance due to the exposure of the underlying choroid and sclera. Sometimes in the normal fundus pigment accumulates in discrete patches in the deeper parts of the retina; the so-called 'cat's paw' pigmentation ('bear's paw' pigmentation in the United States).

It should be noted that a slight darkening of the parafoveal and paramacular areas as compared with the rest of the retina is normal, with the fovea standing out as a glistening white spot.

Abnormal Vascularization

Normally the extensive network of hyaloid vessels which fills the vitreous in the fetus disappears shortly before birth, but occasionally parts of these vessels persist as congenital remnants. A hyaloid artery covered by glial tissue may project from the optic disc into the vitreous (the so-called Bergmeister's papilla).

Embryopathic Pigmentary Retinopathy

A congenital anomaly of the pigment epithelium may follow certain maternal infections (such as syphilis, rubella, and influenza) in the first three months of pregnancy. Involvement of the pigment epithelium in both eyes may result from interference with its normal development (as distinct from destruction of established pigment epithelium in inflammatory conditions); there is irregular pigmentation of the fundus with some areas in which the pigment cells are more or less devoid of pigment and other areas in which they contain an excess of unusually large pigment granules. This anomaly accounts also for the appearance in the fundus of small bluish pigmented spots—the so-called pepper-and-salt changes. It is doubtful if the condition leads to any serious visual disturbance unless the macular area is implicated significantly.

Coloboma

A coloboma of the retina occurs in association with a coloboma of the choroid (chap. 6); sometimes branches from the retinal vessels in other parts of the retina pass over the coloboma.

Retinal Dysplasia

This is a developmental disorder, sometimes of a familial nature, which is present at birth even in term infants. A greyish-white tissue in the vitreous represents the elevated malformed retina which may become adherent to the posterior surface of the lens. The condition is usually bilateral and the eye may be slightly microphthalmic with a shallow anterior chamber. It is frequently associated with other malformations—cardiovascular defects, cleft palate, hare lip, hydrocephalus, mental retardation, polydactylism, and intestinal malrotations. This condition is different from *retinal aplasia* (p. 140).

Injuries

Commotio Retinae (Berlin's Oedema)

Blunt trauma of the eye, for example a hit from a fist or stone may cause an oedema of the retina underlying the area of the injury or of the retina opposite to this area as the result of a contrecoup effect. The affected area appears cloudy and swollen with fine radiating lines of 'tension' on its surface; this appearance is striking when it affects the macular area (the usual site of involvement of the contrecoup effect following an injury to the front of the eye) because the foveal region which does not share in the oedematous process owing to the absence of a nerve fibre layer stands out as a red circular area against the white background of the surrounding swollen retina. Pigmentary changes usually occur in the retina after the subsidence of the oedema and some permanent disturbance of the vision follows macular involvement. Systemic steroids may reduce the extent of the oedmatous process.

Solar Retinopathy

An oedematous condition of the macular may follow exposure to infrared light from the sun; this is induced very rarely by normal exposure, but it occurs more commonly on observing the eclipse of the sun (the so-called *eclipse blindness*).

Battered-baby Syndrome

Retinal haemorrhages, particularly in the form of an extensive pre-retinal haemorrhage involving the central fundus, is a feature of this distressing condition in which the child abuse also causes fractures of the long bones and subdural haematoma, sometimes of a repeated nature. The retinal changes may be so severe as to cause a retinal detachment with haemorrhage in the subretinal space, so that it resembles Coats' disease histologically, and there may be subsequently optic atrophy. Other ocular abnormalities may occur: injuries to the eyelids, posterior subcapsular cataract, peripheral choroideo-retinal atrophy, vitreous haemorrhage and cortical blindness as the result of diffuse cerebral damage. The establishment of the cause of these lesions is often difficult because the history is almost invariably misleading, but the sociological importance of the recognition of the nature of the syndrome is obvious.

Retinopathy

Retrolental Fibroplasia (Retinopathy of Prematurity)

Retrolental fibroplasia in the premature baby almost invariably affects both eyes within a few weeks of birth, particularly when the birth weight is less than 1·35 kg and when there has been exposure to excessive concentrations of oxygen; it is suggested that a concentration of less than 30 per cent in the atmosphere is safe, but the main determining factor is the concentration in the arterial blood. The oxygen causes a sequence of events in the immature retinal vessels; a vasoconstriction which leads to a vasoobliteration during the exposure to oxygen and a vasoproliferation after removal from the oxygen. The earliest ophthalmoscopic changes occur in the periphery of the retina which appears grey with a disappearance of the fine retinal vessels in that area, although these must be interpreted with care because some degree of greyness is normal in the very young, and the retinal vessels do not extend to the most peripheral part of the retina in the premature child. The proliferation of vaso-formative tissue usually progresses to the formation of vascularized fibrous strands from the retina into the anterior part of the vitreous which lead to areas of retinal detachment. Eventually the retina becomes totally detached and disorganized with the formation of a retrolental membrane which obscures any view of the fundus, usually with total blindness. Subsequently new vessels may develop on the surface of the iris and the shallowness of the anterior chamber, a characteristic feature of this condition, favours development of a secondary glaucoma as the result of an obliteration of the filtration angle by peripheral anterior synechiae. Sometimes, however, the early changes in the retinal periphery subside without any invasion of the vitreous so that some visual function is retained although the eye often becomes myopic, and a retinal fold may pass from the optic disc to the periphery of the fundus with a disruption of central vision when it passes temporally through the macular area.

The sequence of events and the characteristic clinical features seldom cause any difficulty in diagnosis, but the conditions which show similar features are *persistent hyperplastic vitreous* and *persistent vascular sheath of the lens* (chap. 10), *retinoblastoma* (p. 142), *endophthalmitis (pseudoglioma)* (chap. 6), and *Coats' disease* (below).

There is no effective treatment, but fortunately it may be prevented by exercising great care that premature babies are not exposed to excessive concentrations of oxygen; this is a difficult policy to enforce in the presence of an acute *respiratory distress syndrome of newborn*, and the avoidance of an undue concentration of oxygen within the oxygen tent (for example, not more than 30 per cent) is not wholly reliable because the only valid criterion is the repeated estimation of the oxygen level in the arterial blood which involves a highly specialized technique in the neonatal period.

MASSIVE RETINAL FIBROSIS

This occurs in early childhood and is a protusion from the retina of a greyish-white fibrous mass as the result of organization of a massive deep retinal haemorrhage which occurs at birth because of some predisposing factor such as prolonged labour, premature delivery, precipitate birth or asphyxia. It does not lead to a true retinal detachment because a proliferation of the retinal pigment epithelium into the mass unites the affected area with the underlying choroid, but a gradual contraction of the lesion progressively involves the surrounding retina. It is an uncommon condition considering the relative frequency of retinal haemorrhage even after a normal delivery (perhaps in the region of 10 per cent). There may be an associated intracranial haemorrhage; death may ensue if this is severe and surviving infants frequently show some permanent malformation of the central nervous system such as cerebral spastic paralysis and mental retardation.

METASTATIC RETINITIS

A metastatic infective embolus may occur in the retina in any septicaemic disease of childhood. It causes a localized inflammatory reaction which may remain undetected because it is often symptomless (except for a loss of vision which is not appreciated by a child), but a subsequent organization of the affected tissue leads to a retinal detachment with the appearance of a white mass behind the pupil. There is usually an associated cloudiness of the vitreous so that the retinal lesion appears as an indistinct white haze.

TOXOPLASMOSIS

The primary involvement of the retina in this inflammatory condition is discussed in Chapter 6.

COATS' DISEASE

Coats' disease is a rare condition which comprises various clinical entities in which a localized retinal detachment, usually in the central part of the fundus, follows an exudative or haemorrhagic extravasation in the outer retinal layers and in the subretinal space. Sometimes it follows a telangiectasis (*retinal telangiectasis of Reese*) or aneurysm formations (*multiple military retinal aneurysms of Leber*) of the retinal vessels. It occurs particularly in male children between the ages of 5 and 15 years, but also sometimes in the female and young adult. It is usually unilateral. The extravasation becomes organized and cholesterol crystals accumulate within the mass; these are regarded usually as a secondary change, but recently it has been suggested that they follow an abnormal effect of the lipoproteins in the blood plasma so that they may have some primary influence. The vision is seriously affected when the macula is involved. Rarely a secondary uveitis or glaucoma develops in advanced cases. The conditions which sometimes show similar features are retinoblastoma (p. 142), pseudoglioma due to an endophthalmitis (chap. 4), angiomatosis retinae (p. 144) and infestation of the retina by *Toxocara canis* (p. 137). There is no effective treatment for the established condition, but photocoagulation of the abnormal retinal vessels may limit the extent of the retinal involvement.

RETINAL VASCULITIS

Retinal vasculitis is essentially an inflammation of the retinal veins (*periphlebitis* or *phlebitis*), but the occasional involvement also of the arteries (*periarteritis* or *arteritis*) dictates the use of the term *vasculitis.* The origin of the disease is unknown and there is little evidence to support the concept of a tuberculous origin. It may be a collagen disease (p. 130).

It is characteristically a condition of young adults, males more than females. The brunt of the disease occurs in the periphery of the retina with irregular dilatation of the retinal veins, the formation of widespread haemorrhages within the retina and near its surface (preretinal haemorrhage), and zones of sheathing along the affected veins. The condition is usually self-limiting after months or even years, but it is only in mild cases that the visual prognosis is reasonably good because of the relative sparing of the central retina; peripheral retinal haemorrhages are liable to extend into the vitreous with subsequent organization of the vitreous haemorrhage by new vessels from the retina (*retinitis proliferans*) which may lead to localized or even extensive areas of retinal detachment. The condition is frequently bilateral but the two eyes may be affected unequally.

More rarely the disease affects the retinal veins within the optic nerve-head with a massive dilatation of the retinal veins along their whole length from the optic disc to the periphery, marked oedema of the retina surrounding the optic disc (papilloedema) and also sometimes of the macular area, but with comparatively few retinal haemorrhages so that vitreous haemorrhage and subsequent retinitis proliferans are unlikely to occur unless there is an associated peripheral form of the disease. Fluorescein angiography indicates that there are two main stages of vascular decompensation. First, this takes the form of a venous decompensation, and the leakage of the dilated retinal veins is shown by perivenous fluorescence, but the capillaries which are also dilated do not show any permeability and there are no microaneurysms. These changes occur when there is only a moderate retinopathy with haemorrhages and cotton wool spots and in the absence of a marked retinal oedema so that the central vision remains good. Second, this takes the form of a capillary decompensation with an extensive leakage of fluorescein. These changes occur when there is a marked retinopathy with an obvious retinal oedema, and a significant impairment of vision particularly when there is a cystic maculopathy. Eventually an elevation of retinal tissue pressure may cause some areas of capillary closure with the development of ischaemic changes. The condition, which is usually confined to one eye, gradually subsides over a period of months but with a persistence of some degree of retinal vein dilatation, some postoedematous blurring of the optic disc, and a variable disturbance of the macular area.

The central form of retinal vasculitis may mimic a central retinal vein thrombosis (p. 125), but in this latter condition the dilatation of the retinal veins and the oedema around the optic disc are associated with widespread retinal haemorrhages and there are often evidences in the unaffected eye of hypertensive or arteriosclerotic changes in the retinal vessels. The two conditions appear, therefore, to be different, but it is suggested that central retinal vasculitis represents a form of central retinal vein thrombosis occurring in the presence of an otherwise normal vascular system so that there is a potential for the development of collateral channels. There are other conditions which show similar features but should not cause confusion; plerocephalic oedema (chap. 8) is bilateral (as a general rule) and the dilatation of the retinal veins is confined to an area around the optic disc, papillitis (chap. 8) is characterized by a marked loss of vision in the acute stage, and a fulminating hypertensive retinopathy (p. 120) is bilateral and shows other obvious features of widespread arterial and venous disease.

Treatment. Systemic steroids reduce the severity of the disease, and it is doubtful if a prolonged sanatorium type of regimen which has been advocated in the past may help to hasten resolution. In the peripheral form of the disease, particularly when one eye is severely damaged by permanent changes, it may be worth while to try and limit the spread of the disease by surface diathermy of the equatorial part of the retina, and whenever possible new vessel formations should be subjected to photocoagulation before the development of vitreous haemorrhage. A vitreous replacement after persistent vitreous haemorrhage is unlikely to be of value in restoring any useful vision because of the associated retinitis proliferans but it may be worth trying as a last resort.

CENTRAL SEROUS RETINOPATHY

In central serous retinopathy there is an oedema of the macular area. It occurs usually in the young adult and is liable to affect both eyes. It causes a general depression of the clarity of the central vision, particularly for colours, but it seldom impairs the level of the visual acuity to a marked extent. The condition clears spontaneously in a few weeks, sometimes completely, but often with some distortion of vision caused by a fine pigmentary disturbance of the macula which follows the oedema, and any recurrence causes a further visual deficit.

Its origin is ill-understood: it has been considered to be the result of a disorder of the retinal capillaries in the macular region, but fluorescein angiography (p. 109) shows evidence of an abnormal leakage of the dye into localized areas of detachment of the retinal pigment epithelium so that it may be the result of a focal choroidopathy.

Treatment. Photocoagulation or laser beam may be of value in limiting the spread of the detachment.

BLOOD DYSCRASIAS

Changes are liable to occur in the retina in various disorders of the haemopoietic system.

Anaemia

In severe anaemia the fundus appears relatively pale and small scattered superficial haemorrhages tend to occur in the retina often in association with a low-grade retinal oedema which increases the pallor of the fundus.

Leukaemia

In leukaemia the retinal veins are usually markedly dilated, but they appear less red than normal and the associated retinal harmorrhages are also less red with sometimes a yellowish tinge. The retina usually shows a moderate degree of retinal oedema, particularly near the optic disc.

Polycythaemia

In polycythaemia the retinal veins are uniformly dilated and appear dark in colour. There are usually associated haemorrhages in the retina and in the advanced stages of the condition the retina becomes oedematous.

Macroglobulinaemia

Macroglobulin within the blood causes an increased blood viscosity with a consequent sludging of the circulation. A well-marked engorgement of the retinal veins is generally associated with papilloedema and retinal haemorrhages, and sometimes the central retinal vein becomes occluded. Pathologically the most striking feature is the development of capillary microaneurysms in the peripheral retina which may be a response to anoxia.

VASCULAR RETINOPATHY

Most of the changes in the retinal arteries and veins in disorders of the cardiovascular system follow an underlying hypertension, but atheroma and involuntary sclerosis may occur in the absence of hypertension.

ATHEROMA

Atheroma may develop in an artery as a patchy subendothelial fatty degenerative lesion, with or without an associated hypertension, particularly in the middle-aged or elderly. Its development may be a response to a diminished blood volume in an artery which is unable to compensate for this because of an associated fibrosis. The patch of atheroma tends to lead to a partial or even total occlusion of the artery as a result of a thrombosis of the atheromatous area. Ophthalmoscopically the affected artery appears as an opaque white mass obscuring part of the blood column.

INVOLUTIONARY SCLEROSIS

Involutionary sclerosis is simply an ageing process in the arteries, not necessarily associated with hypertension, but almost invariably present after the sixth decade of life although sometimes occurring at an earlier age. It affects particularly the larger vessels, but sometimes also the smaller branches. Fibrosis of the larger vessels is followed by a rise in the systolic level of the blood pressure, provided the heart is sufficiently sound to maintain the peripheral circulation, but without any rise in the diastolic pressure because of the absence of any increase in the peripheral resistance (in fact this is reduced because of the relative rigidity of the larger arteries). Ophthalmoscopically the retinal arteries appear relatively straight and diffusely narrow with acute-angled branchings and with a diminution in the intensity of the colour of the blood column but without any obvious loss of transparency of the vessel walls (Plate IV, *upper*); this is in contrast to the normal fundus in which the retinal arteries are wide and sinuous with prominent blood columns and wide-angled branchings. Similar changes in the arteries supplying the optic disc account for the very slight pallor which may occur in an elderly person in the absence of any other disease.

HYPERTENSIVE RETINOPATHY

Hypertension is usually the result of an increased resistance of the peripheral circulation following a generalized and widespread arteriolar hypertonus which is a sustained physiological contraction of the affected vessels, in contrast to a spasm which is a sudden and violent type of contraction of limited duration. It is associated with a rise in the systolic and diastolic levels of the blood pressure, although the increase in the diastolic level tends to be less marked if there is a rigidity of the larger arteries as a result of fibrosis, or if there is a reduction in the area of the peripheral circulation which is capable of exerting hypertonus (also a result of fibrosis) so that to some extent a preexisting sclerosis may diminish the changes which occur in the vessels in hypertension.

It follows that the changes which occur in the arteries vary considerably in different groups of hypertensives and these are reflected in the fundi.

HYPERTENSION IN THE ABSENCE OF A PREEXISTING SCLEROSIS

This usually occurs in the younger age group and the different stages in its development are:

Diffuse Hypertonus. In the early stages the marked hypertonus of the peripheral arteries in conjunction with a resilience of the larger arteries causes a marked increase in the systolic and diastolic levels of the blood pressure. Ophthalmoscopically the normal, fairly wide, sinuous and well-coloured retinal arteries become uniformly narrow, straight and relatively pale (Plate IV, *upper*). There may be some congestion of the retinal veins immediately distal to the point of an arteriovenous crossing, but there is no concealment of the underlying vein.

Hypertrophy and Hyperplasia. In the late stages reactive changes of hypertrophy and hyperplasia occur in the arterial walls; at first they are irregularly placed but later they become more widespread. Ophthalmoscopically the retinal arteries remain narrow and straight but the blood column becomes more pale and shows a slightly irregular outline. There is also concealment of the underlying retinal veins at the arteriovenous crossings (Plate IV, *lower*).

Fibrosis (Arteriosclerosis). This the inevitable outcome of a persistent hypertension so that the abnormal changes of hypertrophy and hyperplasia within the walls of the arteries are affected by a reactive sclerosis, although this fibrosis is seldom evident in the most peripheral retinal branches. Sometimes these changes may be followed by an occlusion of the central retinal artery or of one of its branches. Ophthalmoscopically the affected parts of the retinal arteries become irregularly dilated, curvilinear and red with increased surface reflexes, often termed *copper wiring*, although eventually these changes may become widespread. The most peripheral parts of the retinal arteries usually remain narrow, straight and pale. The appearance of the retina after an occlusion of the central retinal artery is described on page 121.

Fulmination. This usually occurs very rapidly in severe cases of fulminating or malignant hypertension when the peripheral arteries are affected by a marked hypertonus in association with some focal necrosis. Ophthalmoscopically the retinal arteries have a fairly normal calibre near the optic disc, but the blood column is irregularly reduced in size and markedly pale. There are parallel zones of concealment where the arteries cross retinal veins, and later the arteries show marked tortuosity suggesting an elongation of their length. The more peripheral vessels remain straight and narrow. The retinal veins are usually congested with the development of areas of white sheathing within their walls.

There are other changes which may be present in the retina in hypertension.

Haemorrhages. Small haemorrhages of capillary origin occur in the superficial or deep parts of the retina in the more advanced hypertensive cases, and sometimes they lie in radiating lines in the macular area. Occasionally a large haemorrhage occurs at the site of a necrotic arteriole which shows a thrombotic column (straight and deep red in colour) in its proximal part although this is usually separated from the parent stem by a white thread (silver wiring) which persists indefinitely even after a disappearance of the thrombotic column; the distal part of the arteriole is not visible because it is devoid of blood.

Small Round Hard-edged White Exudates. These occur in the deeper part of the retina particularly around the optic disc and in the central fundus. They probably represent haemorrhages which have been altered by phagocytosis.

Soft White (Cotton-wool) Exudates. These occur in the superficial parts of the retina in relation to the thrombosed arterioles (pale infarcts), following focal retinal ischaemia.

Oedema. This occurs in the retina around the optic disc (papilloedema) and often spreads to other parts of the retina. It is particularly noticeable in the macular area ('macular fan').

HYPERTENSION IN THE PRESENCE OF PREEXISTING INVOLUTIONARY SCLEROSIS

This usually occurs in the older age group and the changes in the arteries are irregular; the parts unaffected by fibrosis show hypertonus and the parts affected show dilatation, but the later develop-

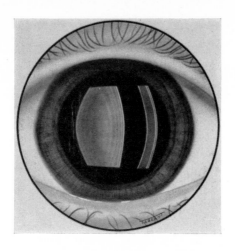

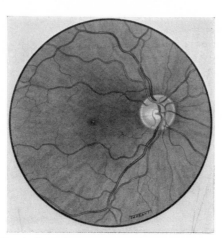

PLATE III (*Upper*) Optical section of the anterior segment of the eye. (*Lower*) Normal fundus of the right eye as seen on direct ophthalmoscopy

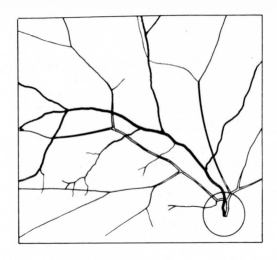

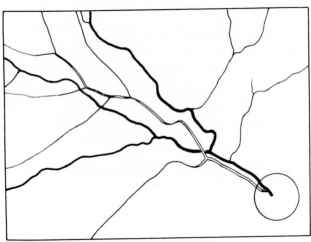

PLATE IV (*Upper*) The fundus in involutionary sclerosis, showing narrowing and straightness of the retinal arteries with a diminution of the blood columns, and with acute-angled branchings. Similar changes also occur in diffuse hypertonus. (*Lower*) The fundus in hypertensive retinopathy. The retinal arteries show different appearances: small, narrow, straight and pale (indicating hypertonus); excessively pale with fine irregularity of the blood column (indicating hyperplasia); and dilated and red (indicating fibrosis). The retinal veins show some congestion and concealment at the A/V crossings ment of hypertrophy and hyperplasia is less extensive because it does not occur in the parts affected by the fibrosis. Ophthalmoscopically the arterioles show irregular changes; the parts unaffected by fibrosis become hypertonic so that the blood column is narrow and less red in colour, and the parts affected by fibrosis become passively dilated so that the blood column is wider and more intense in hue and, because of the elongation of the affected vessel walls, there are areas of localized tortuosity. Eventually the whole arterial system becomes diffusely wide, red and tortuous by a confluence of the fibrotic areas. Conceal-ment of the retinal veins at the arteriovenous crossings is not a prom-inent feature, but the veins immediately distal to the crossings may be dilated, slightly dark and tortuous—features indicative of venous congestion. In the later stages any or all of the changes which have been described in fulminating hypertension may occur, but usually only after a fairly prolonged interval, and the occurrence of arterio-sclerosis provides some defence against necrotizing changes in the arterioles—the so-called defence by sclerosis.

The treatment of hypertension involves many different considera-tions; the state of the cardiac function, the presence of any pulmonary oedema, the possibility of renal disease, etc. Various antihypertensive drugs which decrease the sympathetic control of the blood vessels may be used, some act on the ganglia (ganglionic blockers) and others act on the fibres (adrenergic blockers).

OBSTRUCTION OF THE CENTRAL RETINAL ARTERY

A cessation of the circulation in the central retinal artery affects the vision in a variety of ways. The vision may be lost suddenly, com-pletely and permanently (amaurosis) without any previous visual disturbance, but at other times this may be preceded by transient episodes of blurred vision or even of total loss of vision particularly when it results from a carotid artery insufficiency (see below). Some-times, however, part of the vision may be restored if there is a cilio-retinal artery (a rare occurrence), if a branch of the central retinal artery which leaves the main stem in the deep part of the optic nerve-head is distal to the site of the block (a less rare occurrence), if a re-establishment of the circulation by capillary anastomoses occurs between the uveal and retinal circulations in the optic nerve-head, or if there is a relief of the obstruction of the circulation. These events must become effective before irreparable damage of the retinal ganglion cells, and unfortunately these cells succumb rapidly, certainly within an hour or so.

In the Early Stages

Oedema and Necrosis. Oedema occurs in the retinal nerve fibre layer and necrosis in the retinal ganglion cell layer so that the retina appears cloudy and white because it interferes with the transmission of the normal redness of the underlying choroid; this is particularly marked in the central part of the retina except at the fovea, an attenuated part of the retina without any nerve fibre or ganglion cell layer, which appears unduly red and prominent, the 'cherry-red spot', against the white background of the surrounding retina.

Attenuation of the Retinal Arteries. The retinal arteries often appear obliterated, but there may be some circulation within the attenuated arteries; the poverty of this is demonstrated by the ready production of fragmentation of the blood column (the cattle-trucking effect) on digital pressure to the globe which embarrasses the circulation by causing a slight rise in the intraocular pressure.

The Pupillary Reflex. The direct pupil reaction to light is affected according to the degree of the visual loss, but the consensual reaction is retained provided the unaffected eye is functioning adequately.

In the Later Stages

The Retinal Arteries. These may remain obliterated and appear as white threads, but quite commonly there is a restoration of circulation although seldom with any restoration of useful vision.

Optic Atrophy. Pallor of the optic disc becomes evident within 4 to 6 weeks of the occlusion following atrophy of the nerve fibres as a result of the degeneration of the retinal ganglion cells, and also to some extent of the defective blood supply in the optic nerve-head.

Macular Pigmentation. This usually follows the subsidence of the oedematous changes in the macular area.

Sometimes the early and late changes are limited to certain parts of the retina when the obstruction involves only one or more branches of the artery without involving the main trunk. In such cases only part of the visual field is involved in the form of a sector or quadrant which extends from the region of the fixation spot.

An obstruction of the central retinal artery (or one of its branches) may follow a thrombosis, an embolus or an insufficient circulation.

Thrombosis

A thrombosis may follow arteriosclerotic changes (see above) or inflammatory changes (arteritis).

Giant-celled Arteritis. In this condition the occlusion is usually preceded for several weeks or even months by fleeting attacks of blurred vision, and also by severe unilateral headaches if there is an accompanying temporal arteritis. Retinal haemorrhages sometimes occur in this form of occlusion. It follows a necrotizing arteritis, a form of collagen disorder. The erythrocyte sedimentation rate (E.S.R.) is raised in the active stage.

Embolus

A vegetation from a valve of the heart may form an embolus, or portions of blood clot within the left antrium or within a major artery, such as the carotid artery, may form fibrin emboli which are sometimes multiple and recurrent.

Carotid Artery Insufficiency

This often starts as a transient blurring or loss of vision which may spread from above downwards like a blind being lowered from above, or from below upwards like a blind being raised from below, with a restoration of vision within a few seconds or minutes in the reverse direction. These attacks tend to be repeated every few days or weeks, without any precipitating factors or any accompanying features except occasionally for headache near the affected eye. Rarely the patient is aware of a bruit over the eye. The condition follows a narrowing (and even an occlusion) of the internal carotid artery (involvement of the common or external carotid artery is more rare) which produces a fall in the pressure of the central retinal artery to a level which jeopardizes the integrity of the retina, and sometimes also a diminished blood supply to the ciliary body causing a diminished formation of aqueous humour and ocular hypotension; this may even lead to the development of an anterior segment necrosis (chap. 6). A bruit may be detected with a stethoscope over the stenosed carotid artery (or occasionally over the eye), and the site of the stenosis may be demonstrated by a radiograph after the percutaneous injection of a radioopaque substance into the artery. The diminished pressure in the ophthalmic artery is demonstrated by ophthalmodynamometry; the footpiece of the piston of the dynamometer is applied to the outer surface of the eye after the instillation of a surface anaesthetic, and a gradually increasing pressure is exerted until the retinal arteries show a collapsing pulsation (a measure of the diastolic pressure of the ophthalmic artery), and then until the pulsation just disappears (a measure of the systolic pressure of the ophthalmic artery).

There are sometimes other manifestations of a carotid artery insufficiency: transient attacks of hemiparesis of the arm or leg, dysphasia, and even an acute hemiplegia, resulting from a unilateral reduction of the cerebral circulation.

Spasm

A hypertonus of the arterial wall occurs in hypertension (see above), but it is unlikely that a simple spasm of the central retinal artery is a common cause of obstruction, except in the rare condition called *retinal migraine*. This is transient blindness which may occur in one eye as a result of a vasoconstriction in one or more branches of the central retinal artery in the absence of any disease of the vessels and in the absence of any hypertension. It is suggested that the mechanism of this condition is akin to the changes which occur in the cerebral vessels in migraine.

Treatment. In any obstruction of the retinal arterial circulation it is imperative to improve the circulation as rapidly as possible. This may be achieved by the use of vasodilators (amyl nitrite by inhalation, tolazoline or acetylcholine by subconjunctival or retrobulbar injection), or by reducing the intraocular pressure (the removal of the aqueous from the anterior chamber by paracentesis is an effective method, but simple massage of the eyeball is also of value). It is also necessary to treat any underlying cause, particularly in cases which give prior warnings of an impending obstruction. The treatment of giant-celled arteritis usually involves the use of systemic steroids for a prolonged period. The treatment of carotid artery insufficiency may involve the use of anticoagulants, but this is usually only a temporary expedient and a thrombo-endarterectomy may be necessary or if the thrombus is of long standing a resection of the affected portion of the carotid artery with an end-to-end anastomosis or with a blood vessel graft. The management of hypertension is discussed on page 121.

Vertebro-basilar Artery Insufficiency

A vertebro-basilar artery insufficiency may cause transient episodes of blurred vision of a hemianopic type when one posterior cerebral hemisphere is involved, but if both are involved the blindness is complete (*cortical blindness*), although unlike peripheral blindness it is not accompanied by a sensation of total darkness. These episodes are often accompanied by sensations of flashing lights, dizziness, vertigo or tinnitus. The ischaemic process may spread to the pons and lower midbrain with involvement of the motor nuclei which are concerned with the extrinsic ocular muscles, so that there may be transient paresis and an awareness of diplopia (chap. 13).

POSTHAEMORRHAGIC AMAUROSIS

A loss of vision—partial or complete, transitory or permanent, usually of both eyes—may follow loss of blood, particularly when this occurs over a prolonged period as after the recurrent bleeding of a chronic condition such as haematemesis or haematuria rather than after the sudden and excessive bleeding of surgical or traumatic conditions. Rarely the fundus appears normal, and usually there is some pallor of the optic disc, attenuation of the retinal vessels and oedema of the retina which may be sufficiently marked to cause an obvious papilloedema. Sometimes there are also retinal haemorrhages and 'cotton-wool' exudates so that the picture mimics a renal retinopathy or a malignant hypertensive retinopathy (except for an absence of the usual features of hypertension in the retinal vessels). The oedema and exudates follow a necrosis of the retinal nerve layer owing to ischaemia which is possibly induced by a localized spasm of the retinal arterioles.

THROMBOSIS OF THE CENTRAL RETINAL VEIN

A thrombosis may affect the central retinal vein within the optic nerve-head (near the lamina cribrosa) so that it is *complete*, or it may affect one (or more) branches so that it is *partial*. There is usually an underlying arteriosclerosis and the condition tends to occur in the middle-aged or elderly person.

It may occur without any dramatic visual symptoms except when the macular area is involved by haemorrhage; even then it may not be detected because of the overlap of the vision of the two eyes (unless the unaffected eye happens to be closed), or when the haemorrhage extends into the vitreous. The affected retinal veins are grossly dilated and there are many haemorrhages within the affected parts of the retina; sometimes these extend into the vitreous. The venous circulation in the retina is restored by preexisting or new anastomotic channels in or around the optic disc. The macular area is usually involved by the haemorrhage when the thrombosis is complete, but spared when only partial except when the superior temporal branch is affected. The haemorrhages absorb gradually over a period of months, but their presence in the macular area usually causes permanent impairment of the central vision.

In cases of complete thrombosis new vessel formations (rubeosis iridis) may develop on the anterior surface of the iris after an interval of about three months. These are prone to cause a gradual obliteration of the filtration angle (peripheral anterior synechiae) with the production of an intractable form of secondary glaucoma (*thrombotic glaucoma*).

Treatment. There is no specific treatment for the retinal changes, but attention should be directed to the underlying arteriosclerosis. It is doubtful if anticoagulants are of value once the thrombosis has occurred, but in certain cases they may be used in an attempt to prevent further similar episodes in the same or in the other eye; such treatment demands a careful medical assessment as it may lend to other complications because of the increased risk of haemorrhage. The treatment of rubeosis iridis and of thrombotic glaucoma is discussed in Chapters 6 and 15, respectively.

RENAL RETINOPATHY

The changes in the retina vary according to the type of renal disease.

Acute Glomerulo-nephritis (*Type I Nephritis*)

In this condition a transient hypertension is a common feature at any age, and the retinal arteries become uniformly narrow, straight and relatively pale as a result of hypertonus, but in repeated attacks the changes become more severe with the development of reactive sclerosis so that eventually the affected parts of the arteries become red and dilated.

Nephrosis (*Type II Nephritis*)

This may occur in the absence of hypertension so that the retinal arteries appear normal but the veins are characteristically dilated, tortuous and darker in colour with a slight oedema of the central part of the fundus including the optic disc and macula. If, however, hypertension supervenes, the fundus appearances become typical of a fulminating hypertension (p. 120) although in contrast to the non-renal hypertensive cases this occurs at a much lower level of diastolic pressure and the oedema is more intense with a cloudy quality and a well-marked macular fan; sometimes the oedema may be sufficient to cause the production of small balloon-like areas of retinal detachment of a serous type.

Chronic Nephritis

In this condition the retinal arteries may show the typical appearances of a reactive fibrosis, but when it follows a fulminating type of hypertension the retinal arteries and veins become attenuated and sheathed, fine pigmentary changes appear in the previously oedematous retina, and there is often a gradual absorption of the retinal haemorrhages and exudates.

Uraemia

In a severe uraemia there may be total visual loss (amaurosis) with headaches, vomiting, convulsions, and coma. The amaurosis is not simply the result of the retinal changes (hypertensive and renal retinopathy), but rather the result of a cerebral disturbance (*hypertensive encephalopathy*) which explains the retention of the pupillary light reflex despite the blindness; this is a form of cortical blindness. (A similar amaurosis may occur in eclampsia and lead poisoning.)

DIABETIC RETINOPATHY

Diabetic retinopathy occurs in about one-third of diabetics, particularly in middle-aged or elderly individuals, more commonly in the female, and usually some years after the onset of the disease. It is almost always bilateral, but the two eyes may show different degrees of involvement. It presents as an engorgement of the retinal veins and a hyperaemia of the retinal capillaries, and shortly afterwards with the development of *dot* or punctate retinal haemorrhages which are often widespread although usually more marked in the central retina between the upper and lower macular branches of the retinal vessels; these represent saccular microaneurysms in the venous side (or sometimes in the arteriolar side) of the capillary bed, particularly in the capillaries which join the superficial and deep retinal capillary networks so that they lie mostly within the inner nuclear layer of the retina, as the result of sharply localized degenerative changes in the capillary walls causing the formation of varicose capillary loops, the limbs of which become adherent to one another following the passage of exudate. Later they are the sites of multiple larger *blot* haemorrhages as a result of seepage of blood through their walls and also of multiple small glistening yellow-white exudates caused by a seepage of lipoid and mucopolysaccharide material. Similar haemorrhages and exudates may occur at the sites of degeneration of sclerosed retinal veins sometimes in the absence of microaneurysms. This phlebosclerosis may also produce a partial retinal vein thrombosis, the site of which may be marked by delicate fronds of new vessels which pass into the vitreous (*rete mirabile*).

Sometimes retinal haemorrhages may pass into the vitreous and form the basis of a fibrovascular proliferation (*retinitis proliferans*), but vitreous haemorrhage is particularly prone to arise from retinal new vessel formations; these are detected readily by the method of fluorescein angiography (p. 109), and this also delineates the microaneurysms with precise information about their origin from the venous or arteriolar end of the capillary bed. This is a serious complication because it is liable to cause the development of a localized area of retinal detachment at a later stage and this ultimately may become complete. Exudates may also occur in the retina as a result of areas of neuronal degeneration which, unlike the exudates that follow increased capillary permeability, leave areas of permanent damage with a loss of visual function of the affected parts of the retina.

The retinal arteries are seldom involved in the early stages of diabetic retinopathy, but arteriosclerosis is a feature in the later stages and tends to occur earlier and with greater severity than in non-diabetics so that a hypertensive overlay is common in the progress of the disease. Pathologically it is associated with a subintimal hyalinization which may be so marked in the precapillary terminal arterioles as to cause their gradual occlusion and disappearance. This may be followed by the development of dilated irregular vessels which extend from the neighbouring venous part of the capillaries into the obliterated arterial portion. Occlusive tendencies in the small branches of the retinal arteries which supply the optic disc tissues probably account for the susceptibility of the disc to develop atrophic changes in advanced diabetic retinopathy during the occurrence of any inflammatory condition (like uveitis) or during any rise in the intraocular pressure (glaucoma).

There is an interesting association between diabetic retinopathy and intercapillary glomerulosclerosis (a feature of the Kimmelstiel-Wilson syndrome) in that most diabetics with glomerulosclerosis have retinopathy, and both conditions are closely related histogenetically.

Rarely in the young diabetic an excessive accumulation of fat in the retinal vessels may be visible so that the distended vessels appear pale against the light red colour of the fundus background (retinal lipaemia). Sometimes diabetic retinopathy is associated with new vessel formations on the anterior surface of the iris (*rubeosis iridis*) particularly when the retinal lesions are severe and old-standing; this occurs in other conditions (chap. 6), and is liable to cause a secondary glaucoma.

Treatment. Diabetic retinopathy may develop despite its adequate control, but a rigid maintenance of control is an important factor in diminishing the progress of the retinal changes. Unfortunately the predilection for the haemorrhages to occur in the macular area often results in an early and permanent disturbance of the central vision. A restriction of the intake of animal fat and a reduction in the level of the serum lipids by a diet rich in unsaturated fatty acids may be tried in an attempt to diminish the severity of the damage caused by the retinal exudates. It has been suggested that the progress of diabetic retinopathy is unrelated to the control (or otherwise) of the diabetes but this is incorrect, and a strict maintenance of the health of the patient with a correct diet supplemented when necessary by insulin or hypoglycaemic agents (such as tolbutamide, chlorpromide or aceto-hexamide) which stimulate the function of the pancreas. A reduction of fat intake and the use of vegetable rather than animal fats in the diet are aimed at decreasing the lipid changes in the retinal structures. Sometimes drugs which limit the lipid content of the serum (choline-insitol, methiomine or atromid) may be of value. It has been suggested also that diabetic retinopathy may be influenced favourably by a reduction of pituitary function by hypophysectomy or by a radio-active implant but there are certain criteria which must be verified before considering such drastic treatment: the likely inevitable blindness in the absence of treatment; the presence of reasonable vision in one or both eyes so that there is the possibility of retaining worth-while visual function if the retinal disease is arrested, and the fitness of the patient to withstand the difficult postoperative period because of the widespread manifestations of endocrine dysfunction which require careful control by replacement hormonal therapy. The serious nature of the vitreous haemorrhages which are liable to follow new retinal blood vessel formations determines the attempt to obliterate them by the application of photocoagulation, although its effects tend to be unpredictable. Photocoagulation is sometimes of value also in limiting the spread of the exudative changes in the retina.

TOXAEMIC RETINOPATHY OF PREGNANCY

A toxaemia of pregnancy may occur in the later months of pregnancy (rarely before the sixth month) and the accompanying hypertension leads to a hypertonus of the retinal arteries with the later development of hyperplasia and reactive sclerosis (p. 119) if the hypertension persists after the pregnancy. Sometimes, however, the early response of the retinal vessels to the hypertension is followed rapidly by the changes which occur in a fulminating hypertension (p. 120), but at a much lower level of the diastolic pressure than in nontoxaemic hypertensive cases because of the renal element. The oedema and exudate in the retina are usually abundant and sometimes the formation of subretinal exudate causes a well-marked serous retinal detachment; the affected area shows a characteristic pigmentary disturbance after the subsidence of these oedematous and exudative changes.

THE COLLAGEN DISEASES

In the collagen diseases the connective tissues develop characteristic pathological features—mucoid swelling and fibrinoid necrosis—which are probably the result of some hypersensitivity or autoimmune factor. Several general diseases which may show ocular manifestations—rheumatoid arthritis, disseminated lupus erythematosus, polyarteritis nodosa, Wegener's granulomatosis, dermatomyositis, scleroderma, acne rosacea, giant cell arteritis, and Behçet's syndrome; and several eye diseases—ocular pemphigus, essential atrophy of the iris and choroid, angioid streaks, retinal vasculitis, tenonitis, episcleritis, scleritis and uveitis—may possibly be collagen disorders.

Disseminated Lupus Erythematosus

This disease represents a widespread involvement of the collagen tissues of the body, such as skin, kidneys, spleen, heart. Various ocular tissues may also be involved: conjunctival scarring with subsequent symblepharon formation, deep keratitis, oedematous changes in the lids, and a retinopathy which is characterized by massive fluffy white ('cotton-wool') exudates containing cytoid bodies, haemorrhages and sometimes by peripapillary oedema.

Polyarteritis Nodosa (Periarteritis Nodosa)

This disease is characterized by widespread necrotizing obliterative lesions of the small arteries and arterioles which assume a nodular appearance as a result of granulomatous or aneurysmal changes. It affects young adults, particularly males, with the occurrence of such general manifestations as pyrexia, haematuria, hypertension, and abdominal pain. There may also be involvement of certain ocular structures; the choroid with the production of oedematous foci, the retina with the production of a hypertensive retinopathy in which massive exudates form a characteristic feature, and rarely the extrinsic ocular muscles with some form of paresis or palsy.

Dermatomyositis

This is an acute or chronic inflammatory condition in which involvement of the skin (dermatitis) of the face, particularly the eyelids, with a spread to the upper extremities and trunk, the mucous membranes of the mouth and pharynx, and the muscles (myositis) (chap. 13) may be associated rarely with striking retinal changes; distension of the retinal veins and massive oedematous, exudative and haemorrhagic changes particularly in the macular area.

CYTOMEGALIC INCLUSION DISEASE

An intrauterine infection of the fetus with the virus of cytomegalic inclusion disease may cause chorioretinitis in the newborn with the formation of multiple foci in the more peripheral parts of the fundi sometimes in association with some retinal haemorrhage, but the lesions are often less destructive than those in toxoplasmosis. There are usually also cerebral disorders and an X ray of the skull may show periventricular calcification. Other ocular complications have been described: optic atrophy, cataract, destructive membranous conjunctivitis, keratomalacia and uveitis. There may be widespread involvement of the viscera (liver, lungs, heart, kidney, pancreas), evidences of its blood-borne nature. Inclusion bodies may be isolated in the urine, in gastric washings, in the saliva, and on liver puncture.

TOXIC AMBLYOPIA

Certain toxic substances are liable to affect the retinal ganglion cells particularly those in the macular and paramacular areas, although it is uncertain whether this is a direct effect or an indirect one by an ischaemia of the retinal capillary vessels. There may also be a toxic effect on the macular and paramacular fibres within the optic nerve.

Tobacco Amblyopia

This usually follows prolonged smoking of pipe tobacco following an ingestion (as compared with an inhalation) of the smoking products, so that it does not occur in cigarette smoking except rarely when cigarettes are made from pipe tobacco. Characteristically it occurs in elderly men, but it may occur in younger people who are unduly sensitive to pipe tobacco. Tobacco smoke contains large amounts of

cyanide but normally this is detoxicated safely and efficiently following its conversion into thiocyanate. However, in the presence of a
metabolic defect (perhaps an inborn error of cyanide detoxication)
there is a significantly raised level of cyanocobalamin in the plasma;
this is a metabolically inert substance but its presence in excess is an
indication of an overwhelming of the body stores of vitamin B_{12} by
by cyanide. There is a gradual failure of the central vision in both eyes
and in the early stages this is revealed as a failure of colour perception
particularly in the part of the visual field which lies between the
fixation point and the blind spot (centrocaecal scotoma) which
extends ultimately into the fixation area. Ophthalmoscopic evidence
of optic atrophy is only seen in the advanced stages.

   Treatment. The avoidance of tobacco for several weeks or months
usually results in a restoration of central vision, and this is facilitated
by vitamin B therapy (particularly B_{12}), provided the disease is recognized before permanent changes occur in the ganglion cells. Vitamin
B_{12}, however, is not used simply because of its presumed deficiency.
Indeed the hydroxocobalamin form of vitamin B_{12} has a strong affinity
for cyanide, and this is in contrast to its cyanocobalamin form which
even may be harmful in such cases. The diagnosis may be delayed
because the visual failure may be regarded simply as the result of
'senile' changes (macular degeneration or cataract), and in any elderly
person when the pathological changes within the eyes appear insufficient to account for the visual failure the coexistence of a tobacco
amblyopia should be considered.

Alcohol Amblyopia

   Ethyl Alcohol. This seldom produces a toxic amblyopia on its own
but it may be an additional factor which precipitates the effect of
pipe smoking, and it may also foster a nutritional amblyopia (see
below).

   Methyl Alcohol (Wood Alcohol). This produces widespread and
permanent damage to the retinal ganglion cells so that total blindness
(or total loss of central vision) is almost invariable; death is also
liable to occur because of severe dehydration and prostration.

Quinine Amblyopia

   The effect of quinine is found particularly when there is a sensitivity to the drug. The visual defect follows a retinal ischaemia which
is revealed ophthalmoscopically by an attenuation of the retinal
arteries which affects particularly the peripheral vision.

Chloroquine

This drug is liable to bind itself to melanin so that it affects the integrity of the retinal pigment epithelium with a disturbance of function of the rods and cones. Concentric rings of pigmentation occur around the macular area. It also causes characteristic changes in the cornea (chap. 4).

Filix mas and Salicylates

These drugs may also produce effects similar to those of quinine, although less commonly.

Lead Retinopathy

Lead intoxication may cause a marked retinal arteriosclerosis and periarteritis with an obliterative type of endarteritis which leads to narrowing and sometimes occlusion of the retinal arteries. Similar changes may occur in the cerebral vessels. A lead nephrosis is a cause of uraemia (p. 127). Lead may also cause paralysis of the extrinsic ocular muscles.

NUTRITIONAL AMBLYOPIA

An inadequate diet over a prolonged period, particularly when it is deficient in protein and vitamin B, is liable to cause abnormal changes in the retinal ganglion cells of the macular area, presumably by an interference with their capillary supply. These changes are reversible only when the dietary deficiencies are corrected at a reasonably early stage. It affects the central vision, initially as an undue fatiguability of the close-reading vision but eventually as a central scotoma. Ophthalmoscopically in the early stages there is an oedema of the macular area with occasionally a few small retinal haemorrhages, and in the later stages there is a fine pigmentary disturbance of the affected area. Sometimes there is a partial optic atrophy.

Treatment. This should be aimed at a speedy correction of the defective diet and of any factors which accentuate this, such as an excessive intake of alcohol.

PRIMARY RETINAL DETACHMENT

A primary retinal detachment develops when a break in the integrity of the retina allows fluid from the vitreous to pass into the subretinal space (the space between the optical part of the retina and the pigment epithelium). This break may occur at the site of a degenerative change following a previous oedema or haemorrhage (injury or vascular disorder), following myopic or senile changes, or following an area of abnormal vitreoretinal contact so that retraction of this part of the vitreous pulls on the retina with the formation of a tear; this probably explains the increased incidence of retinal detachment in aphakia because the removal of the lens causes a forwards displacement of the vitreous particularly when the operation is complicated by a loss of vitreous.

There are various forms of retinal breaks—dialysis, crescentic U-shaped tear, and round hole (Fig. 29).

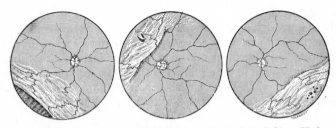

FIG. 29. *Retinal detachment in association with a dialysis* (left), *a U-shaped tear* (centre), *or a round hole* (right)

Dialysis. This is a disinsertion of the peripheral part of the retina at the ora serrata. Characteristically it follows severe contusion of the eye, but it may also follow the rupture of a retinal cyst which occurs usually in the lower outer part of the retina (see below).

Crescentic U-shaped Tear. This follows traction of the vitreous and occurs most commonly in the upper temporal or upper nasal quadrant of the retina in the myopic eye. Its convex border points towards the optic disc and peripheral to the tear there is a darkened area of the retina which represents the site of the vitreoretinal adhesion and forms the operculum (or lid) of the tear.

Round Hole. This occurs particularly in the peripheral parts of the retina near the ora serrata, and there may be more than one hole so that a careful search of the entire retina is essential.

Clinical Features

The retina surrounding the tear becomes detached by the spread of subretinal fluid and the detachment gradually extends to involve most of the retina particularly in the lower part of the eye because the fluid in the subretinal space tracks downwards by the influence of gravity. The detached area is determined readily on ophthalmoscopic examination when it is billowed forwards into the vitreous with the formation of retinal folds, but lesser degrees of detachment are detected by the darkening of its retinal vessels and by the loss of its normal red appearance. The use of the binocular indirect ophthalmoscope is essential in a careful scrutiny of the peripheral retina, particularly when there is some opacity of the media like a partial cataract or vitreous haemorrhage.

The earliest symptoms may be an awareness of flashes of light caused by the pulling on the retina of a vitreous band or an awareness of a floating opacity in the field of vision from an opacity of the vitreous perhaps following a haemorrhage from the retina. Subsequently there is a loss of vision in the part of the visual field which corresponds to the affected area; this may be determined accurately on the perimeter. When the macular area becomes involved in the detachment or in an oedematous process there is a loss or disturbance of central vision.

A retinal detachment is potentially a bilateral disease, except in cases which follow trauma, or a complicated form of cataract extraction, etc., so that the other eye should be scrutinized carefully at frequent intervals for any early signs of an impending detachment.

Treatment. There are several principles involved, although the techniques differ from case to case.

Rest allows the retinal detachment to subside as far as possible for several days before operation; the particular type of posture depends on the situation of the detachment.

The sealing of the retinal tear or tears may be carried out indirectly by applying diathermy or cryotherapy to the sclera overlying the area of the tear, and the accuracy of this application is verified ophthalmoscopically at operation. This produces an exudative reaction of the choroid with the development of an area of choroidoretinal union so that the tear is obliterated within this area. A similar reaction may be obtained by shining an intense light from a photocoagulator into the eye under direct view with a modified ophthalmoscope, but this photoreaction is effective only when the affected area of the retina is in contact with the underlying pigment epithelium.

The removal of the subretinal fluid is achieved by making one or more small openings in the sclera in the region of the detachment with an electrolysis needle, and the evacuation of the subretinal fluid permits the affected area of the retina including the retinal tear to become opposed to the underlying choroid so that the process of retinochoroidal coagulation becomes effective.

A shortening of the eyeball may be achieved by various methods—a lamellar scleral resection over the area of the detachment or an encircling of the equatorial part of the sclera by a silicone strap which surrounds the globe—and it is an essential part of the operation in, for example, myopic or aphakic eyes when a shrinkage of the vitreous is likely to lead to a further area of detachment because the previously detached retina is unable to adapt itself to the normal size eyeball.The aim of an encirclement is also to isolate the defective retinal areas from the more central parts of the retina by the creation of an adequate ridge.

The injection of air or of fresh donor vitreous into the vitreous space may be necessary in certain cases to maintain the retina in appositon to the choroid after the operation, particularly in cases in which there has been a previous loss of vitreous.

SECONDARY RETINAL DETACHMENT

A retinal detachment may occur as a secondary event in many conditions in the absence of a retinal tear; an exudative retinal detachment occurs in Coats' disease (p. 114, toxaemia of pregnancy (p. 129), renal retinopathy (p. 126), Harada's disease (chap. 6) in which there is an associated uveitis and inflammatory changes in the cerebrospinal fluid, when the exudate occurs in the subretinal space between the optical part of the retina and the pigment epithelium. The whole retina may be detached when it is pushed forwards by a mass in the choroid (malignant melanoma) although there is usually also an exudative element in the subretinal space. The retina may be detached also by the contraction of strands of fibrous tissue which pass from the retina into the vitreous (retinitis proliferans) following a vitreous haemorrhage which is associated with new vessel formations from the retina.

RETINAL CYSTS

Cystic degenerative changes in the peripheral retina are not uncommon in the adult although usually so small that they are only detected histologically, but sometimes a large isolated cyst occurs as a congenital anomaly characteristically in the periphery of the outer temporal quadrant of one or often both eyes with a translucent globular detachment which extends to the periphery of the retina without any true hole or dialysis despite the thinness of the cystic retina. These cysts commonly remain unchanged and are detected only on routine examination because they do not cause any obvious visual symptoms, but if the cyst ruptures, or if it causes traction changes in the more central parts of the retina, it requires treatment along the lines of a retinal detachment.

Infestation

Larval Granulomatosis of the Retina

The larva of the *Toxocara canis*, a nematode common in dogs and cats throughout the world may become lodged in the retina with the formation of a creamy-white umbilicated mass, particularly in the central part of the fundus, which protrudes into the vitreous. This mass is composed of fibrous tissue containing areas of fibrinoid necrosis, and there may be some surrounding retinal haemorrhage or exudative retinal detachment, so that the appearance resembles a retinoblastoma, a pseudoglioma (endophthalmitis), or Coats' disease. The disease is usually acquired in childhood at the 'dirt-eating' stage, so that the ova of the *Toxocara* from the faeces of the animal are ingested. The larvae hatch out in the intestine and are liable to be widely disseminated to the liver, lungs, and retina, by way of the bloodstream and lymphatics. The other common manifestations are asthma or urticarial skin eruptions. An eosinophilia is a characteristic feature for several months after the onset. A positive skin test to an intradermal injection of an antigen (1 in 1,000) prepared from an adult *T. canis* is of diagnostic value.

Degenerations

Retinal degenerations may be primary or secondary. The primary, a more involved form, is discussed below. Secondary retinal degeneration may follow any severe disease of the retina (long-standing retinal detachment; extensive retinal vascular disease, etc.) or of the underlying choroid (malignant melanoma, choroiditis, etc.).

PRIMARY RETINAL DEGENERATIONS

Macular Dystrophy

This is an 'abiotrophy' of the visual elements in the macular areas of both eyes and becomes evident at any age, hence the terms *congenital, infantile, juvenile, adolescent, adult (presenile)*, or *senile,*

depending on the time of onset. There are often familial and hereditary factors (*heredomacular degeneration*).

The changes in the macular area are often confined to a slight pigmentary disturbance in the younger age groups, but in the older
person they are sometimes more obvious with the appearance of a
cyst which leads to a partial hole formation, fine haemorrhages,
exudates or colloid deposits. The cases may present with distortion of
central vision or merely with eyestrain following the increasingly
greater efforts which are required for close work. The central vision
may remain reasonably good for many years, but eventually it
becomes impaired, sometimes unequally in the two eyes. The peripheral vision is retained indefinitely.

Macular dystrophy may occur in different ways according to the
site of interference:

Choroid. A degeneration of the choriocapillaris causes a central
areolar choroidal sclerosis (chap. 6).

Bruch's Membrane. Colloid bodies form on Bruch's membrane,
perhaps as a degenerative change in the membrane but more likely
as an abnormal secretion from the retinal pigment epithelium. When
the colloid bodies are profuse the condition may be termed *Tay's
choroiditis* or *Doynce's honeycomb choroiditis*—misnomers because
they are not inflammatory. Large colloid bodies may be termed *drusen*.

Ruptures sometimes occur in the elastic part of Bruch's membrane
which appear as radiating dark red lines resembling to some extent
blood vessels—hence the term *angioid streaks*. Similar changes in the
elastic tissues of the skin constitute the *Groenblad-Strandberg syndrome*. In the macular area they lead to choroidal haemorrhage which
causes a disciform type of macular degeneration (chap. 6), but in this
condition the ruptures of the elastic lamina are apparent only on
histological examination so that these are not visible ophthalmoscopically as angioid streaks.

Retinal Neuroepithelium. Involvement of this part of the retina
leads to various forms of *heredomacular degeneration* (*central tapetoretinal dystrophies*): the *infantile type of Best* (*vitelline dystrophy*), the
juvenile type of Stargardt, the *adolescent type*, the *adult type of Behr,*
the *presenile type*, and *the senile type*. It may also lead to a *central pigmentary dystrophy* in which there may be a profound disturbance of
the central vision, but sometimes an obvious degree of pigmentary
change may be present in the macular area without any significant
visual defect; in fluorescein angiography a series of punctate areas of
abnormal fluorescence may be apparent because of the ready visuali-

zation of the underlying choroidal fluorescence through the damaged pigment epithelium.

Retina as a Whole. In a *cystoid degeneration (cystoid macular oedema)* cavities form within the retina as the result of a disintegration of its neural elements. It may occur in any part of the retina, but with a predilection for the macular area because the avascularity of the region creates difficulties in the resorption of fluid. In fluorescein angiography there is an abnormal fluorescence surrounding the foveal area resulting from a spread of the dye into the retinal tissues in the macular area which assumes a rosette pattern. It occurs in a variety of ways: as a senile degeneration; in any inflammatory condition of the adjacent retina (chorioretinitis) or uvea (posterior uveitis) or sometimes in a remote part of the uvea (pars planitis, chap. 6); in any vascular disorder of the central part of the retina (central retinal vein thrombosis, central retinal artery occlusion, retinal vasculitis, hypertensive retinopathy, diabetic retinopathy, etc.); following various forms of trauma (commotio retinae and solar retinopathy, p. 111); and following a cataract operation, even when this is uncomplicated, usually in an elderly person (chap. 9).

Retinal Ganglion Cells. Lipoid degenerations of the cerebral and retinal ganglion cells (*cerebromacular degenerations*) produce their effects in three characteristic ways at different ages:

1. *Amaurotic family idiocy (Tay-Sachs disease)* is a widespread lipoid degeneration of the cerebral and retinal ganglion cells which becomes evident between the ages of 6 and 12 months when the apparently healthy baby ceases to make progress. There is a white swelling of the retina caused by the engorgement of ganglion cells with lipoid material, particularly in the central region except for the fovea which is devoid of ganglion cells so that it stands out in contrast as a well-defined 'cherry-red spot'. There is eventually an optic atrophy. Death occurs inevitably within about a year of the onset. The condition is not confined exclusively to Jewish children as commonly stated.

2. *Batten-Mayou disease (Spielmeyer-Vogt disease)*, a lipoid degeneration of the retina, cerebral cortex and cerebellum, occurs usually about the age of 3 years with a gradual visual failure and a progressive mental deterioration leading to death in adolescence. There is a diffuse pigmentary change in the central part of the retina. Optic atrophy is not always a conspicuous feature.

3. *Niemann-Pick disease*, the lipoid changes in the retina are sometimes less marked than the widespread changes which occur in the viscera as well as in the central nervous system; the involvement of

the viscera may be determined by a rectal biopsy. It occurs usually about the age of 3 years and death occurs within a few years.

Treatment. This is limited to the provision of suitable reading glasses in the cases which survive, often in the form of telescopic spectacles which are more convenient than a simple hand magnifying lens.

Tapetoretinal Degeneration

This primary retinal degeneration is an abiotrophy of the rods, and also of the cones at a later stage, although the earliest changes probably occur in the pigment epithelium. It is an inherited disease affecting males more than females commonly with a recessive inheritance, sometimes of a sex-linked type so that it is transmitted to the male child by the mother, and rarely with a dominant inheritance. The condition is almost invariably bilateral. The disease is seldom evident before adolescence and its earliest manifestation may be an awareness of defective vision in dim illumination. At this stage there is commonly an annular scotoma in the mid-peripheral ('equatorial') part of the visual field which gradually progresses peripherally and centrally although usually with a sparing of a small island of central vision because of the relative resistance of the cones to the disease; this tubular vision may remain indefinitely but sometimes in middle age it becomes lost.

There are characteristic changes in the eye. Pigment is deposited in the retina, particularly in its peripheral parts, often with branching processes so that each cluster resembles a 'bone corpuscular cell', and this anomaly determines the clinical designation of '*retinitis pigmentosa*'. The pigment sometimes migrates in the perivascular space of the retinal vein so that it forms a zone of sheathing. The retinal arteries become markedly attenuated, and the optic disc becomes gradually atrophic although the pallor has a waxy quality which differs from the usual whiteness of a primary optic atrophy. Cataract affecting initially the posterior cortical part of the lens is a late feature of the disease.

A peculiar form of the condition occurs in infancy (*Leber's congenital amaurosis, retinal aplasia*) or in early childhood, and this is associated usually with a profound disturbance of vision, or even with complete blindness, despite remarkably little abnormality of the fundi on ophthalmoscopic examination. After an interval of months or even years there is a slight attenuation of the retinal arteries and a partial degree of optic atrophy, and eventually these changes become more marked in association with scattered retinal pigmentary deposits so that by adolescence the appearances resemble to some extent a typical retinitis pigmentosa, but inevitably the visual prognosis of this form is extremely poor from an early age.

Sometimes a tapetoretinal degeneration in childhood presents as a macular dystrophy with pigmentary changes in the macular areas and a progressive disturbance of central vision, which is in sharp contrast to typical retinitis pigmentosa in which the macular areas are seldom involved until late. The widespread nature of the condition is only evident after an interval of several years when the typical changes occur in other parts of the fundi, but an early diagnosis may be determined by the ERG which is reduced or absent; this distinction is important because the long-term visual prognosis of a macular dystrophy, in which there is the retention indefinitely of peripheral visual function thus permitting some degree of visual independence, is much better than a generalized tapetoretinal degeneration.

Occasionally tapetoretinal degeneration in the child is associated with other abnormalities—polydactyly (affecting the hands and feet), hypogenitalism, mental retardation (*Laurence-Moon-Biedly syndrome*), or with deafness, and when this is congenital also with dumbness (*Usher's syndrome*). Sometimes an atypical form of retinitis pigmentosa is associated with a chronic polyneuritis leading to an enlargement of the peripheral nerves, ataxia and deafness, the so-called *Refsum's syndrome*.

The two conditions which are regarded as variants of retinitis pigmentosa are:

1. *Retinitis pigmentosa sine pigmento* in which there is no obvious pigmentary disturbance in the retina, but it is unnecessary to regard this is a separate entity because, as described above, a tapetoretinal degeneration may becomes established in the absence of obvious pigmentory changes.

2. *Retinitis punctata albescens* in which there is a widespread distribution of white spots in the retina. This is a true variant and carries a better visual prognosis than the classical retinitis pigmentosa.

Treatment. There is no known effective treatment of tapetoretinal degeneration although many remedies have been suggested, including more recently 'tissue therapy' (the subconjunctival implantation of placental tissue). Removal of the cataractous lens is not associated with any unusual complications, but the final visual prognosis is dependent on the extent of the surviving retina.

Neuroepithelial Dysgenesis

This is a condition akin to tapetoretinal degeneration, but it seems likely that the retinal anomaly is the result of a functional defect of transmission rather than a structural lesion. There is no ophthalmoscopic abnormality, and the nature of the visual disturbance, which is less profound than in tapetoretinal degeneration, is determined by the persistence of a normal EOG despite an abnormal ERG; in tapetoretinal degeneration both the ERG and EOG are abnormal.

Oguchi's Disease

Oguchi's disease is a rare congenital and inherited condition affecting both eyes and results from an excessive number of the cones with very few rods; there may also be an anomaly of the retinal pigment epithelium. The vision is normal in bright illumination but with extreme night blindness in dim illumination, although dark adaptation may occur gradually over a period of several hours. In normal illumination the fundus appears grey or golden in colour, but it assumes its normal red colour after several hours in the dark (*Mizuo's phenomenon*).

Cone Dysfunction Syndrome (see p. 25)

Tumours

Retinoblastoma

The retinoblastoma is the commonest of the neuroepiblastic tumours of the retina and is almost certainly of congenital determination, sometimes with a hereditary factor. It develops as proliferations of 'nests' of cells in the retina, particularly in the inner nuclear layer, which fail to become differentiated and assume malignant properties; it is not a *glioma* but unfortunately this term is frequently used as synonymous with retinoblastoma. The tumour, which develops in the early years of life, usually before the third year, is frequently fairly advanced when detected because it is first noted by the parents as a white mass within the eye, giving the so-called cat's eye reflex, or because it is found by the ophthalmic surgeon during the routine examination of the eyes because of a suspected squint (the squint being the result of the loss of vision in the eye).

In the early stages the lesion appears as a localized white elevation of the retina, sometimes with an obvious dilatation of the retinal vessels supplying the affected area but rarely with any associated haemorrhage. This localized lesion is often followed quite rapidly by the development of other small lesions, sometimes regarded simply as seedling deposits from the main tumour but many represent independent foci (evidence of the multicentric nature of the tumour). The proliferating tumour tissue may extend into the subretinal space, causing a retinal detachment (*glioma exophytum*) with an associated subretinal exudate, or into the vitreous where it forms large masses (*glioma endophytum*); rarely the tumour spreads extensively within the retina so that involvement of the subretinal space or vitreous is delayed. Particles of tumour tissue may pass forward into the anterior chamber with the formation of deposits on the posterior surface of the cornea (resembling large keratic precipitates), or on the iris (resembling inflammatory nodules). Obliteration of the filtration angle by the tumour leads to a secondary glaucoma sometimes with an enlargement of the eyeball as in an infantile glaucoma. A true uveitis may occur in advanced cases. Ultimately the tumour spreads from the eye directly into the orbit by perforating the cornea or sclera or into the brain by passing along the optic nerve with the formation of massive necrotic masses. It rarely forms metastases.

Treatment. Immediate enucleation of the affected eye with removal of as much as possible of the optic nerve is usually the only possible treatment because of the advanced state of the condition on its first recognition. Macroscopic or microscopic evidence of a spread of the tumour through the eyeball or at the cut end of the optic nerve should be followed by irradiation without waiting for clinical evidence of recurrence; an exenteration of the orbital contents may also be considered in such cases, but this is effective only if the disease is confined to the orbit and irradiation has the advantage of being applied over a wider area.

Repeated examinations of the second eye (or of both eyes in a child with a family history of retinoblastoma) permits the detection of the tumour in its early stages so that conservative treatment—external irradiation of the whole retina on the basis of the potential multicentric nature of the tumour, the application of a radioactive cobalt disc to the surface of the sclera overlying an apparently localized tumour, or photocoagulation or laser beam application to the retina surrounding the tumour to prevent its spread and subsequently to the tumour itself—makes possible the retention of useful visual function. Some form of chemotherapy (for example, vincristine and cyclophosphamide) may be of value when the second eye fails to respond to local treatment.

There are other very rare neuroepiblastic tumours which are only locally invasive.

Astrocytoma

Astrocytoma is a tumour of the retinal glial tissue.

Dictyoma and Medulloepithelioma

Both dictyoma and medulloepithelioma are tumours of the ciliary epithelium, which is a prolongation of the optical part of the retina over the ciliary body.

Phakomata

Phakomata are congenital tumours which involve different neuroectodermal tissues, often with familial or hereditary features but rarely with malignant propensities.

Tuberous Sclerosis (Bourneville's Disease). This tumour is derived from neuroglial tissue or neurilemmal cells with the production of multiple small nodules in the skin (adenoma sebaceum), in the cerebral cortex (sometimes causing mental deficiency or epilepsy), in the viscera, and in the heart. The retinal lesions appear as mulberry-like white clusters which project into the vitreous usually in the region of the optic disc; the active nature of these changes is shown sometimes by the occurrence of haemorrhage in the surrounding retina. Drusen of the optic disc sometimes presents a similar appearance (chap. 8).

Angiomatosis Retinae (Von Hippel-Lindau Disease). This tumour is characterized by angioblastomatous formations in the cerebellum, in the medulla oblongata, in the spinal cord and in the viscera (particularly the pancreas and kidney). The retinal lesions appear as isolated dilatations and tortuosities of the retinal arteries and veins with the production of retinal haemorrhages and exudates which may cause haemorrhage into the vitreous or an exudative type of retinal detachment. Sometimes the affected retinal vessels show an arteriovenous communication. A secondary glaucoma may occur as a terminal event. More rarely the retina is the site of more solid angioblastomatous formations.

Treatment. The spread of the retinal lesion may be limited by surface diathermy, photocoagulation or irradiation.

Cephalofacial Angiomatosis (Sturge-Weber Syndrome). This tumour is characterized by angiomatous formations in the skin of the face (naevus flammeus) which is limited usually to the area of distribution of the trigeminal nerve, to the meninges with subsequent calcification, and to the cerebral cortex with the possible production of mental deficiency, epilepsy and hemiplegia. Angiomatous formations may occur in the retina or more commonly in the uveal tract and in the episcleral tissues with the subsequent development of glaucoma. The condition is usually unilateral.

Neurofibromatosis (Von Recklinghausen's Disease). This is usually a widespread disease with the occurrence of firm neurofibromatous nodules in the nerves of the subcutaneous tissues (for example, in the eyelids), in the uveal tract (sometimes leading to glaucoma which may be of the infantile type—buphthalmos), in the retina, in the sclera or in the cornea.

The retina is unlikely to be the site of a *secondary tumour* except by direct spread from adjacent tissues, such as the choroid or optic nerve.

8 | Diseases of the Optic Nerve

Structure and Function

The optic nerve (cranial nerve II) is a direct extension of the brain and, unlike a peripheral nerve, resembles the cerebral white matter; its nerve fibres are myelinated except distal to the lamina cribrosa, its interstices contain neuroglial cells, its external coverings are dura, arachnoid and pia, and there is cerebrospinal fluid in the pia-arachnoid space. The optic nerve fibres arise in the retinal ganglion cells and pass centripetally within the nerve as the afferent visual fibres which terminate in the lateral geniculate body before being relayed to the visual cortex (chap. 16), and as the afferent pupillary fibres which are relayed to the parasympathetic parts of the oculomotor nuclei (chap. 6).

The optic nerve may be considered in four parts.

The first, the *intraocular part* (Fig. 30) begins at the *optic disc* which represents the retinal aspect of the optic nerve as seen with the ophthalmoscope: it marks the exit from the eye of the optic nerve fibres which are slightly elevated at the disc margin (hence the term *optic papilla*). The optic disc has an average diameter of 1·5 mm and is somewhat oval with the vertical meridian slightly larger than the horizontal one. There is a central depression in the optic disc—the *optic cup* (Fig. 30)—through which the branches of the central retinal artery and of the retinal vein enter and leave the eye, usually along the nasal wall of the cup, but rarely along the temporal wall (inversion of the disc or situs inversus). The size of the normal optic cup is variable but it seldom occupies more than 70 per cent of the area of the disc and usually the optic cup of each eye in any one individual is similar in size unless there is a marked difference in the refractive error (for example, one eye myopic and the other hypermetropic). It is usual for the cup to lie in the central part of the optic

146

disc. The depth of the optic cup is variable; sometimes it is sufficiently deep to detect the *lamina cribrosa*, a sieve-like connective tissue structure which passes across the optic nerve at the level of the choroid and sclera. The optic cup appears pale because it is devoid of

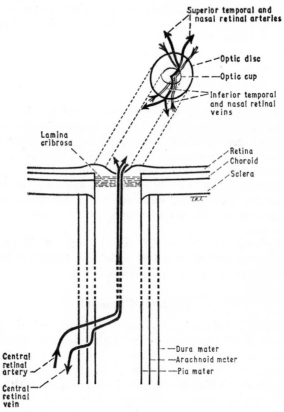

FIG. 30. *Longitudinal section of the optic nerve-head to show the formation of the optic cup and the lamina cribrosa. The ophthalmoscopic appearance of the optic disc is also illustrated ; typical for the right eye, but also for the left eye in situs inversus.*

nerve tissue, but the rest of the disc appears pink because the optic nerve fibres contain a capillary network which is supplied by several small arteries derived probably entirely from the arterial circle of Zinn (or Haller) which lies in the adjoining sclera or from the adjacent

choroid; it is unlikely that there is any component from the branches
of the central retinal artery. Quite frequently the normal disc shows a
slight degree of relative temporal pallor, but almost invariably this is
present equally in the two eyes.

Second, the *orbital part* lies within the muscle cone formed by the
4 recti muscles as they pass from the apex of the orbit to the eyeball.
Its course is tortuous so that the nerve is not stretched unduly during
ocular movement. The central retinal artery (a branch of the ophthalmic artery) enters the optic nerve a short distance (1·25 cm) behind
the eye and travels in the distal part of the nerve before passing to the
retina through the optic cup; the central retinal vein leaves the eye
and the optic nerve in company with the artery. The optic nerve
tissue is supplied mainly by small arteries which pass into the nerve
from the plexus of vessels (derived from the posterior ciliary arteries)
in the pia mater, but also to some extent in its axial region by small
branches from the central retinal artery (or its collateral branch).

Third, the *intracanalicular part* lies within the narrow optic canal
(formed between the 2 roots of origin of the lesser wing of the sphenoid and the body of the sphenoid) and is accompanied by the
ophthalmic artery. The orbital opening of the optic canal lies at the
apex of the orbit.

And, fourth, the *intracranial part* lies between the intracranial
opening of the optic canal and the optic chiasma which is formed by
the junction of the right and left optic nerves.

Congenital Anomalies

Coloboma. A hole (coloboma) may occur in the optic disc, usually,
but not invariably, in association with an inferior coloboma of a sector
of the retina and uvea (chap. 6). More commonly a crescent occurs
along the lower border of the optic disc (*Fuchs' inferior coloboma*)
which should be distinguished from the crescent which occurs in
axial myopia as a degenerative change (this most frequently affects
the temporal border of the disc, chap. 2). Other congenital anomalies
are opaque nerve fibres (chap. 7) and drusen (rarely a congenital
anomaly, see p. 157).

Injuries

The optic nerve is liable to become involved in any fracture of
the bones in the region of the optic canal; directly by a laceration
of the nerve or indirectly by an interference with its nutrient blood

supply or by a pressure on the nerve of surrounding oedematous tissue or haemorrhage. Subsequently there is the development of partial or complete optic atrophy, but the ophthalmoscopic evidence of this is delayed for 4 to 6 weeks after the injury. Sometimes a severe blow on the forehead may lead to a partial or complete loss of function of the optic nerve without any fracture because of a haemorrhage within the optic nerve as the result of its violent concussion against the wall of the narrow bony optic canal or because of a rupture of the nutrient vessels following a sudden displacement of the nerve (contrecoup effects).

An *evulsion* of the optic nerve whereby the nerve is partially or completely torn from the eyeball occurs in deep penetrating wounds of the orbit or, rarely, indirectly in severe contusional injuries of the eyeball as a result of the explosive force which is generated within the eye. In the early stages the central fundus is obscured by haemorrhage, but eventually the previous site of the optic disc is apparent as a 'hole' or as a mass of proliferative scar tissue. The retinal vessels are markedly attenuated and the eye is blind unless the evulsion is only partial, when part of the visual field is retained.

OPTIC NEURITIS

Optic neuritis is an inflammatory condition of the optic nerve in which a process of demyelination is associated with oedematous changes in the surrounding tissues. It is usual to distinguish between two forms—*papillitis* in which the disease occurs in the optic nerve within or near the eyeball, and *retrobulbar neuritis* in which it occurs in some part of the optic nerve away from the eyeball. The condition is commonly initiated dramatically by a sudden loss of vision of the affected eye, although sometimes it is preceded by a vague awareness of discomfort in the eye or by a slight defect of the vision during the previous day or so. The visual loss is usually severe so that there may be merely an appreciation of movement or light (rarely even an absence of light perception), but sometimes the visual loss is limited to the central or paracentral part of the visual field with characteristically a loss of colour perception. It is evident that, although some optic nerve fibres are affected directly, many other fibres are involved only indirectly by the oedema which surrounds the focus of demyelination and this accounts for the relatively good visual prognosis of certain cases. The pupil of the affected eye is characteristically dilated with a sluggish and ill-sustained response to direct light although with a normal consensual response; this is simply an expression of the conduction defect of the afferent visual pathway. In the early stages there may be pain in the affected eye particularly on movement of the eye, and pressure on the upper surface of the eyeball near the insertion of the superior rectus tendon may elicit obvious tenderness (Greeves's sign).

The optic disc in the acute phase may reveal no obvious abnormality or sometimes only a slight oedema, but when the lesion is adjacent to the optic nerve-head (*papillitis*) the disc oedema may be well marked with a few haemorrhages in the peripapillary part of the retina; when the retinal changes are widespread it is termed a *neuroretinitis*.

The subsequent changes which occur in the affected optic nerve depend to a large extent on the nature of the demyelinating process (see below).

Optic neuritis is a feature of several different conditions.

Disseminated Sclerosis (*Multiple Sclerosis*). In disseminated sclerosis scattered foci of demyelination occur in the central nervous system, usually in young adults who are otherwise healthy, with a characteristically variable periodicity so that it tends to run a fluctuating course with acute exacerbations at irregular intervals and with intervening periods of improvement and quiescence before ultimately entering into a more chronic and persistent phase. Optic neuritis occurs in nearly one-third of all cases, typically but not invariably as the first manifestation of the disease, and many years may elapse (5 to 10 years or even much longer) before the next manifestations of the disease (for example, paraesthesia, ataxia, disturbances of bladder control, etc.). Indeed it is reasonable to consider that an optic neuritis may remain as the only manifestation of the disease so that the absence of subsequent manifestations does not preclude the diagnosis of disseminated sclerosis. The optic neuritis is usually confined to one eye initially, but the other eye may be involved similarly some months or years later and sometimes both eyes are involved simultaneously. It is relatively rare for the same eye to be affected more than once. As a general rule there is a gradual restoration of vision within a few weeks of the onset of the optic neuritis with only a small paracentral scotoma or a localized more peripheral field defect as the remaining legacy of the disorder, but sometimes the central vision is permanently affected by a residual central scotoma. The majority of cases shows the development of some pallor of the optic disc, particularly in the temporal region because of the predilection of the papillomacular bundle to be involved in the process.

Encephalomyelitis. Optic neuritis, usually affecting both eyes, may occur as part of an encephalomyelitis in association with one of the exanthemata—measles, chicken pox, herpes zoster, mumps, whooping cough, infectious mononucleosis, one of the virus diseases, or following an undue sensitivity to certain substances (for example, diphtheria, toxoid, smallpox vaccine, triple antigen—diphtheria, tetanus and pertussis vaccine—sulphanilamide, isoniazid, DDT) or the toxic encephalopathic state which occurs in hydrocephalus (p. 157). Sometimes blindness may ensue as the result of an encephalopathy in the absence of an optic neuritis so that it is a form of cortical blindness (chap. 16); this has followed triple antigen.

Neuromyelitis Optica (*Devic's Disease*). In this condition a bilateral optic neuritis occurs in association with a myelitis usually in young children; similar cases which do not show myelitis may be considered as modified forms or as manifestations of encephalomyelitis. The prognosis for a restoration of useful central vision is sometimes remarkably good considering the marked uniform pallor of the optic discs which characterizes the later stages of the condition, but there is inevitably some degree of permanent defect.

Encephalitis Periaxialis Diffusa (*Schilder's Disease*). Optic neuritis is a rare feature of this condition (chap. 16).

Retinal Disorder. A form of optic neuritis may be associated with toxic conditions of the retina (tobacco amblyopia, methyl alcohol amblyopia), but the main lesion lies in the retinal ganglion cells (chap. 7).

Local Inflammatory Conditions. It is suggested that an optic neuritis may be associated sometimes with infection in the neighbouring nasal sinuses or in the surrounding orbital bones (periosteitis), but the evidence for this is inconclusive.

PAPILLOEDEMA

The term *papilloedema* should be used merely to indicate an oedematous state of the optic nerve-head without any aetiological significance because it may occur in various conditions:

1. *Increased intracranial pressure* (*plerocephalic oedema*) is the classical form of papilloedema (or choked disc), and it is produced by an increased intracranial pressure as the result of some intracranial space-occupying lesion; this is usually a tumour, particularly in the posterior cranial fossa (midbrain, cerebellum, occipital lobe), but more rarely it may be an inflammatory focus (abscess or gumma) and sometimes an extensive extradural haemorrhage or severe meningitis

may lead to its production. It is essentially bilateral but sometimes unequally.

Its mechanism is not clearly established, but it is suggested that it is largely the result of a compression of the retinal vein as it passes obliquely through the subarachnoid space of the optic nerve because of a raised pressure of the cerebrospinal fluid. It seems likely, however, that an overloading of the optic disc with blood from the arterial circle of Zinn is also of importance in its genesis whereby the increased resistance to blood flow in the pial plexus causes a diversion of blood from the arterial circle to the tissues of the optic disc. It may occur also because of the high diastolic pressure of the cerebral arteries which follows the increased capillary resistance of the cerebral tissues subjected to a raised intracranial pressure. These theories explain the absence of papilloedema in an atrophic optic disc (which is devoid of an adequate arterial circulation), despite an obvious oedema of the otherwise healthy optic disc of the other eye (Foster-Kennedy syndrome).

2. *Obstruction of the venous outflow from the eye* (*in the absence of an increased intracranial pressure*) may occur in central retinal vein thrombosis, any form of increased blood viscosity such as in polycythaemia and macroglobulinaemia, cavernous sinus thrombosis, carotico-cavernous anastomosis, or any orbital lesion which causes a marked rise in the intraorbital tension (orbital tumour, orbital cellulitis, etc.).

3. *Uveitis* may occur when there is a patch of active choroiditis in the central part of the fundus, particularly in a juxtapapillary situation, and it is also a feature of a panuveitis in association with a generalized retinal oedema.

4. An *optic neuritis* in the anterior part of the optic nerve is associated with papilloedema (papillitis) (p. 149).

5. *Hypertensive retinopathy :* papilloedema is a feature of the malignant form of hypertension retinopathy with involvement of both eyes (chap. 7).

6. In *collagen disorders*, the retinopathy which occurs is usually associated with disc oedema (pp. 115 and 130).

7. *Posthaemorrhagic amaurosis* is discussed in Chapter 7.

8. *Blood dyscrasias* (*anaemia* or *leukaemia*) are associated with retinal oedema (chap. 7), usually in both eyes, when the dyscrasia is severe, but in leukaemia uniocular papilloedema may occur when a mass of lymphomatous tissue disturbs the circulation in the region of the optic nerve-head.

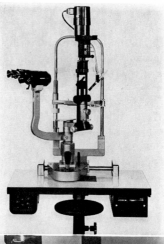

PLATE V (*Upper*) The Haag
Streit slit-lamp microscope (with
attachments for gonioscopy and
applanation tonometry). (*Lower
left*) Romanes magnifier and
(*right*) R.900 Tonometer
(Courtesy of Clement Clarke)

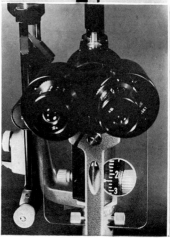

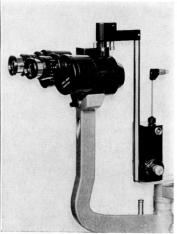

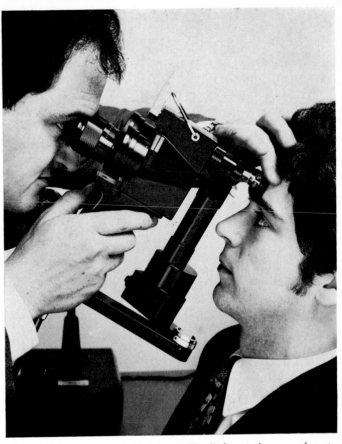

PLATE VI The Kowa hand-held and portable slit-lamp microscope (courtesy of C. Davis Keeler Ltd)

9. *Lead poisoning:* the disc oedema may be produced in various ways; as part of a retinopathy, as a plerocephalic oedema in association with an encephalopathy, or as part of an optic neuritis (papillitis).

10. In *benign intracranial hypertension* which usually affects apparently healthy young people, particularly females, there is a raised intracranial pressure and well-marked bilateral papilloedema (plerocephalic oedema). Ventriculography shows a decreased size ('squeezing') of the ventricles which is the result of an oedema of the brain. Headaches are common, and sometimes giddiness and vomiting may occur; in the female these symptoms may be most marked shortly before menstruation. There may be transient disturbances of the vision; rarely the vision may become permanently impaired as the result of a compression (consecutive) optic atrophy. A paresis of the VIth cranial nerve is also a rare event. Some cases appear to be the result of a thrombosis of a major cerebral venous sinus, but in many cases there is no known aetiology, although it has been suggested that there is some electrolytic imbalance in certain cases.

11. *Hypotony of the eyeball:* rarely a persistently low intraocular pressure, such as may occur in a trephine which is draining excessively, is associated with some disc oedema.

Note: A false appearance of disc oedema may be found in high degrees of axial hypermetropia because of a 'crowding' of the optic nerve fibres at the disc margin (*pseudoneuritis*). Rarely the optic disc margins are markedly elevated as a congenital anomaly.

In papilloedema the dilatation of the vessels on the optic disc surface with extensions on to the surrounding retina causes a hyperaemia, and the increased permeability of these vessels accounts for the oedema which elevates the disc margins, initially on the nasal side, subsequently on the superior and inferior margins and finally on the temporal margin with a reduction in the size or even an obliteration of the physiological cup. The dilatation of the retinal veins and the retinal oedema are limited to the peripapillary region with a spread into the macular region in severe cases, and these changes are followed by the production of varying amounts of retinal haemorrhage. Fluorescein angiography illustrates the presence of the dilated vessels in papilloedema with an early filling of the disc capillaries and there is a leakage of fluorescein in the oedematous areas of the disc with a spread of the dye into the surrounding retina particularly in relation to the retinal vessels. In chronic papilloedema the well-marked vascular network on the surface of the disc is strikingly evident.

There is usually no awareness of any visual impairment, unless the macula is affected, but careful examination of the visual field shows an enlargement of the blind spot. In the later stages the oedema may subside without leaving any obvious ophthalmoscopic signs, but usually there is some permanent blurring of the disc margins and in severe or persistent cases there is some degree of secondary atrophy with a corresponding visual impairment and sometimes even total blindness.

In plerocephalic oedema various other general manifestations—headache, vomiting, visual field defects—occur according to the situation of the intracranial lesion.

Treatment. This depends entirely on the cause of the papilloedema.

It is convenient to distinguish between two forms of optic nerve atrophy—primary and secondary—although these terms have tended to be applied in different ways.

OPTIC ATROPHY: PRIMARY

The term *primary optic atrophy* is applied to an optic atrophy which is the result of a disease process affecting the optic nerve fibres directly within the optic nerve or indirectly because of an involvement of their parent cells (the ganglion cells) in the retina.

Involvement of the Optic Nerve

Congenital. A *coloboma of the optic disc* appears as an atrophic area because of the absence of optic nerve fibres in that region (p. 148).

An *optic disc (optic nerve) hypoplasia* is a developmental anomaly in which there is poverty or absence of optic nerve fibres in the optic nerve-head and usually also in the adjacent part of the optic nerve, although the framework and blood vessels of the nerve are present. It may be unilateral or bilateral, and it is associated almost invariably with a profound visual impairment or even complete blindness. It is apparent ophthalmoscopically as a small excavated optic disc which is grey or white in colour and usually there is some attenuation of the retinal arteries; the significance of the small size of the disc may be overlooked because this is a feature of the hypermetropic disc in early childhood, but on careful observation a faint line is apparent around the hypoplastic disc which represents what would have been the extent of the disc in the absence of the hypoplasia. The hypoplasia may be an isolated event, but sometimes the eye is microphthalmic

(p. 50) or there is an associated neurological disorder such as anencephaly or hydrocephalus (p. 156).

Inherited. An optic atrophy may present in early life as the result of a *dominant* or *autosomal recessive* form of inheritance. In another form of inherited optic atrophy (*Leber's hereditary optic atrophy*) there is a fairly rapid loss of vision in both eyes in the late teen-age period or in early adult life. It is usually transmitted by the female with a recessive and sex-linked mode of inheritance, and at one time it appeared almost exclusively in the male but more recently also in the female. The initial loss of vision may be profound (as in a bilateral optic neuritis), but subsequently there is usually a restoration of peripheral vision although seldom of central vision. The optic discs frequently show a uniform pallor, but sometimes this is limited to the temporal parts of the discs. The condition appears to be the result of an inherent metabolic defect in the conversion of cyanide to thiocyanate (that is, in the detoxication of cyanide) and (chap. 7) the sex distribution which has undergone a change in recent years (at one time exclusively male but now with a significant number of female cases) and the relatively late onset (despite the inherited nature of the condition) may be an indication that environmental factors, especially related to smoking, precipitate the disorder. This is illustrated by the lower thiocyanate concentration in the plasma of smokers with Leber's disease as compared with normal smokers.

Traumatic. Trauma may cause various degrees of optic atrophy following a severance of part or all of the optic nerve fibres, directly or more commonly indirectly following a disruption of the nutrient blood vessels (p. 148).

Also to be noted is the optic atrophy which is found in infancy as the result of brain damage from some obstetric complication, such as a premature separation of the placenta or a slow moulding and compression of the head during labour which lead to a rupture of some of the small veins draining into the longitudinal sinus or which lead to tears in the tentorium cerebelli and falx cerebri with the production of a rupture of the straight sinus or its tributaries. In such cases the optic atrophy is part of the brain damage which follows a disruption of vital structures by haemorrhage, but sometimes the optic atrophy is the result essentially of a state of anoxia in the neonatal period so that it is part of the *respiratory distress syndrome of the newborn* (p. 113).

Inflammatory. Optic neuritis leads to an atrophy of the optic nerve fibres in the affected part of the nerve (p. 149), but a primary form of optic atrophy may occur without any preceding optic neuritis in the neurosyphilitic conditions particularly in association with tabes or general paralysis of the insane; in these conditions the peripheral vision is affected first but later the central vision is involved with sometimes total blindness.

Neoplastic. A glioma of the optic nerve causes a progressive destruction of optic nerve fibres (p. 158).

Involvement of the Retinal Ganglion Cells

Certain retinal diseases are associated characteristically with some degree of primary optic atrophy—toxic amblyopia, tapetoretinal degeneration (Leber's amaurosis, retinitis pigmentosa), Tay-Sachs disease, occlusion of the central retinal artery, posthaemorrhagic amaurosis, etc. Also any advanced form of retinal disease—old-standing retinal detachment, retrolental fibroplasia, etc.—is likely to be associated with some degree of optic atrophy eventually.

OPTIC ATROPHY: SECONDARY

The term *secondary optic atrophy* is applied to an optic atrophy which is the result of an indirect involvement of the optic nerve fibres by a disease process which causes pressure on the optic nerve. It is liable to occur, therefore, in any disorder which increases the intraorbital tension, for example, orbital tumour, orbital cellulitis, thyrotrophic exophthalmos; which exerts localized pressure on the optic nerve in the orbit—meningioma; which restricts the passage of the optic nerve through the optic canal—carcinomatous deposits, Paget's disease of the surrounding bone, oxycephaly, etc.; or which causes pressure on the optic nerve in its intracranial course—pituitary tumours extending into the region of the anterior chiasmal angle, optochiasmal arachnoiditis, etc. It is likely, of course, that these forms of secondary optic atrophy are the result of a pressure effect on the nutrient vessels of the nerve fibres rather than of a direct pressure on the nerve fibres, and the optic atrophy which is associated with a cupping of the optic disc in chronic simple glaucoma and with a plerocephalic oedema is of a similar secondary nature.

Also to be noted is the optic atrophy that occurs in *hydrocephalus* which may be produced in different ways. It may follow a shift in the position of the brain stem so that there is a stretching of the optic nerves or chiasma with a consequent disruption of their nutrient vessels. It may follow a meningitis, which is prone to occur when the ydrocephalus is associated with a meningomyelocele (a form of spinal dysraphism), by a direct spread of infection or by a blood-borne spread as the result of a urinary tract infection, or when the meningitis causes a toxic encephalopathic state with a secondary rise in the intracranial pressure (see above), or when it causes a toxic cardiopathy with the production of a right-sided cardiac failure leading to a further increase in the intracranial pressure in the presence of a Spitz Holter valve because of an interference in the ventriculo-atrial shunt. It may follow a precipitous dilatation of the third ventricle which causes severe pressure on the optic chiasma leading sometimes to a sudden blindness which is permanent unless the pressure is relieved as a matter of urgency; this condition is associated sometimes with a persistent turning down of the eyes (the so-called 'setting-sun phenomenon'). Furthermore, optic atrophy may occur in hydrocephalus simply as the result of a long-standing papilloedema (*consecutive optic atrophy*, see below), and sometimes a severe disturbance of vision or even blindness may ensue in hydrocephalus in the absence of an optic atrophy as the result of an encephalopathy which causes a water-logging of the brain so that it represents a form of *cortical blindness*.

In primary and secondary optic atrophy, there is a gradual loss of the normal pink colour of the disc so that it becomes pale as a result of a loss of the integrity of the arterioles which supply the capillaries of the optic nerve-head, but the margins of the optic disc retain their normal clear-cut outlines. If, however, it follows papilloedema the margins of the disc appear blurred, but this should not be termed necessarily a *secondary* atrophy because it may follow a primary atrophy (as in papillitis) or a secondary type of optic atrophy (as in plerocephalic oedema); the term *consecutive optic atrophy* may be used clinically.

The awareness of a developing optic atrophy by the patient depends to a large extent on the nature of the field defect; a peripheral restriction of the visual field is detected often only in the late stages, but a central or paracentral scotoma is more likely to become apparent in the early stages.

Drusen

This term is applied to translucent glistening bodies composed of concentric laminations of hyaline material which develop on the optic disc as a degenerative condition of an inherited nature with involvement usually of both eyes; rarely they occur as a congenital anomaly. They sometimes proliferate and project into the vitreous, but occasionally they lie buried within the disc so that there may be an ophthalmoscopic appearance suggestive of papilloedema; on fluorescein angiography the absence of any increase in the normal fluorescence of the optic disc and of any extension of the fluorescence into the surrounding retina confirms the diagnosis of buried drusen. They are liable to affect the optic nerve fibres with the production of visual field defects such as an enlarged blind spot or a nerve bundle defect. Tuberous sclerosis of the optic disc may present a similar appearance (chap. 7).

Tumours

The different forms of optic nerve tumour are classified according to their tissue of origin in the nerve or in its surrounding sheaths.

Glioma

This is the commonest form of optic nerve tumour, and it occurs usually in early childhood. It arises from the neuroglial framework of the optic nerve, usually in its orbital part with a possible spread forward to the region of the optic nerve-head or backward to the optic chiasma (with consequent enlargement of the optic canal which is demonstrated radiographically). The main features of the condition are marked visual loss and optic atrophy of the affected eye and not infrequently some degree of visual loss of the other eye when there is involvement also of the optic chiasma. Proptosis is not a common feature in the earlier stages of the condition.

Meningioma

This tumour, which occurs usually in adult life before middle age, arises in the arachnoid sheath with the production of a large growth causing proptosis and diplopia because of the displacement and impaired mobility of the eyeball. Visual defects are seldom evident until the later stages of the condition because the optic nerve tissue is not invaded directly by the tumour. Papilloedema is a characteristic feature and if severe it may lead to some degree of optic atrophy.

Fibroma

This is a relatively benign tumour which arises in the dural sheath in childhood with the production of a slowly increasing proptosis and impaired mobility of the eye in the absence of visual impairment except in the late stages.

Treatment. This consists of local excision of the tumour by a lateral approach (lateral orbitotomy—Krönlein's operation) or by a transfrontal approach, depending on the site and extent of the tumour; in a glioma this entails removal of the optic nerve but in a sheath tumour it may be possible to retain part of the nerve.

9 | Disorders of the Lens

Structure and Function

The lens is a biconvex structure which lies behind the iris (from which it is separated by the narrow posterior chamber) and in front of the vitreous (from which it is separated by the narrow retrolental space). The central part of its anterior surface lies immediately behind the pupil where it forms part of the posterior boundary of the anterior chamber, and the most prominent part of this surface (the anterior pole of the lens) lies about 3 mm behind the posterior surface of the cornea. The lens is composed of three main structures: capsule, epithelium, and fibres.

Capsule

This surrounds the lens and is concerned with the alterations which occur in the shape of the lens during accommodation because it is thicker peripherally than centrally (Figs. 9 and 10), and because it is attached to the ciliary body through the zonule (suspensory ligament). It is also concerned in fluid transference between the lens and the aqueous humour; the lens is dependent on this fluid for its nutrition because of its avascularity, and the capsule is concerned in maintaining the correct amount of fluid in the lens.

Epithelium

The lens is developed from ectoderm and appears at an early stage as a small vesicle. The anterior part of the vesicle forms the lens epithelium, but the posterior part is concerned with the formation of the earliest lens fibres (the embryonic fibres) so that the epithelium is present only over the anterior part of the lens; in the equatorial region the epithelial cells become elongated and are concerned thereafter in the formation of the lens fibres.

Fibres

These comprise the bulk of the lens and are distributed according to their time of formation in different zones; the embryonic fibres which lie in the centre of the lens are surrounded in succession by the fetal fibres, infantile fibres, adolescent fibres and adult fibres (Fig. 31).

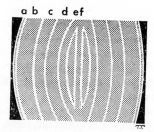

Fig. 31. *Optical section of the lens.* (a) *capsule,* (b) *cortex,* (c) *adult nucleus,* (d) *infantile nucleus,* (e) *fetal nucleus,* (f) *embryonic nucleus*

The embryonic fibres form a homogeneous mass, but the other fibres form characteristic suture lines (such as the Y-shaped sutures of the fetal fibres) which represent the lines of junction between the terminals of the fibres. It follows that the oldest fibres pass toward the centre of the lens where they remain indefinitely, in contrast to the old cells of the skin, also an ectodermal structure, which are shed from its outer surface throughout life. In later life the older fibres form a solid mass of 'dead' fibres—*the nucleus*—which may be differentiated into its embryonic, fetal, infantile, adolescent and adult components, and the newer fibres form a surrounding mass of 'living' fibres—*the cortex.*

The lens is concerned with the transmission and refraction of light rays and its normal transparency is maintained by the clear nature of its structures, by the absence of any blood vessels, and by a correct fluid balance within the lens.

Congenital Anomalies

Ectopia Lentis

In this condition, which is usually bilateral, there is a partial dislocation of the lens resulting from a defective formation of part of the zonule so that the lens is displaced by the remaining intact zonule. The limited action of the zonule causes the lens to become more spherical (thus almost invariably producing myopia) and there is usually also a considerable degree of astigmatism because of a tilting of the lens. The rim of the lens is visible in the defective area on dilatation of the pupil, but in more advanced cases it may encroach also on the undilated pupil so that the patient is aware of two blurred images in each eye; one through the dislocated lens (a phakic image), and the other through the space produced by the dislocation (an aphakic image). The lack of support of the iris by the dislocated lens produces a tremulous wobbling of the iris (*iridodonesis*).

Sometimes ectopia lentis is associated with other developmental anomalies: long spidery hands and feet (arachnodactyly), kyphosis, medial necrosis of the aorta, and occasionally infantilism—*Marfan's syndrome*, or with homocystinuria.

Treatment. As far as possible an attempt should be made to achieve some form of vision by the use of correcting lenses through the phakic (or sometimes through the aphakic) part of the pupil, but eventually it may be necess ary to remove the lens particularly if there is the likelihood of it becoming dislocated into the vitreous; this may be a hazardous procedure because of the difficulty in removing the lens without loss of vitreous.

Coloboma of the Lens

This is a localized indentation of the lens, usually of the lower part in association with defective formation of a small portion of the zonule.

Anterior or Posterior Lenticonus

This is a condition of excessive curvature of the anterior or posterior poles of the lens; it causes a marked increase in the effectivity of the axial part of the lens with the production of high myopia, but there is usually considerable distortion of vision, even after optical correction, because of its localized nature.

Spherophakia

In this condition there is an excessive curvature of both the anterior and posterior surfaces of the lens. It is liable to be associated with cataractous changes and may also lead to a secondary glaucoma because the spherical shape of the lens is liable to block the passage of aqueous through the pupil (pupil-block glaucoma).

Epicapsular Stars
   This condition is discussed in Chapter 6.

Cataract (see below)

Injuries

Cataract may be the result of an injury to the lens and caused by a break in the integrity of the lens capsule (perforating injury) or the result of concussional effects without such a break (blunt trauma), sometimes in association with a ring-shaped deposit of pigment on the anterior capsule of the lens following the imprint of the pigmented posterior layers of the iris on its anterior surface.

Dislocation may also follow trauma.

Exfoliation of the lens capsule may follow exposure to infrared rays, as in the glass-blowing industry, and parts of the capsule become detached so that they project into the anterior chamber or become rolled up like parchment on the surface of the lens; this should not be confused with pseudoexfoliation of the lens capsule (chap. 15).

Cataract

A cataract causes a loss of transparency of the lens following changes in the physical and chemical characteristics of its fibres, for example, because of a denaturation of the lens proteins or an alteration in the hydration of the lens following some abnormality of the lens capsule or of the constituents of the lens.

Cataractous changes may be detected directly by focal illumination when they appear as white opacities within an otherwise clear lens; these opacities may occur in the cortex—*anterior cortical cataract, posterior cortical cataract* or *peripheral cortical cataract*—or they may occur in the nucleus—*nuclear cataract*. They may be detected also indirectly on ophthalmoscopic examination when they appear as black opacities against the background of the red reflex of the fundus. In advanced cases the whole lens becomes opaque so that it prevents the appearance of any red reflex; this absence of a red reflex does not necessarily imply that the cataract is *mature*, a term which is reserved for a cataract which is so complete that the iris fails to cast any shadow on its anterior surface.

Cataract may be considered according to the time of its onset—congenital (or developmental) or senile (sometimes presenile)—or according to its association with some other condition such as ocular disease, ocular trauma, endocrine dysfunction, skin disorders, myotonic dystrophy, mongolism, and inborn errors of metabolism like cystine storage disease (cystinosis) and galactosaemia.

CONGENITAL (OR DEVELOPMENTAL) CATARACT

The term *congenital* is applied to various forms of cataract which are present at birth (thus correctly termed *congenital cataract*) or which appear in the earlier (or even in the later) years of life as a result of some defect which is congenitally determined (thus probably more accurately termed *developmental cataract*). These forms of cataract are the result of hereditary, toxic, nutritional or inflammatory influences.

Anterior Polar Cataract

This is an isolated form of cataract in the region of the anterior pole of the lens following a developmental anomaly in association with strands of persistent pupillary membrane. It may also follow damage to the anterior part of the lens as the result of a contact of the lens with the cornea following perforation of the eye. The opacity usually remains localized and, in the absence of corneal scarring, has little or no affect on the vision.

Anterior Pyramidal Cataract

This is a more obvious anterior polar cataract with a projection of the opaque area into the anterior chamber.

Posterior Polar Cataract

This is an isolated form of cataract in the region of the posterior pole. It is usually the result of a contact with the lens of the hyaloid artery during development, and sometimes a remnant of the artery may project from the affected area into the retrolental space and vitreous.

Nuclear Cataract (Cataracta Centralis Pulverulenta)

This is the result of the formation of fine dots, often of a yellow colour, in the central part of the lens (the embryonic and fetal parts). It seldom interferes with vision significantly.

Sutural Cataract

This is an accumulation of fine white dots in the sutures of the lens fibres, particularly in the Y (or fetal) sutures. They do not affect vision.

Dot and Flake Cataract (Fig. 32)

Fine dot opacities which appear blue (*blue-dot cataract*) or larger flake opacities which appear white (*coronary cataract*) are common features in the more peripheral parts of the lenses. They lie between

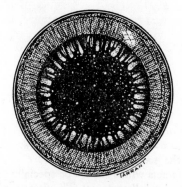

FIG. 32. *Dot and flake (coronary) cataract*

normal lens fibres and represent areas of degeneration of isolated fibres. They are often present in youth and may increase in number with age, but seldom interfere significantly with vision until later life when they become associated with senile lens changes.

Lamellar (or Zonular) Cataract (Fig. 33)

This cataract affects only a particular zone of the lens with a concentric layer of opacity, sometimes narrow but often very extensive, within an otherwise clear lens except for fine lines of opacity which pass from the circumference of this layer towards its centre like the spokes of a wheel. The congenital form is sometimes due to an inherited trait, usually of a dominant type, and is frequently bilateral, but it may be associated with the rubella syndrome or it may occur as an acquired form after injury, in association with some other ocular disease, or as a result of parathyroid deficiency (p. 174).

Coralliform Cataract

This appears as a collection of opacities in the nuclear part of the lens resembling a mass of coral.

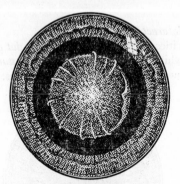

FIG. 33. *Lamellar cataract*

Axial Fusiform Cataract

This appears as a narrow spindle-like cataract extending from the anterior pole to the posterior pole.

Two other cataracts which should be specially noted are: *galactosaemic cataract* and *rubella cataract*. The first may become apparent in the early weeks of life as a refractive ring ('drop of oil' as seen by the ophthalmoscope) in centre of the lens leading to complete opacification of the lens unless lactose is eliminated from the milk diet. The early recognition of the cataract is also of great importance because of the serious general disorders which follow the malnutrition.

The *rubella cataract* is essentially of a congenital nature because it is the result of maternal rubella (German measles) during pregnancy, particularly during the first 8 weeks. The cataract is frequently complete but sometimes of the lamellar type. It commonly affects both eyes, but may be strictly unilateral. Live rubella virus may persist in the cataractous lens for two or more years after birth and this is an important factor in the management of such cases (see below).

Maternal rubella may be responsible for other abnormalities of the eyes: microphthalmos, buphthalmos, embryopathic pigmentary retinopathy (chap. 7), and defective development of the dilator muscle of the iris so that there is a persistent miosis. It may cause other general abnormalities such as congenital heart defects and perceptive deafness and their association with cataract constitutes the *rubella syndrome*.

Treatment of Congenital Cataract. Complete bilateral congenital cataracts require early surgical treatment because of a failure to use the eyes in the early weeks or months of life causes a stimulus depriva- tion amblyopia (chap. 13) and a loss of central fixation which make negligible responses to later treatment. These complications are still more prone to occur in a unilateral complete (or even partial) cataract

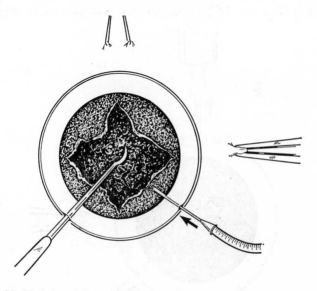

FIG. 34. *Discission of the anterior lens capsule with a Ziegler's needle; note the preplaced needle which is attached to a saline reservoir so that the anterior chamber is maintained throughout the operation*

and the prognosis for a restoration of central vision is invariably poor unless the operation is performed in the first few weeks of life and followed by occlusion of the unaffected eye and the provision of a con- tact lens to correct the aniseikonia which is inevitable in uniocular aphakia. Partial bilateral cataracts, particularly of the lamellar type are often best left alone because they may be compatible with adequate vision in the distance and remarkably good close reading vision. In such cases the optical disadvantages of aphakia and the long-term risks of an ocular complication like retinal detachment, uveitis or secondary glaucoma outweigh the advantages of an improved level of distant vision following a cataract operation.

A congenital cataract is removed most readily by *aspiration* after *discission.* The anterior chamber is maintained throughout the operation with saline by means of a preplaced needle, and, after an adequate opening of the anterior lens capsule (discission) with a Ziegler's needle (Fig. 34), the lens material is aspirated through a large bore needle (such as the Scheie needle which enters the anterior chamber by a subjunctival approach at the limbus (*ab externo approach*) (Fig. 35). Alternatively, the lens material may be irrigated

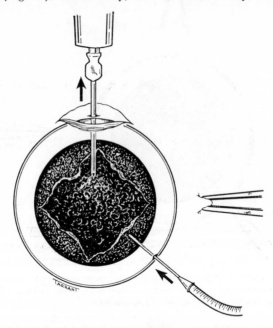

Fig. 35. *Apiration of lens material by a Scheie needle which is inserted into the anterior chamber by an ab externo approach at the upper part of the limbus; note the preplaced needle which is attached to a saline reservoir so that the anterior chamber is maintained throughout the operation*

from the anterior chamber after the discission, but this is sometimes less effective. Certainly there is no indication to confine the operation to a simple discission with a reliance on a subsequent spontaneous absorption of the lens material because this is liable to create the need for multiple discission operations and the liberated lens material is prone to cause uveitis; this applies particularly in the rubella cases when an intense endophthalmitis may destroy the eye despite intensive anti-inflammatory measures. It follows that the surgical treatment of a complete rubella cataract which must be early (to avoid stimulus deprivation amblyopia) demands the immediate removal of as much as possible of the liberated lens material (because it contains live virus); if, however, a destructive endophthalmitis occurs in the first eye the cataract on the second eye should be delayed until at least the age of 2 years.

It is essential in the surgical treatment of congenital cataract to avoid any interference with the posterior capsule of the lens because of the frequency of an abnormal attachment of the vitreous to this part of the capsule; it follows that an intracapsular extraction is contraindicated because it is prone to cause a loss of vitreous which greatly increases the risk of a subsequent retinal detachment. In bilateral congenital cataracts which are confined to the more central parts of the lenses an adequate level of vision may be obtained by securing some degree of mydriasis (for example, by the use of atropine $\frac{1}{16}$ per cent drops once daily), or sometimes by carrying out an optical iridectomy in the lower outer segment of the eye.

SENILE CATARACT

The term *senile* is applied to all forms of cataract which develop spontaneously in the absence of any congenital disorder, ocular disease, ocular trauma, or associated systemic disorder, and, although it is prone to occur in the elderly, it may occur at an earlier stage so that it is sometimes termed *presenile*. Presenile cataract may occur in certain families as isolated events, sometimes showing a certain degree of 'anticipation' so that the cataract occurs slightly earlier in each succeeding generation, but it occurs classically in Werner's syndrome which is a heredofamilial condition with posterior cortical cataract which usually affects one eye more than the other, premature greying of the hair, premature baldness, scleroderma affecting particularly the face and the extremities, chronic ulceration of the legs and feet, hypogonadism and, sometimes, osteoporosis, blue sclerotics and peripheral arterial calcification. There are various forms of senile or presenile cataract.

Nuclear Sclerosis

Changes in the nucleus of the lens are to some extent natural because some gradual hardening and loss of elasticity is inevitable, but when marked it causes distortion of the vision particularly for distant objects and a greater effectivity of the refractive power of the lens with an increased myopia (or decreased hypermetropia). This accounts for the myopia which develops in some elderly people who are then often able to read small print without glasses—a surprising event to an elderly person who has required reading glasses for many years.

Nuclear Cataract (Fig. 36)

It is usual for nuclear sclerosis to progress to true cataract formation so that the central part of the lens becomes opaque. This type of cataract is not particularly noticeable on straightforward examination

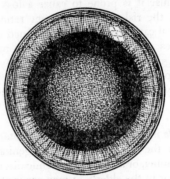

FIG. 36. *Nuclear senile cataract*

because the pupil remains 'black' owing to the clarity of the surrounding cortical parts of the lens, but it may be detected readily by focal illumination or by ophthalmoscopic examination.

Cortical Cataract

Stage of Incipient Cataract. In the early stages of cortical cataract there is an abnormal accumulation of fluid between the lens fibres (perhaps as a result of an increased permeability of the lens capsule) so that, although the lens appears somewhat cloudy, there is no true opacification.

Stage of Immature Cataract. Changes occur in the lens fibres which produce irregular white opacities and these are usually distributed within the periphery of the cortex in a radial manner (*cuneiform cataract*) (Fig. 37), but sometimes they assume a more uniform distribution in the posterior cortex (*cupuliform cataract*). Occasionally these changes are associated with a marked increase of fluid within the lens which may even cause swelling of the lens (*intumescent cataract*) with a consequent embarrassment of the filtration angle which may lead to secondary glaucoma.

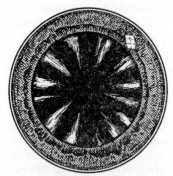

FIG 37. *Cuneiform senile cortical cataract*

Stage of Maturity. The whole lens becomes opaque with a disappearance of the iris shadow which is normally apparent on the anterior surface of the lens and with an absence of any red reflex. The vision becomes reduced to a vague awareness of hand movements (H.M.) or even to a mere perception of light (P.L.) but with retention of the ability to discern the direction from which the light is coming; this *normal projection of light* is tested by shining a bright light from different areas of the visual field into the eye and asking the patient to point to the various sources of the light. Failure of perception of light (No P.L.) is evidence of some additional lesion within the eye—vitreous haemorrhage, retinal detachment, optic atrophy, etc. Defective projection of light in a particular direction is evidence of some more localized lesion within the eye, a finding which necessitates a guarded prognosis for a restoration of useful vision after the cataract operation.

Stage of Hypermaturity. This should be avoided by the treatment of a cataract before it becomes completely mature because hypermaturity is liable to cause various complications.

Morgagnian cataract—the cortical cataract becomes liquefied and the hard nucleus sinks to the lower part of the capsule. This is frequently associated with a tremulousness of the iris on movement of the eye (*iridodonesis*).

Dislocation of the lens—the cataractous lens becomes dislocated into the vitreous (or more rarely into the anterior chamber) because of an associated degeneration of the suspensory ligament of the lens. This is also associated with iridodonesis.

Phacolytic glaucoma—this follows a leakage of lens material through the defective capsule into the anterior chamber where it accumulates within phagocytic cells; these cells may block the filtration angle causing a secondary glaucoma (chap. 15).

Lens-induced uveitis—this follows a leakage of lens material through the capsule causing a uveitis in an eye previously sensitized to lens protein (chap. 6).

COMPLICATED CATARACT

Complicated cataract is the result of various forms of long-standing ocular disease, such as recurrent severe uveitis, a retinal detachment which has failed to respond to treatment, and it is likely that it is the result of a general metabolic disorder of the diseased eye. It forms characteristically in the posterior cortical part of the lens, sometimes with striking colour changes in the affected region as a result of the diffraction of the light rays by the tiny opacities (*polychromatic lustre*).

TRAUMATIC CATARACT

Any break in the integrity of the lens capsule following a perforating injury (for example, the all-too-frequent perforation in the young child with scissors or some sharp-pointed toy, or the entry of a metallic fragment in the industry worker) or following inexpert instrumentation during an intraocular operation (for example, a penetrating keratoplasty or certain glaucoma operations) is followed by cataractous changes. This may remain localized if the opening in the capsule becomes sealed rapidly, but otherwise the whole lens becomes cataractous. If the opening in the capsule is large the persistent permeation of aqueous into the lens results in the gradual dissolution and eventual absorption of the lens material, but sometimes this liberation of lens material into the anterior chamber causes an anterior uveitis or a secondary glaucoma by an impairment of the drainage of aqueous through the filtration angle.

Cataract may also follow injury of the eye in the absence of any perforation of the lens capsule, for example, severe contusion of the eye (*concussion cataract*), exposure to irradiation, exposure to radar waves or to infrared rays; this usually takes the form of small opacities in the anterior or posterior subcapsular parts of the cortex, but some times larger leaf-like zones of opacity radiate out from the centres of these areas (the so-called *rosette cataract*).

TOXIC CATARACT

Cataract may follow the systemic administration of various drugs, such as chlorpromazine, ergot and the corticosteroids, or even the topic administration of drugs of the anticholinesterase group (DFP and Phospholine iodide); the opacities usually start in the anterior or posterior subcapsular regions. Some metals given for therapeutic reasons (topically or systemically) or absorbed by frequent contact in certain industrial processes may lead to a pigmentation of the anterior lens capsule with eventually the development of anterior subcapsular opacities; silver (*argyrosis*), mercury (*mercurialentis*), copper (*chalcosis*) and iron (*siderosis*).

ENDOCRINE CATARACT

Diabetes Mellitus

True diabetic cataract is rare because of the early diagnosis and treatment of diabetes. It is more likely to occur in adolescents and progresses rapidly in both eyes with the formation of subcapsular opacities, particularly posteriorly, and then with complete opacification and intumescence. Sometimes this is reversible provided the diabetes is controlled before the oedematous lens changes are followed by an irreversible denaturation of the lens proteins. Senile cataract in diabetics is similar to that which occurs in nondiabetics, although there is some evidence that it may occur more frequently and more early and that it may progress more rapidly in diabetics. An increased tendency to haemorrhage and a more marked liberation of pigment from the posterior surface of the iris are two features often noted during a cataract extraction in diabetics, but the greater liability to postoperative infection is not now common because of the improved control of the disease and the use of antibiotics.

Transient changes in the refraction of the eye are common features in diabetes during periods of faulty control of the disease. Hyperglycaemia causes a decrease in hypermetropia (or an increase in myopia) and hypoglycaemia causes an increase in hypermetropia (or a decrease in myopia), changes which are caused by alterations in the water content of the cortical and nuclear parts of the lens with an increased or decreased effectivity of the lens, respectively.

Parathyroid Deficiency

Hypoparathyroidism, which is characterized by an increased excitability of the neuromuscular system (*tetany*) as a result of a hypo-calcaemia, may be associated occasionally with a localized subcapsular cataract late in the disease. This may remain localized so that some years later it appears as a lamellar cataract. Spasmodic movements of the eyelids may occur in tetany.

Hypothyroidism

Cataract in the form of subcapsular opacities may occur rarely in cretinism.

ATOPIC CATARACT

Certain severe skin conditions, such as generalized eczema in children or scleroderma, are associated rarely with cataract formation, following a disturbance within the lens which is akin to that occurring within the skin. In *Rothmund's syndrome* the development of cataract in early childhood is associated with poikiloderma and with various forms of vascular disturbance.

CATARACT IN MYOTONIC DYSTROPHY

Anterior and posterior subcapsular flaky opacities may occur in myotonic dystrophy—a condition of generalized muscular disturbance affecting particularly the hands, arms and legs with the production of a peculiar form of weakness in which the affected muscles, after a delayed and relatively weak contraction, exhibit an inability to achieve a spontaneous relaxation (this is detected readily in the handshake of such patients). These subcapsular changes gradually extend to involve the whole lens in a presenile type of cataract. Ptosis may occur in this condition (chap. 11).

CATARACT IN MONGOLISM

Fine opacities within the fetal (Y) sutures and blue-dot and coronary opacities within the peripheral parts of the lens are commonly found to a much greater degree in mongolism than in the normal population. A localized arcuate opacity within the lens is also a feature of some cases, and this is a distinctive change.

Treatment. The absence of any accepted medical method of pre-venting or treating cataract, despite innumerable claims over the years, determines the necessity for surgical treatment, but each case must be assessed carefully before advising operation:

An estimation of the corrected distant and near visual acuities of the affected (or more affected) eye. Certain forms of cataract, such as a nuclear cataract, may be compatible with quite reasonable vision, although the interpretation of 'reasonable' varies with the intellec-tual capacity and occupation of the individual. For example, an elderly person may be content with poor distant vision if the near vision is reasonably good, whereas a younger person may have entirely different requirements. Sometimes in cataract the vision may be improved for a time simply by a change of spectacle lenses (for example, as compensation for increasing myopia in a nuclear lens sclerosis) or by preventing a too marked constriction of the pupil by the use of dark glasses or by a mydriatic which is sufficiently weak to allow the retention of some accommodation (for example, atropine $\frac{1}{16}$ per cent once daily).

An estimation of the corrected distant and near visual acuities of the unaffected (or less affected) eye. It is not possible with conventional spectacle lenses to obtain the use of the two eyes together (binocular vision) after a cataract operation on one eye owing to the marked size difference (aniseikonia) of the two retinal images; this difficulty may be overcome by a contact lens or by an acrylic lens implant in the anterior or posterior chamber, but these latter procedures are not free from risks—an anterior chamber implant may affect the corneal endothelium leading to a corneal dystrophy or a bullous keratopathy, although this is avoided when the implant is attached to the anterior surface of the iris, and a posterior chamber implant may become dislocated subsequently into the vitreous. It follows that a cataract operation may be postponed often until the second eye shows some degree of visual impairment unless the cataract of the affected eye is mature because of the complications which may follow hypermaturity (see above).

An estimation of the potential visual function of the affected eye after operation. This entails a determination of any coexisting ocular dis-ease, such as vitreous haemorrhage, retinal detachment, senile mac-ular degeneration, diabetic retinopathy, optic atrophy, and, when the cataract is immature, this is possible after the instillation of a my-driatic. If, however, the cataract is extensive reliance must be placed on indirect methods:

1. The relation of the corrected visual acuity to the degree of cataract; a reduction in acuity which is greater than would be expected from the cataract is suggestive of some coexistent lesion, and, as discussed above, even a mature cataract never reduces the vision beyond a level of 'perception of light with accurate projection'.

An examination of the visual field by simple confrontation or by the perimeter (chap. 16) may indicate some other abnormality.

3. An examination of the less affected eye; the recognition of a condition which tends to affect both eyes, such as macular degeneration, makes it possible that it is present also in the cataractous eye.

4. A determination of any childhood squint which may have caused an amblyopia and sometimes a loss of central fixation with or without an eccentric retinal fixation (chap. 13); in such a case the central vision would be improved to only a limited extent after a cataract operation. This is excluded best by a careful history because the presence of a squint of the cataractous eye is not necessarily an indication of a childhood squint because it may have followed simply the dissociation of the two eyes by the defective vision of one eye. This applies particularly to a congenital (or developmental) cataract when it is confined solely or largely to one eye because the affected eye is usually amblyopic following its disuse, often with a loss of central fixation.

5. The detection of any abnormality of the eye which might progress after the operation thereby affecting the visual prognosis. For example, an early corneal dystrophy, particularly affecting the corneal endothelium as in Fuchs' dystrophy (chap. 4), tends to advance rapidly following the inevitable trauma to the cornea during the removal of the lens, or the evidence of a previous uveitis is an indication of an increased likelihood of a postoperative uveitis, particularly if soft lens material is liberated at the operation. Evidence of an active uveitis is usually a contraindication to operation, except when the uveitis is of the lens-induced type (pp. 95 and 172), or in a child with uveitis of the form which occurs in Still's disease (p. 92) when a persistence of some degree of uveitis is inevitable.

6. An assessment of retinal function by electrodiagnostic tests (chap. 7).

An estimation of the maturity of the lens. A mature cataract usually demands early treatment irrespective of other considerations because of the complications which tend to follow hypermaturity (see above).

Cataract Surgery

The Preparation of the Patient

It is important to exclude or treat before operation any general condition which might cause adverse complications (haemorrhage, infection, iris prolapse). These include diabetes, cardiovascular disease, renal disorders, focal sepsis and bronchitis.

The Preparation of the Eye

It is essential to eliminate any surface infection by an appropriate antibiotic when a routine culture of the conjunctival sacs determines the presence of pathogenic organisms even in the absence of any obvious infection, but some surgeons rely on the routine use of powerful topical antibiotics (for example, penicillin and streptomycin) to deal with any such organisms. It is necessary also to determine the absence of any infection within the lacrimal sac or obstruction within the nasolacrimal duct by syringing through the upper and lower canaliculi; if the sac is infected (dacrocystitis) it should be removed before performing the cataract operation. It is essential also to exclude any unsuspected glaucoma by routine tonometry (chap. 15).

The Operation

This depends on the particular form of cataract. The surgical treatment of congenital cataract which occurs in early life has been discussed previously (p. 167).

Extracapsular Extraction. The anterior capsule of the lens is divided by a capsulotomy needle or removed partially by capsulectomy forceps so that the solid nucleus and as much as possible of the soft cortical lens fibres are expressed from the eye through the upper limbal incision; any residual lens material is washed out by saline irrigations, because it tends to cause irritation and even uveitis. This operation does not interfere with the integrity of the posterior lens capsule and sometimes it is necessary to cut a small hole in this capsule (a *needling* or *capsulotomy*) some weeks or months later to provide clear vision. It may also be necessary to divide the residual anterior capsule if this becomes thickened over the original gap.

Intracapsular Extraction. The lens is removed intact within its capsule by grasping the capsule with special noncutting forceps (intracapsular forceps), by the use of a suction apparatus (erysiphake), or by cryosurgery whereby the tip of the cryoprobe is securely attached to the capsule and the underlying lens fibres by the formation of a blob of ice. The difficulty of dislocating the lens from its zonular attachments to the ciliary body without rupturing the capsule, particularly when unduly resistant as in the younger patient or in an immature cataract, may be overcome by a partial digestion of the zonule with a solution of alpha chymotrypsin (zonulysin) behind the iris a few minutes before the removal of the lens. The intracapsular method is the operation of choice in all forms of presenile and senile cataract.

Complications

A disturbance of the vitreous is one of the main complicating features of a cataract extraction and is more likely in the intracapsular extraction. Vitreous loss is serious because it predisposes to the development of uveitis or a retinal detachment, but a forwards displacement of vitreous into the anterior chamber, even in the absence of vitreous loss, may also be serious by leading to glaucoma by obstructing the flow of aqueous (pupil block or filtration difficulties) or to corneal degenerative changes when in contact with the endothelium. Several procedures help to maintain the vitreous in its correct place during and after the operation: the prevention of spasm of the orbicularis oculi muscle of the eyelids during the extraction by facial akinesia, the prevention of spasm of the extrinsic ocular muscles during the extraction by retrobulbar anaesthesia, but these two procedures only apply when the operation is performed under local anaesthesia and as a general rule general anaesthesia is preferred unless there is some contraindication, the restoration of the anterior chamber after the extraction by the insertion of air which is retained because of adequate direct suturing of the limbal incision, and the facilitation of the circulation of aqueous within the eye after the operation by providing one or two small holes in the peripheral parts of the iris (peripheral iridotomies or iridectomies).

Haemorrhage into the anterior chamber (hyphaema) after the operation usually absorbs within a few days, but rarely it has to be removed by irrigation because of the development of secondary glaucoma. Rarely severe haemorrhage occurs within the eye during the extraction (*expulsive choroidal haemorrhage*) in an elderly person with defective choroidal vessels because of the sudden reduction of the intraocular pressure which follows the removal of the lens;

preliminary massage of the eye, before commencing the operation, lowers the intraocular pressure and diminishes this risk, but the lowering of the intraocular pressure by an osmotic agent like glycerol is more certain and should be adopted as a routine when there is any doubt about the intraocular pressure or in the presence of a high degree of myopia which increases the risk of vitreous loss.

A prolapse of iris into or through the limbal incision may occur in a restless patient, sometimes after severe coughing, but its incidence is reduced by the adequate closure of the limbal incision with direct sutures and by the restoration of the anterior chamber with air after the extraction. An iris prolapse should be abscissed, but sometimes it may be replaced provided the prolapse is only within the wound without any true exposure and is of recent onset so that a uveitis (which might lead to a sympathetic ophthalmitis—chap. 6) is unlikely.

Sometimes a cystoid degeneration of the macula may occur spontaneously after a cataract operation, even when this is uncomplicated, usually in an elderly person so that there may have been a predisposition to its development, but vitreous traction is often an important factor.

Dislocation of the Lens

This follows a defect in the zonule:

1. Congenital anomaly (p. 161).
2. Trauma (p. 163).
3. Degenerative conditions, such as a mature cataract secondary to an old-standing retinal detachment or in advanced infantile glaucoma (buphthalmos) when there is an enlargement of the eye but not of the lens.

The dislocation may be incomplete (as in ectopia lentis) or complete so that the lens becomes dislocated anteriorly into the anterior chamber or posteriorly into the vitreous.

Anterior Dislocation. This is almost invariably followed by such complications as secondary glaucoma (due to obstruction of the filtration angle by the lens), corneal degeneration (due to contact of the lens with the posterior corneal surface), or anterior uveitis. The only effective treatment is usually removal of the lens, although sometimes the lens may be restored to its normal position after pupillary dilatation (by the instillation of a mydriatic) where it is maintained thereafter by pupillary constriction (by the instillation of a miotic).

Posterior Dislocation. This has little effect initially except visually because of the aphakia, so that a correcting lens is necessary in the interests of clear vision. There are, however, many later complications; adhesion of the lens to the lower peripheral part of the retina by an inflammatory exudate, intense uveitis, secondary glaucoma, or retinal detachment. It is usually advisable therefore to remove such a lens, although this involves the loss of some of the vitreous during the opening of the eye at the corneoscleral junction (because of the vitreous which entered the anterior chamber at the time of the dislocation) and during the removal of the lens (because of the vitreous which surrounds the lens), so that the results of the operation are sometimes inevitably poor, and in certain circumstances it is expedient to adopt a 'wait-and-see' policy in such cases.

10 | Disorders of the Vitreous Body

Structure and Function

The vitreous body is a clear transparent gel-like substance which fills the space between the posterior surface of the lens and the inner surface of the retina. It is formed by fibrillar micellae composed of a protein substance, related to but perhaps not identical with collagen, and also of hyaluronic acid, so that it has some form of structural framework which accounts for its tensile strength and elasticity. The vitreous body is surrounded by a *hyaloid membrane* which is essentially a surface condensation; its disruption in an intraocular operation or in a perforating injury is followed by a prolapse of the vitreous. The vitreous lies in apposition to the inner surface of the retina without any true attachment except anteriorly to the ciliary epithelium and posteriorly to the margin of the optic disc. Its anterior surface appears on slit-lamp microscopy to be separated from the posterior surface of the lens by a narrow capillary space (*retrolental space*), but in fact this contains a homogeneous type of vitreous which has a narrow circular zone of tenuous attachment to part of the lens. Sometimes this attachment is unduly strong as in certain forms of congenital cataract, so that an attempt to perform an intracapsular cataract extraction in such an eye is liable to be associated with vitreous loss. A narrow 'canal' (Cloquet's canal) passes through the vitreous from the central part of the lens to the optic disc, but it is not a true space because it contains modified vitreous; it represents the site of the hyaloid artery which is present in the developing eye but disappears before birth. The vitreous maintains the optical part of the retina in contact with the underlying retinal pigment epithelium. This is a purely mechanical effect and it follows that any loss of vitreous during an intraocular operation or perforating injury of the globe may predispose to a later retinal detachment, as may also a spontaneous detachment of the posteriod hyaloid membrane.

Congenital Anomalies

Persistent Hyaloid Remnants

Small persistent remnants of the hyaloid artery or its branches constitute vitreous 'floaters' (*muscae volitantes*) (see below). Sometimes a persistent hyaloid artery may ramify in a remnant of the posterior fibrovascular sheath which lies behind the developing lens in intrauterine life with the formation of a *persistent tunica vasculosa lentis*.

Persistent Hyperplastic Primary Vitreous

In this condition active hyperplastic changes originate in the anterior part of the vitreous after birth in association with a persistent tunica vasculosa lentis so that a mass of vascularized tissue forms behind the lens in a localized area or over the whole posterior surface and sometimes passing round the equator of the lens to its anterior surface. This tissue varies in thickness from a thin membrane to a thick mass extending into the anterior part of the vitreous. The anterior chamber usually becomes shallow with a consequent narrowing of the filtration angle. Characteristically the ciliary processes become elongated, atrophic and drawn out to become incorporated in the mass; zonular fibres may also extend into the mass. Usually the peripheral retina is involved in these changes so that it becomes disorganized and detached and the development of a uveitis or secondary glaucoma is a likely terminal event. The condition may be unilateral or rarely bilateral. There is no effective treatment; an attempt may be made to incise the mass of tissue but there is unlikely to be any visual improvement because of the other changes in the eye.

Disorders of the Vitreous

Increased Fluidity of the Vitreous

The normal vitreous has a certain degree of fluidity but this may become accentuated in advancing age, myopia or any form of long-standing intraocular disease such as uveitis. A fluid vitreous is usually associated with the appearance of vitreous opacities and sometimes also with a lowering of the intraocular pressure.

Shrinkage of the Vitreous

A shrinkage of the vitreous may occur in advancing age with the production of a detachment of the posterior part of the vitreous so that it becomes separated from the inner retinal surface; a subjective awareness of flashings of light or of floating opacities may coincide with this separation. This form of vitreous detachment may precipitate a retinal detachment particularly if a haemorrhage occurs in the underlying retina.

Opacities in the Vitreous

Small particles may occur in the vitreous gel (the *muscae volitantes*) as the result of congenital remnants or as the result of coagulations of protein material usually in association with an increased fluidity of the vitreous. Sometimes they remain undetected by the patient unless they are viewed against a bright background, but they are visible particularly when they lie in the central part of the vitreous and are more clearly defined when they lie near the retina; to some extent they are most troublesome in the introspective type of person, The opacities, which appear subjectively as black spots or threads. shift on movements of the eye, but this change in position is not precise so that on attempting to view them against a particular part of the background they flit rapidly away; this is in contrast to the scotoma which follows a retinal lesion, such as a macular haemorrhage, which may be viewed precisely in any desired direction. The opacities may be observed with the ophthalmoscope or, when anteriorly placed, with the slit-lamp microscope, but sometimes they are too small to be readily visible.

There are other primary opacities in the vitreous which are seldom associated with any subjective awareness; peculiar small white particles which are composed of calcium soaps—the so-called *asteroid bodies*—occur rarely in old age, even sometimes in the absence of any obvious ocular disease and usually as a unilateral phenomenon, and numerous clusters of glittering golden cholesterol crystals—*synchisis scintillans*—occur after long-standing uveitis or vitreous haemorrhage and they cascade through the degenerate fluid vitrous.

There are also other vitreous opacities which are essentially of a secondary nature; collections of inflammatory cells or exudates as a result of a uveitis, free haemorrhage from the retina, strands of organized haemorrhage from the retina (retinitis proliferans, chap. 7), or new vessel formations within the vitreous in the absence of pre-existing haemorrhage (rete mirabile, chap. 7).

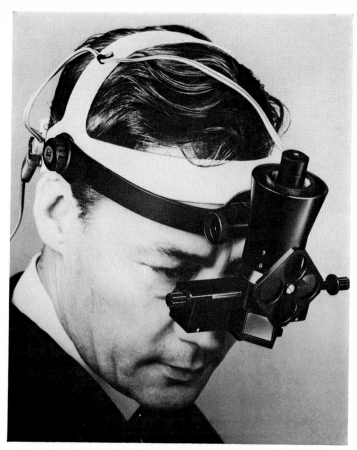

PLATE VII Binocular indirect ophthalmoscope (courtesy of C. Davis Keeler Ltd)

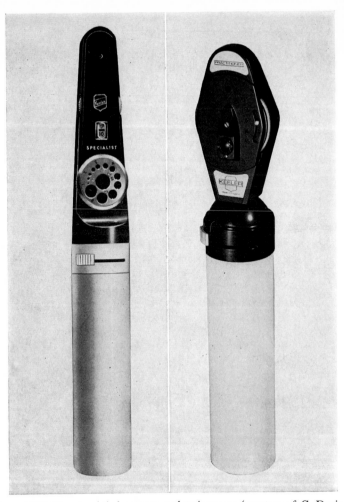

PLATE VIII Direct ophthalmoscope and retinoscope (courtesy of C. Davis Keeler Ltd)

11 | Diseases of the Eyelids

Structure and Function (Fig. 38)

The upper and lower eyelids are modified folds of skin consisting of orbital and palpebral portions which are continuous with one another across the superior and inferior orbitopalpebral folds. In the upper eyelid the orbital portion extends down from the eyebrow to cover the upper part of the orbit and the palpebral portion covers

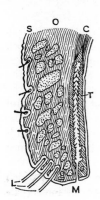

Fig. 38. *Section of the eyelid to show skin (S), orbicularis oculi muscle (O), palpebral conjunctiva (C), tarsal plate (T), containing a Meibomian (tarsal) gland which opens at the lid margin (M), and the eyelashes (L)*

the upper part of the eye. In the lower eyelid the orbital portion extends up from the cheek to cover the lower part of the orbit and the palpebral portion covers the lower part of the eye. The eyelids in the subcutaneous layer contain the orbicularis oculi muscle which is innervated by the facial (VIIth cranial) nerve and forms an oval sheet of concentric muscle fibres surrounding the eyelids. The palpebral parts of this muscle, particularly of the upper lid, are utilized in gentle lid closure, and the orbital parts are also brought into play in forcible lid closure. The closure of the lids is associated reflexly with an upwards movement of the eye which is effective before the full closure of the lids (Bell's phenomenon). The orbicularis muscle is concerned also in the drainage of the tears (chap. 12). The closure of the upper lid by the orbicularis muscle is opposed by the combined actions of the levator palpebrae superioris muscle and its associated muscle the superior palpebral muscle (of Müller) which retract the lid. The levator is a voluntary muscle which is innervated by the oculomotor (IIIrd cranial) nerve and extends into the upper lid from its origin in the apex of the orbit. It has a widespread insertion but its main part is attached indirectly to the upper border of the tarsal plate by way of the involuntary superior palpebral muscle which is innervated by the cervical sympathetic nerve; this is an unusual anatomical feature whereby a striated muscle adopts a smooth muscle to carry out its main action.

The palpebral opening is the entrance into the conjunctival sac which is bounded by the upper and lower lid margins; these margins terminate laterally in an acute angle (the *lateral canthus*) which is attached laterally to the bony orbit by the *lateral palpebral ligament* and medially in an elliptical junction (the *medial canthus*) which is attached medially to the bony orbit by the *medial palpebral ligament*. When the eyelids are opened in the normal way with the eyes directed straight ahead it is usual for the upper margin of the cornea to be covered slightly by the upper lid margin and for the lower margin of the cornea to be at the same level as the lower lid margin, but in the infant the upper lid margin is often above the cornea (with the appearance of a *upper scleral rim*) and in the adult there is a tendency for the lower lid margin to lie below the cornea (with the appearance of a *lower scleral rim*).

The lid margin is a narrow zone (about 2 mm in width) which separates the outer (skin) surface of the eyelid from its inner (palpebral conjunctival) surface; the junction of the medial sixth and lateral five-sixths of the lid margin is represented by a papilla which contains the lacrimal punctum (chap. 12). There are other structures on the lid margin:

1. Two or three irregularly placed rows of short stout hairs (the *eyelashes* or *cilia*) which are more numerous in the upper than in the lower lids are placed anteriorly on the lid margin. The eyelashes are renewed rapidly after epilation, reaching their normal size within about ten weeks. They provide some degree of protection to

the eyes and are associated directly with sebaceous glands (of Zeis) and indirectly with sweat glands (of Moll).

2. The *intermarginal sulcus* lies behind the lashes and is visible clinically as a 'grey line'. It is important surgically because it represents the line of division of the lid into its anterior portion (skin and orbicularis muscle) and its posterior portion (tarsal plate and conjunctiva).

3. The openings of the ducts of the Meibomian (tarsal) glands, 30–40 in the upper lid and 20–30 in the lower lid, lie immediately behind the grey line. These large sebaceous glands lie within the tarsal plate, a dense formation of connective tissue within each lid which provides the palpebral portion of the lid with some degree of rigidity, and their sebaceous secretions on the lid margins prevent an overspilling of the normal tear flow from the conjunctival sac. The secretions also form the surface layer of the precorneal fluid thus preventing an undue evaporation of the tears from the surface of the cornea.

Congenital Anomalies

Epicanthus

This is a semilunar fold of skin which passes from the medial part of the eyebrow in a crescentic manner towards the lower lid so that it tends to obscure the medial canthus and to increase the apparent breadth of the nose. It occurs to a minor degree in most young children, but usually disappears spontaneously as the bridge of the nose becomes formed in the early years of life except in certain races, like the Mongols, in which it remains as a permanent feature. It is usually bilateral although not always symmetrical. Epicanthic folds tend to give a false appearance of a convergent squint (chap. 13). A more severe form of epicanthus occurs in association with a congenital ptosis and sometimes also with a marked narrowing of the palpebral fissure (*blepharophimosis*); this condition requires correction by a plastic operation.

Coloboma

A notch in the lid margin, usually at the junction of the middle and inner thirds of the upper eyelid, may occur as a developmental anomaly. It may be corrected by a plastic operation for cosmetic reasons and for protective reasons if the notch is sufficiently large to cause undue exposure of the cornea even during closure of the lids.

Ankyloblepharon

Rarely a small area of adhesion between the upper and lower lid margins may occur as a congenital anomaly, evidence of the fact that the lids are adherent to one another at an early stage of development; such an adhesion is treated by simple division.

Ptosis

A drooping of the upper lid may occur as a congenital anomaly of the levator muscle; it may be unilateral or bilateral and is sometimes associated with a weakness of the extrinsic ocular muscles, particularly those concerned with elevation of the eye. Most of these defects are caused by a failure in the development of the affected muscle or muscles so that they are of myogenic origin, but a few cases are of neurogenic origin. The degree of ptosis is variable, usually it is largely a cosmetic defect because it is not sufficiently marked to prevent the eye from functioning visually, but in severe cases the affected eye is likely to develop a stimulus deprivation amblyopia as a result of its disuse, although this is avoided in bilateral cases because of the necessity to tilt the head backwards to achieve any form of vision.

Marcus Gunn Jaw-winking Phenomenon. In this form of unilateral congenital ptosis the ptosis is replaced by a marked retraction of the affected lid during the opening of the jaw (so that it is recognized by the mother at an early stage of life during the act of sucking): this retraction increases on deviating the jaw away from the affected eye and decreases on deviating the jaw towards the affected side. The condition is probably the result of an abnormal nervous connection of the oculomotor nerve to levator muscle with the motor part of the trigeminal nerve. As a general rule the phenomenon becomes less obvious when the child becomes older, and operative treatment is seldom if ever indicated because it would necessitate the elimination of levator function by a myectomy (to avoid the retraction of the lid) and the subsequent correction of the persistent ptosis by the utilization of the frontalis or superior rectus, as discussed below.

The detection of ptosis is obvious on simple inspection of the eyelids, but an assessment of the degree of levator function demands the prevention of any upwards movement of the eyebrow by pressing on it with the finger so that the frontalis muscle is not allowed to exert an indirect elevating influence on the lid.

Treatment. The surgical correction of congenital ptosis is seldom carried out before the age of 3 years unless the ptosis is sufficient to prevent the development of central vision; after that age it is easier to assess the extent of the operation because in the early years of life there may be some degree of spontaneous improvement. There are several types of operation:

Levator resection is usually the most effective procedure and the muscle may be approached through the skin (*Everbusch's operation*) or through the conjunctiva (*Blaskovics's operation*).

Utilization of the superior rectus provides a link between part of the superior rectus muscle and the tarsal plate of the upper lid (*Motais's operation* or *Greeves's operation*) so that the lid is lifted during upwards movements of the eye but it is of no value when there is an associated weakness of the superior rectus, and is contra-indicated when there is binocular function because it usually causes some hypotropia of the operated eye with consequent diplopia.

Utilization of the frontalis muscle provides a link between the frontalis muscle and the upper lid by the insertion of fascial slips so that the patient raises the eyebrow to reduce the ptosis.

Distichiasis

Rarely the Meibomian glands fail to develop and are replaced by extra rows of eyelashes which turn inwards so that they rub on the cornea. They should be removed by electrolysis puncture which destroys the follicles of the aberrant eyelashes.

Injuries

Lacerations

A laceration requires immediate suturing to ensure healing of the lid without subsequent structural deformity; this applies particularly when the lid margin is involved, because unless great care is exercised in suturing the cut ends into perfect opposition the lid margin becomes notched.

Burns

A superficial burn is treated simply by eliminating any infective agent with an application of cetrimide 1 per cent lotion to the affected area and then applying some form of antibiotic powder until healing is complete. A severe burn involving a large area of the lid or its whole thickness demands urgent and effective treatment because the exposure of the eye which follows the failure of the lid to protect the eye may result in serious damage to the eye. A tarsorrhaphy may provide sufficient protection, but an early plastic repair is the most satisfactory procedure.

Abnormal Positions of the Lid Margins

The integrity of the eye is dependent to some extent on a correct positional relationship between the margins of the eyelid, particularly the lower one, and the eyeball. This is upset in two conditions —*ectropion* and *entropion*.

Ectropion

In this condition the lid margin is everted so that it fails to be in contact with the surface of the eye with exposure of the palpebral conjunctiva and persistent epiphora. It may be produced in different ways:

Atonic conditions, a marked weakness of the orbicularis oculi, occur in a facial palsy with a sagging and ectropion of the lower lid, usually termed *lagophthalmos* because of the inability to close the eyes properly. An atonic condition of the skin and its fascial tissues in the elderly also predisposes to the development of an ectropion which is increased by the tendency for the patient to wipe the lower lid persistently in a lateral direction because of an associated epiphora. The treatment of this type of ectropion depends on its severity; a true lagophthalmos may be lessened by decreasing the extent of the palpebral aperture by a lateral tarsorrhaphy (union of the lateral parts of the upper and lower eyelid margins) or by supporting the lower lid with a fascial sling. An ectropion may be relieved by a wedge resection of the part of the lid affected most severely, but when the ectropion is of small degree and confined to its medial part so that epiphora is the main symptom the epiphora is relieved simply by opening the punctum and the adjacent part of the canaliculus (three-snip operation) in conjunction sometimes with a cauterization of the adjacent palpebral conjunctiva to try and oppose the lid to the eyeball.

Cicatricial conditions, the occurrence of scarring in the eyelids following trauma (gunshot wounds, burns), severe inflammation or neoplastic disease, may cause an ectropion of the upper or lower lids. The treatment involves excision of the scar tissue and the restoration of the defective area by a skin graft.

Entropion

In this condition the lid margin is inverted so that the lashes rub against the eyeball causing irritation of the eye, and sometimes fine abrasions of the lower part of the cornea which may lead to ulceration. It may be produced in different ways:

Spastic conditions, a spasm of the orbicularis oculi which accompanies the irritation of any inflammatory condition of the surface of the eye or follows a simple bandaging of the eye, may cause an entropion of the lower lid particularly in elderly people who have a loss of the normal elasticity of the connective tissues of the lower lid. Sometimes the entropion is relieved simply by removing its cause, or by applying a strip of adhesive plaster from the lid margin towards the cheek. In other cases a series of cautery punctures through the skin and orbicularis muscle immediately below the lid margin may cause sufficient areas of scarring in the muscle to prevent the excessive spasm. In more severe cases correction of the entropion is achieved by removing a strip of skin and underlying muscle, the 'skin-and-muscle operation', but this suffers from the disadvantage of causing a shortening of the lid so that some degree of ectropion may occur later, and a more satisfactory procedure is to provide a pressure effect on the lower border of the tarsal plate by transplanting or shortening a large strip of the overlying orbicularis muscle (Wheeler's operation or one of its modifications) thus preventing the upper border of the tarsal plate from rotating inwards.

Cicatricial conditions: an entropion may follow any form of scarring of the lid (traumatic, inflammatory or neoplastic) and it is treated by a plastic repair.

A simulated form of entropion may occur in early childhood when the fold of skin which is present immediately below the lower eyelid margin is unduly prominent (*epiblepharon*) so that on a downward movement of the eye the lid margin becomes inverted and the lashes rub on the cornea causing discomfort. The condition usually resolves spontaneously but in severe cases the fold of skin may be excised (without any removal of the underlying orbicularis oculi muscle) and the edges of the wound united with fine silk sutures.

ABNORMAL MOVEMENTS OF THE EYELIDS

Blepharospasm. Spasm of the eyelids may occur in any inflammatory condition of the eye, particularly when there is photophobia, so that it is an exaggeration of the normal protective mechanism of the eye. It occurs sometimes on attempting to examine the eye in children and may then be associated with an eversion of the lids so that the conjunctival surfaces of the lids become exposed, thus preventing any view of the eyeball; in babies it is sometimes necessary to open the lids with a special retractor.

Myokymia. This refers to fine rhythmical contractions of an involuntary nature which occur from time to time within a small portion of the orbicularis muscle of either lid. There is a marked subjective awareness of this phenomenon, but the contractions are scarcely visible on inspection. It is essentially a functional condition which is produced by fatigue and eyestrain. Rarely these involuntary movements are more marked and widespread, as in a tic, sometimes with an associated trigeminal neuralgia (tic douloureux).

Ptosis

Ptosis (drooping of the upper lid) is commonly a congenital anomaly (p. 188), but it may also be an acquired condition.

Myasthenia Gravis

Ptosis is frequently the presenting feature of this disease and the weakness of the levator muscle follows a failure of the transmission of the efferent motor nervous impulses across the myoneural junction because of the presence of an abnormal substance with a curare-like action. Other muscles may also be involved, e.g. the extrinsic ocular muscles, the pharyngeal muscles, and more rarely the skeletal muscles. The disease runs a progressive course, often with apparent remissions and characteristically with an increase of the condition at times of fatigue so that it is obvious towards the end of the day. The diagnosis is confirmed by the temporary amelioration of the paresis after the administration of prostigmine or edrophonium chloride (Tensilon), but electromyographic studies are a more sensitive register of early cases. The disease usually responds to treatment with prostigmine; in severe cases thymectomy may be of value.

Horner's Syndrome

A small degree of ptosis follows a paresis of the smooth muscle of the upper lid as the result of an involvement of the cervical sympathetic nerve in such conditions as syringomyelia, aortic aneurysm, lesions of the upper part of the lung, trauma, etc. The ptosis is associated with a slight upwards displacement of the lower lid so that a narrowed palpebral aperture is a characteristic feature; this accounts for the suggestion of some degree of enophthalmos, but this is a false appearance. There is also some constriction of the pupil (miosis) because of a loss of tone of the dilator muscle of the pupil, and a decreased sweating of the affected side of the face.

Neurogenic Lesions

Any lesion of the oculomotor nerve (IIIrd cranial nerve) may be associated with ptosis (p. 246). Rarely the Marcus Gunn phenomenon (p. 188) may occur as an acquired condition.

Myopathic Lesions

Ptosis is a characteristic feature of an ocular myopathy (progressive external ophthalmoplegia, chap. 13), and it may occur in myotonic dystrophy although cataract is the more usual ocular complication (chap. 9). The ptosis which occurs in thyrotrophic exophthalmos (exophthalmic ophthalmoplegia) may be the result of changes within the levator muscle, but it is also mechanical because of the swelling of the upper eyelid (chap. 14).

Mechanical Lesions

Any abnormal tissue within the upper lid which increases into bulk (haemorrhage, oedema, trachomatous scarring, neoplastic deposits, etc.) may cause a ptosis.

Traumatic Lesions

The ptosis which follows trauma is usually the result of an involvement of the oculomotor nerve or of the cervical sympathetic nerve, but the levator muscle may be affected directly by a traumatic lesion of the upper lid, for example, following the surgical exploration of the upper part of the orbit.

Treatment. This is essentially treatment of the condition which is causing the ptosis, and correction of the ptosis by operation (p. 189) is less frequent than in the congenital form of the condition. Sometimes spectacles with a metal crutch which presses backwards against the junction of the palpebral and orbital parts of the upper

lid are of value, but they tend to cause discomfort and a special
form of haptic contact lens which supports the upper eyelid is more
effective.

Lid Retraction

Lid retraction is discussed in Chapter 14 in relation to endocrine
exophthalmos.

Inflammatory Conditions

Blepharitis

It is customary to consider two types of blepharitis, *squamous* or
nonulcerative, and *ulcerative*, but the marked decrease of ulcerative
cases in recent years is an indication that to a large extent they
merely represent cases of nonulcerative blepharitis in which there
is a secondary infection; this is usually avoided by the use of topical
antibiotics. The squamous type is characterized by a hyperaemia of
the lid margins, some swelling and redness of the eyelids, fine
powdery deposits or scales on the eyelashes, and sometimes by a
tendency for an increased loss of the eyelashes. It is usually chronic
and the abnormal changes are accentuated by a tendency to rub
the eyelids. It is essentially a seborrhoeic condition, hence its increased incidence in childhood, particularly in early adolescence, but
it may be induced also by constant exposure to some form of irritant
such as smoke or cosmetics. The occurrence of any secondary
infection, usually of a staphylococcal nature, increases the severity of
the condition with obvious sepsis in the region of the eyelashes so
that in the later stages permanent distortions (*trichiasis*) of the eyelashes may cause some of them to run on the cornea with an increased irritation of the eyes and with the development of corneal
ulceration. It is obvious that the ulcerative form of blepharitis is
prone to occur in dirty surroundings and in conditions of malnutrition or in association with other diseases, such as the exanthemata,
when there is a lowered resistance to infection so that its incidence is
greatest in childhood.

Treatment. The immediate treatment consists of maintaining the
eyelid margins as free as possible from discharge, powdery deposits
or scales by the application of cotton wool soaked in a bland lotion
like saline, and the elimination of any secondary infection by the
use of an appropriate antibiotic ointment; the isolation of the infec-

tive agent and an assessment of its sensitivity to various antibiotics determines the particular drug. The elimination of any associated dermatitis or seborrhoeic condition of the face, and scalp is also of value. The long-term treatment is aimed at eliminating the conditions of poor hygiene and malnutrition which foster its continuance. In recalcitrant cases an autogenous vaccine may be of value. Ingrowing eyelashes may be removed with epilation forceps, but they regrow almost invariably within a few weeks and it may be necessary to destroy the follicles of the offending lashes by electrolysis puncture.

A blepharitis may be associated sometimes with a dermatitis (eczema) of the eyelids; this may be of an infective or allergic nature.

Infective Dermatitis
The lids may be affected by a variety of infective agents; bacterial conditions like furunculosis, sycosis barbae and impetigo contagiosum; fungal conditions like tinea (ringworm) and actinomycosis; parasitic conditions like the crab louse, scabies and myiasis (fly maggots); and virus conditions like herpes simplex, herpes zoster ophthalmicus, vaccinia, verruca, and molluscum contagiosum. Dermatitis of the eyelids is a feature of dermatomyositis (chap. 7).

Herpes Simplex
This is discussed in Chapter 4.

Herpes Zoster Ophthalmicus
This unilateral condition causes a swelling of the eyelids, particularly the upper one, with a characteristic vesiculation of the skin and with a similar involvement of the skin of the affected side of the face and scalp within the distribution of the ophthalmic division of the trigeminal nerve (cranial nerve V). The other ocular complications are keratitis (chap. 4), uveitis (chap. 6), secondary glaucoma (chap. 15), internal ophthalmoplegia (chap. 6) and external ophthalmoplegia (chap. 13).

Vaccinia
A typical vaccination pustule may develop in the skin of the eyelid following the direct transmission of the virus from a smallpox vaccination on the arm or leg. It is associated with a marked

redness and swelling of the lids and an enlargement of the preauricular and submaxillary glands.

Verruca

This is an infective type of simple wart; it may be single or multiple on the eyelid, particularly near the lid margin.

Molluscum Contagiosum

This forms a raised globular mass on the lid, usually in the region
of the lid margin, which shows a characteristically umbilicated
centre; this appearance may suggest a basal cell carcinoma (rodent
ulcer), but it lacks the nodularity which is evident on palpation of
such a lesion. Sometimes the lesion extends very rapidly. A simple
excision of the mass should be followed by a cauterization of its
base to prevent recurrence.

Allergic Dermatitis

The lids are prone to be affected by external agents which produce
an allergic response resulting in a moist eczema and oedematous
swelling. There are many such irritants, for example, drugs such as
atropine, cosmetics such as mascara and nail varnish (which is
transferred to the eyelids from the finger nails by rubbing the eyes),
various chemicals used in industry, various metallic substances such
as nickel which characteristically causes the 'spectacle' form of
dermatitis because of its use in some spectacle frames, and plants
such as the Primula. The lids may also show an allergic response in
certain systemic conditions such as the ingestion of shellfish in
hypersensitive individuals.

Treatment. The main aim of treatment is to eliminate the offending agent. The local reaction may be relieved by the administration
of topical steroids, but sometimes antihistamine drugs are necessary
to combat the condition.

Stye (External Hordeolum)

This is an infective condition of the follicle of the eyelash or its
associated sebaceous glands of Zeis. It is usually acute with considerable pain and tenderness of the eyelid. The affected part of
the lid margin becomes swollen, red and tense with the production
of a yellow 'head' which points along the line of an eyelash before
finally discharging its purulent contents, and there is a surrounding
oedematous reaction. Sometimes a stye may be chronic and recurrent

sties may be associated with a blepharitis as part of a seborrhoeic diathesis.

Treatment. The most effective treatment is to hasten its discharge by the application of heat usually in the form of hot spoon bathings; this involves the use of a large wooden spoon (*wooden* simply because the handle of a metal spoon becomes too hot to hold) to which is attached a large wad of cotton wool by a bandage and, after dipping it into a bowl of boiling water, the pad is gradually brought near the eye (which is kept closed) so that the steam from the pad circulates around the eye until finally the pad is sufficiently cool to allow it to be held against the eye. This process is repeated several times over a period of 10 to 15 minutes. Rarely it is necessary to incise the stye at the lid margin to facilitate the discharge of the pus.

Chalazion (*Internal Hordeolum* or *Meibomian Cyst*)

This is an enlarged tarsal gland which results from an accumulation of its sebaceous products because of a failure of their expulsion through the tarsal duct owing to some obstruction by a foreign material such as a particle of dirt. The affected gland ceases to enlarge after a few days or weeks because the accumulated material obliterates the formative basal cells of the gland. The cyst usually forms a round painless projection on the conjunctival surface of the lid or a pouting of the blocked duct on the lid margin. Subsequently the cyst becomes organized with the formation of a relatively solid mass. Sometimes a carcinoma may show a similar appearance. More rarely there is a secondary infection of the cyst with the production of pain and oedema of the surrounding parts of the lid; this oedema is particularly marked when the infected tarsal cyst lies near the lateral or medial canthus and in this situation the cyst may be difficult to palpate although its presence is determined by an area of tenderness on gentle prodding with a glass rod. A generalized infective condition of the tarsal glands (meibomitis) is associated sometimes with blepharitis.

Treatment. Sometimes a chalazion subsides spontaneously within a few weeks, but usually it is necessary to evacuate its contents by curettage after making a vertical incision over the conjunctival surface of the cyst which is secured by a special clamp. In long-standing cases it is also necessary to excise part of the thickened wall, but care should be taken to retain the overlying conjunctiva so that a mass of scar tissue on the inner surface of the lid is avoided.

Cysts

Cyst of Moll

A cyst of Moll forms a small translucent cyst at the lid margin which protrudes in the region of an eyelash. Simple puncture is usually followed by a recurrence and the cyst should be excised.

Sebaceous Cyst

Sebaceous cysts may assume different forms in the eyelid; a simple cyst of one of the sebaceous glands of the skin is excised in the usual way if sufficiently large, multiple small white spots which are slightly elevated above the surface level (*milia*) may be shelled out if necessary, and the conditions which may arise in the specialized sebaceous glands (glands of Zeis and tarsal glands) are discussed above.

Syphilitic Conditions

A *primary chancre* of the eyelid presents as an acute inflammatory swelling with an associated preauricular and submaxillary adenitis in the primary stage of the disease, a *skin rash* may involve the eyelids in the secondary stage of the disease, and a *gumma* may involve the deeper tissues of the lid, particularly the tarsal plate (so that it mimics a chalazion), in the tertiary stage of the disease.

Oedematous Conditions

Oedema of the eyelids is a common feature in a wide variety of conditions of the lids or of their adjacent structures, for example, traumatic, inflammatory, or allergic disorders. It is also a feature of any condition which causes an increased pressure within the orbit (such as endocrine exophthalmos, proptosis resulting from an orbital tumour), and of certain systemic conditions like renal dysfunction and cardiac failure.

Blepharochalasis

Blepharochalasis is the term applied to the redundant folds of skin which occur sometimes in the upper lid, and also, more rarely, in the lower lid, of the elderly person. It may be treated in certain cases by simple excision but usually its correction requires treatment of the whole skin of the face (the plastic operation of 'face-lift').

Tumours

Papilloma

This is a benign wart which may assume various forms; usually it appears as a raised vascular mass, but it may remain relatively flat particularly in the elderly person. Rarely it becomes pigmented. Sometimes a cutaneous horn may form on its surface. A wart may be treated by simple excision.

Angioma

This is a benign malformation of the blood vessels of the skin. It may appear as a bright red area owing to a proliferation of capillary vessels (capillary angioma or telangiectasis) or as a blue-coloured area due to the formation of abnormal venous channels (cavernous angioma). An angioma of the eyelid may be associated with a similar condition of the face ('port wine' stain) or with angiomata elsewhere (as in the Sturge-Weber syndrome—chap. 7). An angioma of the lid in a baby is often noticed first when the child cries, because it then becomes larger. Treatment is seldom indicated in the young child, unless the angioma is sufficiently large to prevent adequate opening of the eye so that a stimulus deprivation amblyopia is likely to occur, because an angioma almost invariably becomes less obvious as the child grows older. Surgical excision of an angioma is liable to cause considerable fibrosis. Irradiation may cause some decrease in the size of the lesion.

Xanthelasma

This is a benign tumour which develops in unicellular sebaceous glands which are present in the medial parts of the upper and lower eyelids with the formation of several yellowish slightly raised masses. They may be removed by simple excision for cosmetic reasons.

Molluscum Sebaceum (Keratoacanthoma)

This is a benign condition, but it may simulate a squamous cell carcinoma clinically because of its destructive nature and also sometimes even histologically.

Carcinoma

This is a malignant tumour which assumes different forms:

Squamous-cell carcinoma (*epithelioma*) may arise spontaneously or rarely as a result of malignant change in a papilloma. It causes a localized nodular tumour which eventually breaks down centrally to form an area of ulceration with destruction of the affected tissues of the lid. It is liable occasionally to form metastases.

Basal-cell carcinoma (*rodent ulcer*) is the commonest form of carcinoma of the eyelid and occurs characteristically at the lid margin, particularly of the lower lid, or in the skin around the medial canthus. It forms a nodular lesion which readily and repeatedly breaks down with crust formations in its central ulcerated zone. The surrounding nodular part of the lesion gradually spreads with extensive involvement and destruction of the neighbouring tissues but without any tendency to form metastases.

Basosquamous carcinoma. Clinically it is sometimes difficult to distinguish between the squamous-cell and basal-cell types of carcinoma, and it is not surprising, therefore, that an intermediate form exists which shows features of both types.

Intraepithelial carcinoma (*Bowen's disease*), a rare form of carcinoma of the lid, is discussed in relation to the conjunctiva in Chapter 3.

Treatment. In all cases of suspected carcinoma the histological examination of a biopsy specimen is essential and this routine procedure avoids the erroneous recognition of some of these lesions as chalazion, molluscum sebaceum, etc. The surgical excision of a lid carcinoma demands the removal of sufficient surrounding healthy tissue to ensure its complete removal. This is a difficult task when the lesion involves the whole thickness of the lid or the region of the lid margin and it is necessary to carry out elaborate plastic procedures to repair the defect in the lid after the removal of the tumour. In many of these cases irradiation provides a more satisfactory result.

Melanoma

The various forms of melanomata which involve the lid are discussed in relation to the conjunctiva in Chapter 3.

12 | Diseases of the Lacrimal Apparatus

Structure and Function

The lacrimal apparatus consists of the structures which are concerned in the production and drainage of the tears.

THE PRODUCTION OF TEARS

Tear production occurs in the *lacrimal gland* which lies in the upper and outer corner of the orbit in a recess immediately behind the orbital margin so that it is seldom possible to palpate the normal lacrimal gland. The main (or orbital) part of the gland (the *superior lobe*) is continuous behind with the smaller (or palpebral) part (the *inferior lobe*) which curves forwards to end in the region of the superior fornix. The tears which are secreted in both parts of the lacrimal gland pass into the eye by openings from the inferior lobe in the superior fornix; this secretion is regulated by the secreto-motor fibres of the greater superficial petrosal nerve which is derived from the facial nerve. There are also scattered nodules of lacrimal gland tissue (the *accessory lacrimal glands*) in various parts of the conjunctiva. It should be noted that tear formation is very scanty in the first few weeks of life and becomes reduced in advanced age.

THE DRAINAGE OF TEARS

This takes place along the lacrimal passages which are lined by a mucous membrane and which are in continuity with the nasal mucous membrane so that they are liable to catarrhal affections (Fig. 39).

The Lacrimal Puncta

There are two puncta (superior and inferior), one for each eyelid, which represent small circular openings on the lid margins near their medial ends. The upper punctum functions much less efficiently than the lower one for purely mechanical reasons.

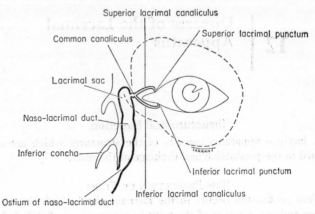

FIG. 39. *The structures which are concerned with the drainage of tears—the upper and lower puncta, the upper and lower canaliculi, the common canaliculus, the tear sac and the nasolacrimal duct*

The Lacrimal Canaliculi

Each punctum opens into a canaliculus which runs for a short distance vertically before passing horizontally in a medial direction to the region of the medial canthus where the two canaliculi (superior and inferior) join to form the *common canaliculus.*

The Lacrimal Sac

The common canaliculus opens into the lacrimal sac which lies in a recess (the *lacrimal fossa*) between the most medial part of the lower orbital margin (the *anterior lacrimal crest*) and the *posterior lacrimal crest*).

The Nasolacrimal Duct

The lower part of the lacrimal sac is continuous with the naso-lacrimal duct which passes downwards (and very slightly backwards and outwards) to open into the inferior meatus of the nose with a valvular mechanism at its opening. In the fetus the duct is initially a solid cord of cells which becomes canalized later; sometimes in the newborn there is a failure of this canalization or a failure of the valvular mechanism at the opening of the duct to become effective, but usually these defects are only temporary.

The drainage of tears is an active process involving the mechanism of the *lacrimal pump* which is dependent on the integrity of the orbicularis oculi muscle of the eyelids; closure of the lids draws the lacrimal fluid from the puncta and canaliculi into the sac by a suction effect, and opening of the lids forces the lacrimal fluid from the sac into the nasolacrimal duct and then into the nose through the lower end of the duct the valvular mechanism of which opens during this movement.

The main function of the tears is to maintain a normal degree of moisture of the eyes, and this is essential for the health of the surface tissues, particularly the cornea; the lacrimal fluid is one of the constituents of the precorneal fluid (chap. 4). The tears also contain an enzyme (lysozyme) which has an important antibacterial effect so that, in the absence of any active inflammation, a culture of the conjunctival sac is often negative. The presence of this enzyme determines the fact that repeated irrigations of the eye, which dilute its influence, are unwise procedures in any inflammatory condition except to remove a copious discharge from behind the eyelids.

The patency of the lacrimal passages is assessed by the following methods:

Syringing. This consists of irrigating the tear sac with saline after passing a cannula into the lower canaliculus through the lower punctum and the process is repeated with a cannula in the upper canaliculus through the upper punctum; the entry of the cannula is facilitated by dilating the punctum and the early part of the canaliculus with a dilator (Nettleship's). Free entry of the fluid into the nose (and into the throat when the patient is lying flat) implies a patency of all the passages. No entry of fluid into the nose and a regurgitation of fluid from the canaliculus which is not being syringed, as well as from the canaliculus which is being syringed, implies some obstruction beyond the point of formation of the common canaliculus, that is in the lacrimal sac or nasolacrimal duct. No entry of fluid into the nose and a regurgitation of fluid only from the canaliculus which is being syringed, usually implies some obstruction in the canaliculus before the formation of the common canaliculus.

Radiographic Examination. Irrigation of the lacrimal passages with a radiopaque substance, such as Lipiodal, provides a radiograph which gives an accurate picture of the site of the obstruction.

Fluorescein Test. The detection of fluorescein in the nasal secretions after instillation of the drug into the conjunctival sac is of diagnostic value provided the result is positive; a negative result is not conclusive evidence of an obstruction because the dye may fail to pass into the nose in sufficient quantities to be detected readily.

The volume of tear production is measured by Schirmer's test—one end of a strip of filter paper (4 mm in width) is inserted into the lateral part of the inferior fornix of each eye with the main part of the paper projecting over the lid margin and down the cheek. The extent of the passage of tears down the paper is measured over a short period (up to 5 minutes); in normal eyes the rate of formation is very variable—sometimes it is most profuse because of the mechanical stimulus of the filter paper—but when it is less than 15 mm over a period of 5 minutes the flow may be regarded as subnormal.

Excessive Watering of the Eyes

Excessive watering of the eyes may be the result of an overabundant production of tears (*lacrimation*) or of a failure of adequate drainage of the tears (*epiphora*).

EXCESSIVE LACRIMATION

This may be induced by any noxious stimulus of the eye such as inflammatory conditions (such as conjunctivitis, keratitis, uveitis), traumatic conditions (such as foreign bodies, chemical agents, ingrowing eyelashes), closed-angle glaucoma, which all exert their effects by a reflex action relayed by afferent stimuli through the trigeminal nerve and then by efferent stimuli through the greater superficial petrosal nerve. It is also induced by excessive exposure to bright light so that the afferent part of the reflex is the afferent visual pathway. Excessive lacrimation also follows various emotional stimuli.

Treatment. The main aim of treatment is to correct the underlying defect, and only rarely is it necessary to consider excision of part of the lacrimal gland in an attempt to reduce the formation of tears; indeed the indications for such an operation must be assessed with great care because a later spontaneous reduction in the residual tear formation may lead eventually to an undue dryness of the eye, a much more serious state than one of excessive moisture.

EPIPHORA

This occurs because of some failure of the adequate drainage of tears:

1. A failure of the punctum of the lower lid to lie in correct apposition to the eyeball caused by an ectropion or entropion of the lid; the treatment is the rectification of the eyelid defect (chap. 11).

2. A failure of patency of the punctum or canaliculus of the lower lid. This may be the result simply of a small foreign particle or of an eyelash so that the epiphora is relieved by removal of the obstruction. It may occur also by an accumulation of infective material—usually in the form of fungi (actinomyces) which proliferate to form a thick yellowish-white cheese-like material so that the epiphora is relieved by removing the infective material, if necessary after opening the punctum and the associated part of the canaliculus (the 'three-snip' operation), and by treating the affected epithelium with silver nitrate 1 per cent or weak iodine. It also follows injury of the medial part of the lower lid involving the punctum or canaliculus directly or sometimes indirectly as the result of a later reparative fibrosis; fibrosis of the punctum may respond to a 'three-snip' operation, but a fibrosis of the canaliculus requires more elaborate surgical treatment (p. 207). Sometimes, however, it is possible to prevent this fibrosis by a plastic repair shortly after the injury; for example, a severance of the lower canaliculus may be repaired by inserting a nylon thread into the cut ends of the canaliculus, if it is possible to identify them, before suturing the torn lid, with its subsequent removal once healing is complete and this necessitates leaving the free end of the thread beyond the punctum at the time of the operation. Damage to the punctum is usually easier to repair.

3. A failure of the lacrimal sac and nasolacrimal duct to drain the tears as a result of some form of obstruction.

Congenital Stenosis of the Nasolacrimal Duct

A failure of the nasolacrimal duct to become canalized or a failure of the valvular mechanism of the lower end of the duct to become effective results in an accumulation of the lacrimal and conjunctival secretions within the sac; this stenosis is liable to foster the occurrence of infection (dacryocystitis). Sometimes the infective element is the primary and not the secondary event so that a narrow but patent duct may become blocked by the occurrence of inflammatory changes in the mucous membrane of the duct. The regurgitation of the contents (mucous, mucopurulent, or purulent) of the lacrimal sac into the conjunctival sac is associated with a conjunctivitis. The condition is sometimes unilateral.

Treatment. The control of any infective element by local antibiotics (as for conjunctivitis, chap. 3) is the first essential, and this may relieve the obstruction in the duct by permitting its final canalization. This process may be aided by instructing the mother to press on the lacrimal sac (pressure on the skin of the most medial part of the lower lid immediately behind the anterior lacrimal crest) in the hope of expressing the contents of the sac down the nasolacrimal duct. If the obstruction persists it is necessary to relieve the obstruction, and this may be achieved by a simple syringing with saline through the punctum of the lower eyelid particularly if the cannula is inserted just beyond the common canaliculus to achieve a more forcible entry of the fluid into the duct; this manoeuvre also serves to verify that the lower canaliculus is not the site of the obstruction. If the syringing fails to relieve the obstruction a fine lacrimal probe should be passed down the length of the nasolacrimal duct, and this is approached by way of the upper punctum and upper canaliculus; this route is favoured because the probe may damage the epithelial lining of the canaliculus leading to the development of an obstruction, an unfortunate complication in the lower canaliculus but of much less importance in the upper one. It is seldom necessary to perform this probing before the age of 4 months, but it is unwise to delay it much beyond the age of 6 or 8 months otherwise the relief of the obstruction may only be temporary. The probing is carried out under a short general anaesthesia.

Dacryocystitis

This may occur in the infant, as described above, but it is usually a disease of adults, particularly after middle age and in the female. The infection of the tear sac may arise from the direct spread of infective material from the conjunctiva into the sac or from the retrograde spread of infective material from the nasopharynx, but it is usually the result of an infection following a stagnation of tears within the lacrimal sac as the result of an obstruction of the lower end of the lacrimal sac where it joins the nasolacrimal duct, or within the duct particularly in an area of narrowing in conjunction with some catarrhal swelling of the mucous lining of the duct. This causes an accumulation of pus or mucopus within the tear sac which regurgitates into the conjunctival sac through the canaliculi and puncta particularly after pressure over the lacrimal sac. A rapid control of the infection by local and systemic antibiotics may relieve the obstruction, although it may be necessary after the resolution of the acute stage to obtain proper patency by a syringing of the sac. Sometimes, however, the obstruction at the lower end of the sac persists with the development of a distended sac (a *mucocele*) which contains a mucous type of fluid often without any infective constituent. If, however, the lacrimal sac is extensively involved in the infection and particularly if the infection continues for a prolonged time, the so-called *chronic dacryocystitis*, the sac becomes shrunken because of fibrosis.

In other cases the chronic infection of the sac is followed by an *acute dacryocystitis*. This presents suddenly with a tense swelling which projects from the lacrimal fossa with redness and oedema of the overlying and surrounding skin. The condition may respond to intensive treatment with systemic antibiotics, but sometimes there is an abscess formation with a subsequent discharge of pus spontaneously or after incision; in either event the obstruction at the lower end of the sac is unrelieved and the sac remains infected. A chronic dacryocystitis is usually associated with a recurrent conjunctivitis and even sometimes with a septic type of keratitis; it may be of particular danger during the conduct of an intraocular operation because it predisposes to a purulent endophthalmitis, but this is a less likely complication in the antibiotic era.

Treatment. The obstruction of the nasolacrimal duct is very seldom relieved by a *probing,* except as discussed above in the early months of life, and any occasional success is usually only shortlived.

The removal of the tear sac (*dacryocystectomy*) may be advised after an acute dacryocystitis to prevent further infection, but this does not relieve the epiphora; the main indication for such an operation is in the elderly patient who is not fit for general anaesthesia, and sometimes the subsequent epiphora is not unduly troublesome because of the natural reduction of tear production in old age. The most effective treatment is to perform an anastomosis between the medial half of the lacrimal sac and the nasal mucosa which lines the middle meatus of the nose (dacryocystorhinostomy). A stenosis of the lower canaliculus is difficult to relieve surgically, but an effective method is to break down the obstruction by a probe during the conduct of a dacryocystorhinostomy and then to pass one end of a thin plastic tube from the opened tear sac into the lower canaliculus, out of the lower punctum, into the upper punctum, along the upper canaliculus to the sac where it is then passed with the other end of the tube through the opening in the nasal mucosa to the lower part of the nose just behind the nostril; if possible this tube is retained for several weeks or even months to ensure the patency of the previously obstructed canaliculus, with subsequent repeated syringings for a few weeks.

Carcinoma of the Lacrimal Sac

This may follow a chronic dacryocystitis, or a spread of a carcinoma from the neighbouring nasopharynx and it causes epiphora because it results in an obstruction of the sac or duct. The extent of the lesion may be determined by radiographic examinations and by surgical exposure (which will also provide material for a biopsy examination), but postoperative irradiation is almost certainly necessary because the diffuse nature of the lesion usually prevents its complete removal.

Diminished Watering of the Eyes

A diminished supply of tears is the result of two main conditions: a reduction in the formation of tears, or a decreased ability of the tears to reach the eye. A reduction in the formation of tears occurs in any destructive process of the lacrimal gland—tumour formations, inflammatory conditions, and atrophic conditions such as Sjögren's disease, although sometimes this reduction is preceded by a short period of increased tear formation, or in any defect of the afferent part of the lacrimation reflex because of an impairment of the trigeminal nerve. A decreased ability of the tears to reach the eye occurs in any severe chronic inflammation of the conjunctiva that causes an obstruction of the channels which are concerned in the passage of tears into the conjunctival sac from the lacrimal gland, for example, in trachoma, or sometimes as the result of trauma, for example, a lime burn.

Riley-Day Syndrome (Familial Dysautonomia)

This condition becomes evident in infancy, usually in the Jewish child, with difficulty in swallowing, recurrent respiratory infections and failure to thrive. There is a marked tendency to dehydration with excessive perspiration, but characteristically with an absence of tears which may lead to corneal ulceration.

Treatment. The eyes should be kept moist with artificial tears (methyl cellulose drops), but recently the hydrophilic acrylic soft contact lens has proved to be of value.

Dacryoadenitis

Acute Dacryoadenitis

This causes a painful swelling of the lacrimal gland which becomes easily palpable and is associated with considerable oedema of the overlying part of the upper lid. Abscess formation is rare. It is seldom the result of a local ocular infection. Sometimes it is a feature of mumps.

Chronic Dacryoadenitis

This causes a painless swelling of the lacrimal gland and usually has a granulomatous origin (for example, tuberculosis, sarcoidosis). Sometimes both lacrimal glands are involved together with the salivary glands and this symptom-complex is termed *Mikulicz's syndrome*. Ultimately the condition may regress spontaneously, but sometimes a granulomatous response may mask a malignant condition of the gland.

Tumours of the Lacrimal Gland

These are not common, but the *pleomorphic adenoma* and the *adenocarcinoma* constitute the majority of such tumours; the pleomorphic adenoma is akin to the mixed tumour which occurs in the salivary gland and may be regarded as epithelial in origin but adenomatous in nature. Lacrimal tumours tend to occur in early middle age. The tumour usually arises in the orbital part of the gland with the formation of a slowly growing hard mass in the upper outer part of the orbit. The eye becomes displaced in a forwards and downwards direction (*proptosis*) and shows a limitation of movement particularly on elevation with consequent diplopia. There is usually a reduction of tear formation, after an initial period of increased lacrimation. The growth may be removed by local excision after its exposure through a lateral orbitotomy; the histological finding of malignancy is an indication for postoperative irradiation, particularly if there is a local recurrence, and it is noteworthy that most adenomas have some degree of malignancy.

More rarely the lacrimal gland may be involved in one of the reticuloses (such as lymphoma, lymphosarcoma), sometimes as an isolated event but at other times in association with general manifestations of the disorder. The localized lesions usually respond to irradiation, but if the lesions become widespread some form of general anticancer therapy (cytotoxic drugs, chemotherapy) is necessary in an attempt to control the disease.

Cysts of the Lacrimal Gland

These are essentially retention cysts of the lacrimal gland fluid and they occur most often in the palpebral part of the gland so that they are visible in the superior fornix after eversion of the upper lid. Simple incision usually only gives a temporary effect, and excision of the whole cyst is necessary to avoid a recurrence.

below in front of the equator. It rotates the eye back and outwards, the eye, and raises the eye inwards (adduction).

13 | Disorders of the Extrinsic Ocular Muscles

Structure and Function

There are six extrinsic ocular muscles concerned with the rotatory movements of each eye (uniocular movements). These movements take place around a variable centre of rotation and are distinct from translatory movements which represent movements of the eye from side to side, up and down, and backwards or forwards in the absence of any rotation (chap. 14).

Lateral Rectus (Fig. 40)

This arises near the apex of the orbit and passes forwards on the lateral side of the eye to be inserted on the lateral surface of the sclera in front of the equator of the eyeball. It runs in the horizontal meridian of the eye and rotates the eye outwards (*abduction*).

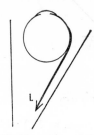

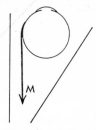

FIG. 40. *The action of the right lateral rectus muscle (L) in the primary position (abduction)*

FIG. 41 *The action of the right medial rectus (M) in the primary position (adduction)*

Medial Rectus (Fig. 41)

This arises near the apex of the orbit and passes forwards on the medial side of the eye to be inserted on the medial surface of the

211

sclera in front of the equator. It runs in the horizontal meridian of
the eye and rotates the eye inwards (*adduction*).

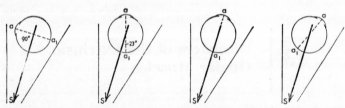

FIG. 42. *The actions of the superior rectus (S) in 67° of adduction (adduction and
intorsion), in the primary position (elevation, adduction and intorsion), in 23°
of abduction (elevation), and beyond 23° of abduction (elevation, abduction and
extorsion) (aa, = the vertical meridian of the eye)*

Superior Rectus (Fig. 42)

This arises near the apex of the orbit and passes forwards and
outwards above the eye to be inserted on the upper surface of the
sclera in front of the equator. It runs in the line of the orbital axis

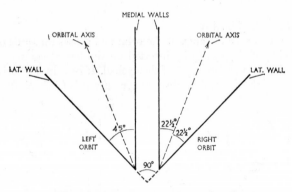

FIG. 43. *The direction of the orbital axis*

(Fig. 43) thus forming an angle (usually regarded as 23°) with the
vertical meridian of the eye in the primary position* so that in that
position it rotates the eye upwards (*elevation*), rotates the eye inwards (*adduction*) and twists the eye inwards (*intorsion*). When the

* The *primary position* is the position of the eye when it is directed straight
ahead (so that there is an absence of any horizontal and vertical deviation),
with an absence also of any torsional deviation and with the head held
vertically erect.

eye is in a position of 23° abduction the muscle causes only elevation because it runs then in the vertical meridian, and when the eye is in a position of 67° adduction it causes only adduction and intorsion because it runs then at 90° to the vertical meridian. When the eye is abducted beyond 23° it continues to cause *elevation*, but it also causes *abduction* and *extorsion* (twisting outwards).

Inferior Rectus (Fig. 44)

This arises near the apex of the orbit and passes forwards and outwards below the eye to be inserted on the lower surface of the sclera in front of the equator. It runs in the orbital axis and with

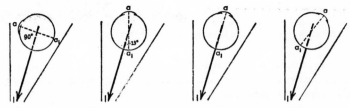

FIG. 44. *The actions of the inferior rectus (I) in 67° of adduction (adduction and extorsion), in the primary position (depression, adduction and extorsion), in 23° of abduction (depression), and beyond 23° of abduction (depression, abduction and intorsion). (aa, = the vertical meridian of the eye)*

the eye in the primary position it rotates the eye downwards (*depression*), rotates the eye inwards (*adduction*) and twists the eye outwards (*extorsion*). When the eye is in a position of 23° abduction it causes only depression because it runs then in the vertical meridian, and when the eye is in a position of 67° adduction the muscle causes only adduction and extorsion because it runs then at 90° to the vertical meridian. When the eye is abducted beyond 23° it continues to cause depression but it also causes abduction and intorsion.

Superior Oblique (Fig. 45)

This arises near the apex of the orbit and passes forwards on the upper and medial surface of the eye to the anterior part of the roof of the orbit where it hooks round a pulley (the *trochlea*) before passing backwards and outwards above the eye at an angle of 54° with the vertical meridian in the primary position to be inserted on the upper and outer surface of the sclera behind the equator. This

partial reversal of its line of pull causes it to rotate the eye downwards (*depression*) despite its situation above the eye, and it also
rotates the eye outwards (*abduction*) and twists the eye inwards
(*intorsion*). When the eye is in a position of 54° adduction it causes

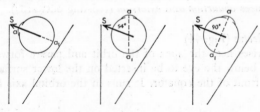

Fig. 45. *The actions of the superior oblique (S) in 54° of adduction (depression),
in the primary position (depression, abduction and intorsion), and in 36° of
abduction (abduction and intorsion) (aa, = the vertical meridian of the eye)*

only depression because it runs then in the vertical meridian, and
when the eye is in a position of 36° abduction the muscle causes only
abduction and intorsion.

Inferior Oblique (Fig. 46)

This arises from the anteromedial part of the floor of the orbit
and passes backwards and outwards below the eye at an angle of
51° with the vertical meridian in the primary position to be inserted

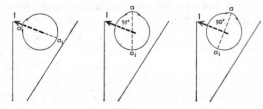

Fig. 46. *The actions of the inferior oblique (I) in 51° of adduction (elevation), in
the primary position (elevation, abduction and extorsion), and in 39° of abduction
(abduction and extorsion). aa, = the vertical meridian of the eye)*

on the lower and outer surface of the sclera behind the equator. This
pull of the muscle from in front causes it to rotate the eye upwards
(*elevation*) despite its situation below the eye and it also rotates the
eye outwards (*abduction*) and twists the eye outwards (*extorsion*).
When the eye is in a position of 51° adduction it causes only elevation

because it runs then in the vertical meridian, and when the eye is in a position of 39° abduction it causes only abduction and extorsion.

BINOCULAR MOVEMENTS

These movements of the two eyes together may be of a *conjugate* or *disjunctive* nature.

Conjugate Movements

These are coordinated movements of the two eyes in the same direction (*version movements*) which occur in the following 6 main directions (the *cardinal positions* of the eyes) with one muscle in each eye concerned primarily in the movement:

1. *Dextroelevation* (up and to the right)
Right superior rectus
Left inferior oblique
2. *Dextroversion* (to the right)
Right lateral rectus
Left medial rectus
3. *Dextrodepression* (down and to the right)
Right inferior rectus
Left superior oblique
4. *Laevoelevation* (up and to the left)
Right inferior oblique
Left superior rectus
5. *Laevoversion* (to the left)
Right medial rectus
Left lateral rectus
6. *Laevodepression* (down and to the left)
Right superior oblique
Left inferior rectus

This illustrates that in any movement of the eyes, paired muscles which are synergists (*agonists*) contract together, and it should be noted also that paired muscles which are *antagonists* simultaneously relax (in an active way) by the phenomenon of reciprocal innervation; for example, in a movement of dextroelevation the right inferior rectus and left superior oblique act as antagonists with the right superior rectus and left inferior oblique acting as agonists.

The range over which conjugate movement is possible is termed the *binocular field of fixation*, and it forms a circle of about 45° to

50° from the primary position except below when it is restricted on both sides to about 35° by the nose (Fig. 47), but its full extent is seldom used because head movements are usually brought into play when there is more than about 20° rotation.

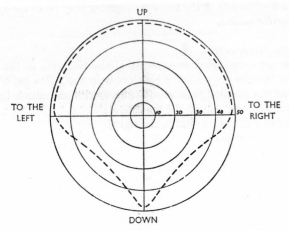

FIG. 47. *The binocular field of fixation*

Disjunctive Movements

These are coordinated movements of the two eyes in opposite directions (*vergence movements*) which occur in two directions; *convergence* (or *positive convergence*) when each eye is turned inwards, and *divergence* (or *negative convergence*) when each eye is turned outwards from a convergent position.

THE NERVOUS CONTROL OF OCULAR MOVEMENT

The extrinsic ocular muscles are influenced by three main systems; the afferent system, the efferent system and the extrapyramidel motor system.

The Afferent System

The afferent system has several components:

Visual stimuli travel in the afferent visual pathway so that the visual awareness of an object may induce a particular form of ocular movement; part of the psychooptical reflex.

Proprioceptive stimuli arise in the labyrinth (the semicircular canals provide information about movements of acceleration or deceleration of the head, and the utricle and saccule provide information about the position of the head in space), in the neck muscles and in the extrinsic ocular muscles; the *postural reflexes*.

Auditory stimuli arise in the inner ear.

The Efferent System

The *efferent* part of the motor system has several components:

Cortical centres,* the *frontal centres*, are concerned with the production of binocular movements as a result of a voluntary desire or in response to a command, and the occipital centres are concerned with the production of binocular movements in response to a visual stimulus so that they are part of the psychooptical reflex pathways. The right cerebral hemisphere is concerned with movements to the left, and the left hemisphere with movements to the right.

Intermediary centres, or supranuclear centres, are described in the tectal part of the midbrain in the region of the superior colliculi for vertical movement, in the pretectal region for convergence, and near the VIth cranial nerve nuclei for lateral movement, but the evidence for these is essentially clinical which is at variance with experiemntal evidence based on precise stereotaxic methods and sensitive recording devices; these show several reactive areas in the brainstem near the midline or within the median plane for vertical movements, and also several reactive areas in the brainstem (the tegmentum of the midbrain and pons, the central grey matter, the vestibular nuclei, the paramedian zone and the reticular activating system) which represent a vast mass of interrelated neurons in the tegmental part of the central core of the brainstem for lateral movements. It is evident, therefore, that the true location of the intermediary centres is at present ill-understood.

Cranial nuclei III, IV and *VI* and their cranial nerves are also included. The IIIrd cranial nucleus which lies on each side of the midbrain controls four extrinsic ocular muscles—*medial rectus, superior rectus, inferior rectus* and *inferior oblique*. The IVth cranial nucleus which lies on each side of the midbrain controls one extrinsic ocular muscle—the *superior oblique*. The VIth cranial nucleus which lies on each side of the pons controls one extrinsic ocular muscle— the *lateral rectus*. The *medial (posterior) longitudinal bundle*

* The term *centre* may be incorrect because recent experimental evidence indicates that wide areas of the cerebral cortex may exert such motor effects.

(fasciculus) which runs through the brainstem forms a nervous link between these three paired cranial nuclei.

The Extrapyramidal Motor System

The motor system of the eye is controlled also by the *extrapyramidal motor system*, which is a complex nervous mechanism (comprising *cortical centres, basal ganglia, nuclear masses in the midbrain* and the *reticular formation*, and the *cerebellum*). These are concerned in the maintenance of proper degrees of muscle tone and rhythm which are essential for the conduct of precise ocular movement, and the reticular formation appears to function as a master control mechanism because of its ability to modify and integrate the vast assortment of conflicting sensory impulses.

The movements of the eyes are influenced also by the *fascial tissues* of the orbit (chap. 14).

THE DEVELOPMENT OF BINOCULAR VISION

Binocular vision is achieved by the use of both eyes together so that the separate images arising in each eye are appreciated as a single image by a process of fusion. This achievement is an acquired ability, not simply an inborn one, and is built up gradually during the early months and years of life provided there is a proper coordination of various abilities:

1. The ability of each retina to function properly from a visual point of view, particularly the central part of the retina (the fovea), and this necessitates a reasonably intact retina and an absence of any significant defects in the transparent structures of the eye (the cornea, the anterior and posterior chambers, the lens and the vitreous).

2. The ability of the visual areas of the brain to promote fusion (bifoveal fixation) of the two separate images which are transmitted to them from each eye so that a single mental impression is achieved of the object. This is made possible by the forwards direction of the eyes in man so that the visual field of one eye almost completely overlaps the visual field of the other eye (*the binocular field of vision*) (see Fig. 56, chap. 16), and within the parts of the retina of one eye which are concerned with this binocular field are countless visual elements which correspond with similar visual elements in identical parts of the retina of the other eye. In this way any small object in the binocular field of vision may be regarded as producing a stimulation of corresponding retinal points, although this has a

physiological rather than an anatomical significance. The association of the visual fibres from corresponding retinal points is achieved in the brain by the rearrangement of these fibres from each eye at the optic chiasma (chap. 16).

3. The ability of each eye to lie correctly in its bony orbit so that the *visual axis* (the line which passes from the object of fixation to the fovea) of each eye is directed to the same object at rest and during movement (*central fixation*). The control of the position of the eye demands carefully integrated controlling mechanisms which may be considered in three groups—mechanisms which give information to the brain (*the fixation reflexes*), mechanisms which produce the movement (*the motor responses*) and mechanisms which steady the movement (*the steadying influences*).

The Fixation Reflexes. These are concerned with informing the brain about the positions of the eyes and they may be of two types, visual or postural. *Visual information* is the result of the possession of each retinal receptor of a projection in a particular direction in space so that stimulation of a receptor by an object gives information on the position of that object, quite apart from the detail of the object which is seen visually. The central point of the retina (the fovea) has a straight-ahead type of projection (the principal visual direction of the fovea) so that it is concerned with direct fixation of an object, whereas the other retinal receptors are concerned with objects in the paracentral and peripheral parts of the field of vision. This is the psychooptical reflex which is composed of the *fixation reflex* (the fixation of an object by one or both eyes), the *refixation reflex* (the change in fixation from one object to another object or the maintenance of fixation on a moving object by one or both eyes), the *conjugate fixation reflex* (the fixation of an object which involves a conjugate movement of both eyes), the *disjunctive fixation reflex* (the fixation of an object which involves a disjunctive movement of both eyes), and the *corrective fusion reflex* (the maintenance of fusion in the primary position and during conjugate and disjunctive movements by the strength of the fusional influences (*fusional vergence reflex*) despite a tendency to develop a squint (heterophoria).

Postural information is of a more primitive kind and is the result of the existence within the muscles of the eye, head and neck of specialized structures (muscle spindles and tendon organs) which record the amount of contraction and relaxation of each muscle so that the position of the eyes in relation to one another and in relation to the position of the head is known. It is the result also of impulses

from the labyrinthine mechanisms (see above). These postural
reflexes are responsible for the fact that the eyes continue to move
together even when one eye is totally blind although there is usually
an associated deviation of the blind eye.

The Motor Responses. The influence of the complex efferent motor
systems is discussed above p. 217.

The Steadying Influences. The influence of the extrapyramidal
motor system is also discussed above p. 218.

4. The ability of the mechanism which turns the eyes inwards to
a near object (convergence) or outwards from a convergent position
to a distant object (divergence or negative convergence) and the
focusing mechanism of the eye (accommodation) to achieve an
adequate degree of harmony. The mechanism of accommodation
has been discussed (chaps. 2 and 6). The mechanism of convergence
is essentially of a reflex nature with three components in addition
to reflex accommodative convergence; tonic reflex convergence
which implies the existence of some inherent tonus of the medial
recti, proximal reflex convergence which is induced simply by the
presence of a near object, and fusional reflex convergence which is
exerted to maintain fusion of an object of fixation.

There is a close relationship between the mechanisms of accommodation and reflex convergence whereby a unit of accommodation
(A), one dioptre—1 (D), is accompanied inevitably by the stimulus
to induce an appropriate degree of accommodative-convergence
(AC) (in prism dioptres—Δ); this is the accommodation convergence and convergence relationship (the AC/A ratio). During the
binocular fixation of an object one metre (1 M) from the eyes so that
each eye exercises 1D of accommodation there is a total convergence
of the two eyes of 6Δ in the presence of an average interpupillary
distance of 60 mm. Thus in emmetropia and orthophoria the
theoretical AC/A ratio is (6Δ/1D), but in practice the normal ratio
is about 4, and a lower than normal ratio is necessary in uncorrected
hypermetropia (because accommodation must exceed convergence)
and a higher ratio in uncorrected myopia (because convergence must
exceed accommodation) if binocular vision is to be maintained at
different distances of fixation by the influences of the fusional
vergence reflex. The AC/A ratio may be measured in different
ways; the *heterophoria method* which compares the differences in the
latent deviation of the eyes (the phoria) at distant and at near
fixation; the *gradient method* which compares the change in the
phoria at a fixed point of fixation during the application of convex

spherical lenses (which reduce accommodation) and concave spherical lenses (which increase accommodation); the *graphic method* which measures the convergence response of the eyes to different concave spherical lenses on the synoptophore and compares these with the normal responses graphically; and the complicated *fixation disparity method* which is concerned with the disparity (retinal slip) which may occur within Panum's areas in a phoria in certain circumstances.

Orthophoria

The development of binocular vision permits the visual axes of the two eyes to be directed to a particular object in the primary (straight-ahead) position, during all forms of conjugate and disjunctive movement, and at all distances of fixation (near and far); this ideal state is termed *orthophoria* and it should be maintained rigidly even when the eyes are dissociated from one another by occlusion of one eye which prevents the normal controlling influences of the fusion mechanism, but this is often an unrealized ideal even in normal persons.

THE DEVELOPMENT OF SQUINT (STRABISMUS)

Squint is the condition in which there is a failure of the visual axis (the line which passes from the fovea to the fixation object) of one eye (the squinting eye) to be directed at the same time to the object which is being observed by the other eye (the fixing or non-squinting eye), although this failure may occur only under certain circumstances. In general a squint is the result of a failure in the development of normal binocular vision, and the 'obstacle' which induces this failure may arise in any of the complex mechanisms which have been discussed above.

1. The obstacle may arise because one eye has a defective form of central vision as the result of some structural anomaly of the cornea, lens, retina, etc.

2. The obstacle may arise because of a difficulty in promoting fusion. Fusion is obviously defective if the vision of one eye is poor, but fusion is prevented, even when the corrected vision of each eye is good, if there is a significant difference (usually more than 5 per cent) between the sizes of the retinal images transmitted to the brain (a condition termed *aniseikonia*, chap. 2), usually the result of a marked difference in the refractions of the two eyes (anisometropia),

but sometimes because of a difference in the retinal mosaic in the central parts of the two eyes. A weakness of the fusion mechanism may be the result of some severe general illness or of certain psychological states affecting the stability of the cerebral mechanisms. In general, however, a weakness of the fusion mechanism is most often the result of the squint so that the failure of the eyes to be directed at the same time to the same object inhibits the promotion of the fusion mechanism.

3. The obstacle may arise in some defect which prevents the eyes from maintaining the correct positions relative to one another at rest or during movement; these defects may be of a structural nature (for example, a defect in the shape of the orbit), of a neurogenic nature (this accounts for the paretic or paralytic type of squint), or of a myogenic nature (this accounts for many of the squints of congenital origin, but also of acquired origin as in exophthalmic ophthalmoplegia), as discussed later in this chapter.

4. The obstacle may arise in some defect which prevents the establishment of a harmony between the accommodation and convergence reflexes so that there is an abnormal AC/A ratio. The frequent occurrence of fairly high degrees of hypermetropia in a young child leads to an excessive use of accommodation with a tendency to overconvergence thus favouring the development of a *convergent* squint, the so-called *accommodative squint*, but a convergent squint may occur also in the absence of excessive hypermetropia when there is a high AC/A ratio (the convergence excess esotropia). Conversely, in myopia there is a diminished use of accommodation which may lead to a decreased convergence of the eyes thus favouring the development of *divergent squint*.

It is apparent that many factors affect adversely any part of the complex mechanisms responsible for the development of binocular vision with the production of a squint, but it must be appreciated that these adverse effects vary greatly; in the very young child with poorly developed binocular vision, a relatively trivial defect may cause a squint particularly when the child is unwell, but in the older child with good binocular vision such a squint may be avoided.

Adaptations to the Development of Squint

It might be assumed that the development of a squint is the final event in a chain of events which leads to a failure in the proper establishment of binocular vision, but in fact the squint only represents the beginning of a new series of events which take place because of the occurrence of double vision. Double vision is the direct result of the squint which causes the visual axes of the two eyes to be directed to two different objects thereby causing a superimposition of two different images (this form of double vision is called *confusion* and is the result of a stimulation of corresponding retinal points by two different objects, Fig. 48), and which also

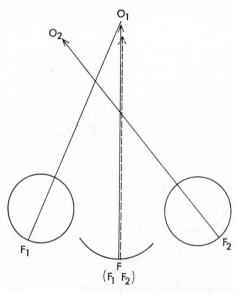

FIG. 48. *The occurrence of* confusion *in a right convergent squint; the stimulation of corresponding retinal points in each eye (F_1 and F_2) by two different objects (O_1 and O_2) causes a superimposition of the two images which are projected straight ahead from the fovea of the binoculus (F)—the binoculus is a perceptual concept which represents the single eye (the median eye) which is common to the two eyes*

causes the stimulation by one object of retinal areas in the two eyes which do not correspond with one another thereby causing a separation of the two images (the true image and the false image) of the object (this form of double vision is called *diplopia*, Fig. 49). The nature of confusion and diplopia is illustrated with relation to the *binoculus*; this is a perceptual concept which represents the single eye (the median eye) which is common to the two eyes. Certainly in the normal binocular act there is no mental impression of a synthesis of two separate images and it seems that the binocular image is projected from somewhere behind the eyes.

The changes which follow the development of double vision represent attempts by the brain to overcome its troublesome effects and may be called adaptations which are produced subconsciously

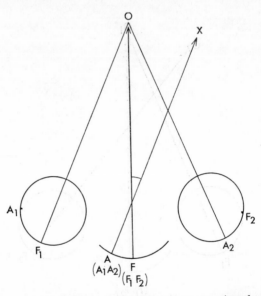

FIG. 49. *The occurrence of* diplopia *in a right convergent squint; the stimulation of noncorresponding retinal points in each eye (F_1 and A_2) by one object (O) causes a separation of the two images, one of which (the left one) is projected straight ahead from the fovea of the binoculus (F) and the other (the right one) is projected to the right of the straight-ahead position from a peripheral point of the binoculus (A). It should be noted that the angle between the projection from F on the binoculus (which represents F_1 in the left eye) and the projection from A on the binoculus (which represents A_2 in the right eye) is equal to the angle of the squint.*

particularly in the young child. The following adaptations may occur:

Suppression. The vision of the squinting eye may be ignored by a process of active neglect of the eye by the visual cortex (suppression), but this is a temporary phenomenon which occurs only when both eyes are given the opportunity of acting visually; it is a feature of the early stages of a uniocular squint and persists in an alternating or intermittent squint, but on transferring fixation from one eye to the other spontaneously or by covering the fixing eye there is an immediate cessation of the suppression. Suppression is a feature also of normal binocular vision whereby the diplopia of objects nearer to or farther from the object of fixation (*physiological diplopia*) is ignored (Fig. 50).

Amblyopia. The vision of the squinting eye may be ignored by a process of active neglect of the eye by the visual cortex, but unlike suppression this cortical inhibition is a progressive and permanent phenomenon (in the absence of treatment) so that it persists during an enforced fixation of the squinting eye (*strabismic amblyopia*). It follows that in an amblyopic eye there is a loss of central vision which cannot be explained wholly on the basis of a structural defect of the eye or of the afferent visual pathways. In this context it is appropriate to consider other related forms of amblyopia:

1. *Stimulus deprivation ambylopia (amblyopia ex anopsia)* occurs when an eye is deprived of visual stimuli at an early stage of life (as in congenital cataract (chap. 9) or in complete ptosis), and the amblyopia is intense and accompanied by a loss of fixation. Experimental work on kittens and monkeys indicates that this form of amblyopia is related to a lack of integration of the complex visual pathways in the cortex which seems dependent on adequate stimuli in early life.

2. *Anisometropic amblyopia* is the result of an inhibition of the vision of one eye because of a significant difference in the refractive errors of the two eyes so that one eye is favoured at the expense of the other.

3. *Ametropic amblyopia* occurs in the presence of an uncorrected refractive error of sufficient magnitude so that a correction of the refractive error at some later stage only produces a partial improvement in the vision. It may occur in both eyes.

4. *Nystagmic amblyopia*, a defective form of vision, occurs in nystagmus which is frequently unrelated to any structural defect of the eye (p. 259).

Eccentric Retinal Fixation. The fixation of the squinting eye may become abnormal by the development of an eccentric type of retinal fixation. In many cases of squint the retinal elements may retain their normal projections despite a marked amblyopia of the squinting eye, but sometimes, particularly when the squint occurs at an early age and when there is a prolonged interval between the development of the squint and the start of effective treatment, this ability is lost and some other retinal area assumes the principal visual

226

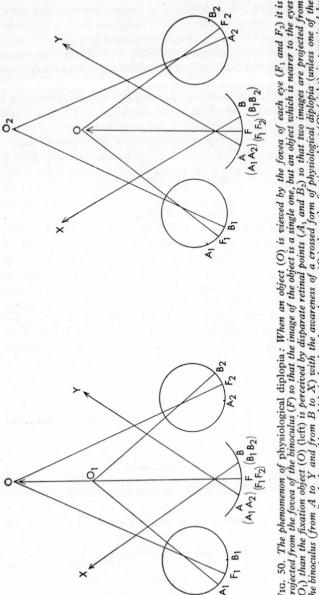

FIG. 50. *The phenomenon of physiological diplopia: When an object (O) is viewed by the fovea of each eye (F_1 and F_2) it is projected from the fovea of the binoculus (F) so that the image of the object is a single one, but an object which is nearer to the eyes (O_1) than the fixation object (O) (left) is perceived by disparate retinal points (A_1 and B_2) so that two images are projected from the binoculus (from A to Y and from B to X) with the awareness of a crossed form of physiological diplopia (unless one of the images is suppressed). And, an object which is farther from the eyes (O_2) than the fixation object (O) (right) is perceived by disparate retinal points (B_1 and A_2) so that two images are projected from the binoculus (from B to X and from A to Y) with the awareness of an uncrossed form of physiological diplopia (unless one of the images is suppressed).*

direction so that it becomes a point of eccentric retinal fixation. The nature of the eccentric fixation may be designated according to the position in the retina of the eccentric point; parafoveal (within 3° of the fovea), paramacular (within 4° to 5° of the fovea), and peripheral (beyond 5° of the fovea), and in each case the eccentric fixation may be steady or unsteady. There is also a *wandering fixation* in which there is no fixed point of retinal fixation (central or eccentric).

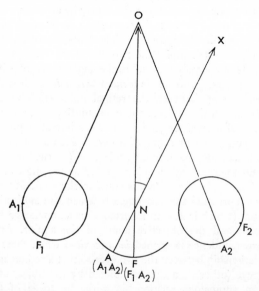

Fig. 51. *The phenomenon of harmonious anomalous retinal correspondence in a right convergent squint; the stimulation of noncorresponding retinal points (F_1 and A_2) by the fixation object (O) would create two projections from the binoculus (from F to O and from A to X) in the presence of normal retinal correspondence, but in a harmonious anomalous retinal correspondence A_2 in the right eye assumes an anomalous relationship with F_1 so that both projections are from F on the binoculus in a straight-ahead direction to O. The angle between the normal and abnormal projections of $A_2(ONX)$ represents the angle of anomaly; it is identical with the angle of the squint (ONX), and the angle of anomaly may be regarded also as the difference between the subjective angle of the squint (which is zero) and the objective angle of the squint (ONX).*

Anomalous Retinal Correspondence (Abnormal Retinal Correspondence). The eyes may develop an anomalous association with one another in order to obtain a form of binocular vision (albeit of an anomalous type) despite the presence of a squint; this implies that the retinal area of the squinting eye which is stimulated by the object of fixation assumes an anomalous relationship with the fovea of the nonsquinting eye so that it is projected anomalously from the fovea of the binoculus. It should be noted that the retinal area of the squinting eye which assumes the anomalous relationship with the fovea of the nonsquinting eye is not necessarily a point of eccentric fixation because in anomalous correspondence (a sensory anomaly of a binocular nature) there may be no eccentric fixation (a sensory anomaly of a uniocular nature) or there may be an eccentric fixation which is not compatible with the anomalous correspondence during the use of the squinting eye alone. Sometimes, however, in a small angle esotropia (microtropia) the two conditions are compatible so that the angle of anomaly is equal to the angle of eccentricity.

Anomalous correspondence is termed *harmonious* when there is a precise relationship between the retinal point stimulated by the fixation object and the fovea of the nonsquinting eye, and the angle between the abnormal projection of the stimulated point of the squinting eye (in the presence of a harmonious anomalous retinal correspondence) and its normal projection (in the presence of a normal retinal correspondence) is regarded as the angle of anomaly (Fig. 51). The angle of anomaly is equal to the angle of the squint, and it also represents the difference between the subjective angle of the squint (which is zero in a harmonious anomalous retinal correspondence) and the objective angle of the squint. Anomalous retinal correspondence is termed *inharmonious* when there is a less precise relationship between the two eyes so that a retinal area of the squinting eye (other than that stimulated by the object of fixation assumes an anomalous relationship with the fovea of the non-squinting eye; in this way the angle of anomaly is less than the angle of squint, and the subjective angle of the squint is no longer zero although it is less than the objective angle (Fig. 52); the subjective and objective angles of a squint are equal only in a normal retinal correspondence. It is most unlikely that the inharmonious type of anomalous retinal correspondence exists in everyday seeing, and it is found more or less only in certain diagnostic tests which introduce an element of dissociation of the eyes (such as, the method using the major amblyoscope).

Compensatory Head Posture (*Abnormal Head Posture*). This may be adopted in certain forms of incomitant squint, usually when it involves one of the vertically acting muscles, in order to avoid diplopia particularly in the primary position and on looking down.

There are two main components in this abnormal posture: *face turning* (up, down, right or left) in order to turn the eye as far away as possible from the field of action of the affected muscle—this involves turning the face into the direction of this field of action

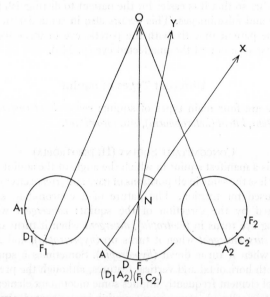

FIG. 52. *The phenomenon of inharmonious anomalous retinal correspondence in a right convergent squint; the stimulation of noncorresponding retinal points* (F_1 *and* A_2) *would create two projections from the binoculus (from F to O and from A to X) in the presence of normal retinal correspondence, but in an inharmonious anomalous retinal correspondence* C_2 *in the right eye assumes an anomalous relationship with* F_1 *so that the projection from* A_2 *is from D on the binoculus to Y in contrast with the projection from* F_1 *which is from F on the binoculus in a straight-ahead direction to O. The angle between the normal and abnormal projections of* A_2 (YNX) *represents the angle of anomaly; it is less than the angle of squint* (ONX), *and the angle of anomaly may be regarded also as the difference between the subjective angle of the squint* (ONY) *and the objective angle of the squint* (ONX)

because the eye then turns automatically into the opposite direction, and *head tilting* (right or left) to diminish the vertical separation of the true and false images and to compensate for any abnormalities of torsion which are usually the result of a weakness or overaction of one of the oblique muscles. Sometimes, a compensatory head posture is adopted in a concomitant squint if there is an associated A or V phenomenon (p. 241).

Increase in the Angle of Squint. Sometimes the development of a
small degree of squint may be followed by a much greater degree
of squint (the *purposive* squint) because diplopia is less troublesome
when the two images of the one object are widely separated from
one another so that it is easier for the patient to distinguish between
the true and false images. This occurs also in some paretic squints
when the patient may fix with the paretic eye to make use of the
secondary deviation of the unaffected eye (p. 244).

Different Types of Squint

There are four main types of squint: *concomitant* (*heterotropia*),
intermittent, latent (*heterophoria*), and *incomitant*.

Concomitant Squint (Heterotropia)

This is a manifest squint in which the angle of the squint remains
more or less the same in all positions of gaze and irrespective of which
eye is used for fixation. The nature of a concomitant squint is
designated by the direction of the squint: *convergent* when the
squinting eye turns in (*esotropia*), *divergent* when it turns out (*exotropia*), *sursumvergent* when it turns up (*hypertropia*), and *deorsum-
vergent* when it turns down (*hypotropia*). Sometimes a squint may
show both horizontal and vertical features, although the presence of
a vertical element frequently implies some incomitant element in the
squint originally. A concomitant squint is designated also by the
terms *right* or *left* according to the eye which is the *squinting* one
(as distinct from the *fixing* one) or by the term *alternating* when
either eye may squint in turn or indiscriminately. The development
of a concomitant squint is essentially the result of some obstacle in
the development of normal binocular function as discussed above.
The only presenting symptom is an awareness of confusion and
diplopia, but these are seldom appreciated except by the older and
more introspective child and are rapidly eliminated by the mechanism of suppression. The complications of concomitant squint—
amblyopia, eccentric retinal fixation and anomalous retinal correspondence—are discussed above.

False Squint (*Pseudostrabismus*). Quite frequently there is a false
appearance of a convergent squint in early childhood because of
the presence of well-marked folds on either side of the nose (*epicanthic folds*) which, in conjunction with the characteristically flat base

of the nose in early childhood, combine to give an impression of a convergent squint; much more rarely a narrowing of the lateral canthi causes a false appearance of a divergent squint. The cover test (see below) is of great value in determining the absence of any squint, and this is confirmed by a positive response to the prism vergence test; when a prism (usually 12 Δ) is placed base out in front of one eye there is a movement of convergence to eliminate the diplopia which is induced by the prism in the presence of binocular vision.

The Management of Concomitant Squint

The methods of investigation and treatment should proceed as soon as possible after the onset because the aim is to restore binocular function whenever possible. Obviously in very young children some methods are inapplicable, but this is no valid reason for deferring certain forms of examination in all cases.

History of the Squint. This is important because an accurate determination of the age of the child at the time of onset of the squint, of the length of time during which the squint has remained only occasional before becoming constant, and of any previous form of treatment is of great value in assessing the chances of obtaining a binocular result after treatment.

Diagnosis of the Type of Squint. This is achieved by the following methods of examination:

1. *An observation of the corneal reflexes.* The presence of a squint may be established by careful judgement of the positions of the reflexes which are visible on the cornea of each eye when a light shines on the eyes. In the absence of a squint these reflexes lie on symmetrical parts of the cornea of each eye, but in a convergent squint the reflex on the cornea of the squinting eye is displaced towards its outer side and in a divergent squint the reflex is displaced to its inner side. A vertical type of squint is associated similarly with an alteration in these reflexes.

2. *The cover test.* This test is composed of two parts: the *cover and uncover test* and the *alternate cover test*. The *cover and uncover test* consists of covering each eye in turn with the hand or some form of occluder during the fixation of the other eye on a target; in the absence of any squint there is no movement of either eye during this test, but if a convergent squint is present on removing the cover from one eye and transferring it to the other eye the uncovered eye moves outwards to take up its correct central position because

it turned inwards during the time it was covered, or conversely, if a divergent squint is present on transferring the cover the previously covered eye will move inwards from an outwards position to become straight. A vertical type of squint is determined also by this method.

The alternate cover test consists of rapidly and repeatedly transferring the hand from one eye to the other so that there is a dissociation of the eyes, and this reveals a latent squint which is controlled only by the corrective fusion reflex (p. 219); the rapidity of recovery on removing the dissociating influence is a measure of the strength of this reflex. The extent of the deviation (manifest or latent) may be measured by the *prism and cover test* when prisms of increasing strength are placed before one eye (with the base of the prism in a direction which is opposite to the direction of the squint, that is, base out in a convergent squint, etc.) until there is an absence of any deviation.

The cover test is of supreme value in early childhood when reliance must be placed solely on an objective assessment, but it is of equal value in a rapid evaluation of any form of squint, at any age, particularly as it is a reliable test which requires no form of instrumentation.

3. *Ocular movements.* This should be carried out in all directions of gaze for each eye separately and for both eyes together. In a concomitant squint the range of movement of each eye is usually normal. Sometimes, however, there is a weakness of movement of the squinting eye in a direction away from the squint; for example, in a right convergent squint there may be an apparent weakness of the right lateral rectus muscle because of habitual disuse of the eye in a position of full abduction, and the absence of any true paresis is demonstrated by the recovery of movement which follows a short period of occlusion of the left fixing eye unless contractural changes have developed in the right medial rectus muscle (the ipsilateral antagonist). A weakness of movement of the squinting eye also occurs in a squint which becomes concomitant after starting originally as an incomitant one (p. 243).

4. *The nature of the potential binocular function.* This is assessed most readily by the synoptophore (major amblyoscope) which involves the principles of the stereoscope. In this instrument there is an eyepiece for each eye and the position of the eyepieces may be adjusted to compensate for the angle of the squint; this adjustment is correct when the examiner observes that the corneal reflections

on the eyes are in central and symmetrical positions and it provides an *objective* measurement of angle of the squint. Pictures on slides are then presented to each eye and the patient adjusts the eyepieces to obtain a superimposition of these pictures; this provides a *subjective* measurement of the angle of the squint. Various types of pictures are used to provide information on the grades of binocular vision:

Grade I—simultaneous macular perception is the simplest form of binocular vision and implies the ability of each eye to superimpose two dissimilar objects—the classical example is to put the bird (seen with one eye) into the cage (seen with the other eye) (Fig. 53). A

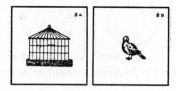

FIG. 53. *The slides for testing simultaneous macular perception on the synoptophore*

failure to see one of the objects indicates suppression or amblyopia. The concept of simultaneous macular perception is essentially an instrumental one and its presence implies some form of fusion.

Grade II—fusion is a more elaborate form of binocular vision and implies the ability of the eyes to produce a composite picture from two similar objects each of which is incomplete in one detail—

FIG. 54. *The slides for testing fusion on the synoptophore*

the classical example is the rabbit with a tail but without a bunch of flowers and the rabbit without a tail but with a bunch of flowers (Fig. 54). The range of fusion is then tested by moving the arms of the synoptophore so that the eyes have to converge and diverge to maintain fusion; under normal conditions this should be possible over at least 25° of convergence and 3° of divergence, and it is obvious that simple fusion without any range of fusion is of little or no practical value.

Grade III—stereopsis is the highest form of binocular vision and implies the ability to obtain an impression of depth by the super-imposition of two pictures of the same objects which have been recorded from very slightly different angles so that there is a small degree of dissimilarity—the classical example is the bucket which is appreciated in its true dimensions (Fig. 55).

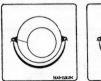

FIG. 55. *The slides for testing stereopsis on the synoptophore*

The synoptophore also provides accurate information on the state of retinal correspondence; when there is a normal retinal correspondence the subjective and objective angles are equal, but when there is an abnormal retinal correspondence the subjective angle is less than the objective angle and this difference is termed the *angle of anomaly*.

A Determination of the Health of Each Eye. It is important to establish the fact that each eye is free from any disease which would affect its visual function, for example, a scar of the cornea, a cataract or some retinal disorder like a retinoblastoma. This is a further reason why all infants with a suspected squint must have an early examination.

Determination of the Refraction of Each Eye. It is an essential part of the treatment of squint to carry out an accurate refraction in order to prescribe glasses if these will be in any way helpful in ensuring that the vision of each eye is brought up to as normal a level as possible and in ensuring that a satisfactory relation is achieved between the mechanisms of accommodation and convergence. This necessitates the estimation of the refraction by retinoscopy (chap. 2) after the use of a cycloplegic drug, and when possible, the recording of the uncorrected and corrected vision of each eye for distance and for near vision.

Treatment of Defective Vision of the Squinting Eye by Occlusion. If the vision in the squinting eye is defective despite the wearing of spectacle lenses it is essential to try and improve it by covering the nonsquinting eye, usually totally, for sufficiently long periods, often for several weeks or even months. It is, however, necessary before starting this occlusion to be certain that the fixation of the squinting eye has not become eccentric otherwise the covering of the nonsquinting eye will merely serve to establish still further the abnormal fixation of the squinting eye without any return of useful vision; the nature of the retinal fixation is determined by a special type of ophthalmoscope (the visuscope) by observing the area of the retina which fixes a target incorporated in the beam of light. In cases of established eccentric fixation a period of prolonged covering of the squinting eye should be carried out in the hope of obtaining a disappearance of the abnormal fixation simply by preventing any abnormal visual impressions from reaching the visual cortex, although this is successful only in a limited number of cases. In cases in which the eccentric fixation of the squinting eye is unsteady it is essential to carry out a preliminary occlusion of the nonsquinting eye and this should be continued as long as there is an alteration in the fixation of the squinting eye towards a more normal type so that ultimately there may be a restoration of a central form of fixation. This preliminary occlusion of the nonsquinting eye is also justified in an apparently steady form of eccentric fixation, but it should be discontinued in a few days if there is no change in the fixation because further occlusion merely enhances the establishment of the eccentric retinal point.

Treatment by Orthoptic Methods. This is carried out by Orthoptists who are Medical Auxiliaries concerned in all the different aspects of the diagnosis and treatment of squint. There are many different instruments which are designed specifically for binocular training (for example, the synoptophore) and the foveae of the two eyes are associated with one another by repeated stimulations in an attempt to maintain or to reestablish binocular function despite the presence of the squint.

A more recent form of orthoptic treatment (*pleoptic treatment*) is designed to correct eccentric retinal fixation by the creation of an after-image within the squinting eye which is projected from the eye incorrectly in the early stages of treatment but correctly after the reestablishment of a normal type of retinal fixation. This treatment, however, is only applicable to children over the age of 5 years because of the concentration and cooperation which it demands, and it is often necessary to continue the treatment at frequent intervals for several weeks and even months; the restoration of central fixation in the squinting eye is followed by the usual treatment to improve the vision of the squinting eye. It is obvious that pleoptic treatment has only a limited application in cases of squint which occur in early childhood, and the whole emphasis on treatment must be on the prevention of such complications as an establishment eccentric fixation by early treatment of the squint. Pleoptic treatment, however, is of distinct value in obtaining an improved form of vision in an amblyopic eye in later life when the vision of the good eye is lost as the result of some injury or disease.

Correction of the Squint Surgically. In some cases the use of glasses may be sufficient to correct the squint, but in many cases it is necessary to correct the deviation by carefully planned surgical treatment on one or more of the eye muscles of one or both eyes sometimes in more than one stage. It is important to take regard of any difference in the extent of the ocular deviation on near as compared with distant fixation; this is discussed in relation to latent squint (see below). As a general rule children stand up to this operation very well; the child leaves his bed in hospital for the operating theatre in a relaxed state because of the use of modern sedatives, the operation is carried out under a general anaesthetic, and the operated eye as a rule only requires to be covered for a few hours or often not at all, particularly when an operation is carried out on both eyes. Ideally this surgical treatment enables the restoration of binocular function, but the operation is justified purely on cosmetic grounds because a person with an obvious squint creates problems of a psychological nature for himself, or, in the case of a child, for the parents, quite apart from the fact he may be prejudiced in obtaining many forms of employment in later life.

Use of Miotic Drugs. Drugs like pilocarpine, and DFP (di-isopropylfluorophosphonate) and phospholine iodide, which cause a constriction of the sphincter of the pupil (miosis), also induce a contraction of the ciliary muscle so that the peripheral accommodation is enhanced and the necessity to produce accommodation by central impulses is reduced with a corresponding reduction in the convergence of the eyes. These drugs are of value, therefore, in the accommodative type of squint in which the deviation is controlled for distant fixation but not for near fixation. DFP 0·01 to 0·05 per cent drops or phospholine iodide 0·06 or 0·12 per cent drops are more effective than pilocarpine and only need to be instilled once every 24 hours (preferably in the morning so that their greatest effect is during the day), but if they cause pain and irritation because of their powerful effect they may be instilled before going to sleep.

Use of Bifocals

Bifocals are of value in the accommodative type of squint when the deviation is controlled by ordinary glasses for distant fixation but not for near fixation because of the extra accommodative effort which is then required, provided the reading segment (which may be as much as +3 dioptres stronger than the distant segment permits a control of the deviation for near. It is essential to make the reading segment sufficiently large so that the child is forced to use it for all close work and is not tempted to rely simply on the distant segment.

In general the aim of the treatment of a manifest squint is to achieve a functional result so that there is the establishment of binocular function, rather than simply an amelioration of a cosmetic blemish. When the squint is of relatively late onset, when it shows a prolonged intermittent phase, or when treatment is applied at an early stage it may be possible to restore normal binocular function (bifoveal fixation), but quite frequently even when various lines of treatment result in a scarcely perceptible residual deviation (microtropia) there is evidence on critical methods of examination of an anomalous retinal correspondence; in certain circumstances, however, this is a perfectly satisfactory result because it provides an adequate form of binocular association with an anomalous form of fusion which is usually sufficient to stand up to the rigours of the visual demands on the eyes in adult life.

INTERMITTENT SQUINT

This is a squint which is present only at certain times and, by convention, it is reserved for the squint which is manifest at one distance of fixation but latent at another distance of fixation. The term is applied largely to the esodeviations (convergent squints) and the exodeviations (divergent squints), and these may be classified according to the position of fixation in which the deviation is manifest.

Intermittent Convergent Squint (Intermittent Esotropia)

1. *Convergence excess esotropia*—the esotropia is manifest on near fixation, but latent on distant fixation.

2. *Divergence weakness esotropia*—the esotropia is manifest on distant fixation, but latent on near fixation.

Intermittent Divergent Squint (Intermittent Exotropia)
   1. *Divergence excess exotropia*—the exotropia is manifest on distant fixation, but latent on near fixation.
   2. *Convergence weakness exotropia*—the exotropia is manifest on near fixation, but latent on distant fixation.

The various forms of vertical squint (hypertropia and hypotropia) may also show intermittent phases.

The methods of diagnosis and treatment of intermittent squint are essentially based on those applied to manifest squint (discussed above) and to latent squint (discussed above).

LATENT SQUINT (HETEROPHORIA)

This is a condition in which there is an imbalance of the extrinsic ocular muscles so that under conditions of stress there is a failure of the fusion mechanism to function adequately with the development of a squint. The nature of the latent squint is designated by the direction of the occasional squint; a tendency for the eye to turn in (*esophoria*), which is of three main types—*convergence excess* when the deviation is greater for near than for distant fixation, *divergence weakness* when the deviation is greater for distant than for near fixation, and *basic* when the deviation is more or less equal on near and distant fixation; to turn out (*exophoria*), which is also of three main types—*divergence excess* when the deviation is greater for distant than for near fixation, *convergence weakness* when the deviation is greater for near than for distant fixation and *basic* when the deviation is more or less equal on near and distant fixation; to turn up (*hyperphoria*), to turn down (*hypophoria*), to wheel-rotate in (*incyclophoria*), or to wheel-rotate out (*excyclophoria*). These imbalances are produced by the same obstacles which cause a manifest squint, but in the latent squint they are sufficiently minor to be controlled (compensated), often in the absence of any feeling of strain, except under conditions of stress, illness, advancing age, etc., when they tend to become uncontrolled (decompensated) so that the latent squint becomes converted to a manifest one. It follows that some forms of heterophoria are associated with symptoms (unlike a heterotropia), when an effort is required to maintain control of the latent deviation, which are essentially those of eyestrain:

headache, ocular discomfort, redness of the eyes, blurring of vision at certain times, or even intermittent diplopia, particularly after intensive use of the eyes.

Diagnosis

The diagnosis of a case of heterophoria is dependent on inducing the latent deviation by a dissociation of the eyes and this is achieved in various ways:

The Alternate Cover Test. This test (p. 232) is of great value because it dissociates the eyes so that a latent deviation becomes converted into a manifest one during the rapid transference of the cover from one eye to the other; the rapidity of the recovery of the eyes to a binocular position after the removal of the cover is a useful method of assessing the strength of the fusional vergence and, therefore, the degree of the control of the latent deviation in normal circumstances. The maximum extent of the latent deviation may be measured accurately by placing prisms of increasing strength (with the base of the prism in a direction opposite to that of the deviation) until there is no further breakdown—the so-called *prism and cover test*—and the test is carried out for near fixation ($\frac{1}{3}$ m) and for distant fixation (6 m) because of the marked difference which may occur in these positions.

The Maddox Rod Test. The Maddox rod is an optical appliance which consists of a series of red-coloured glass rods which converts the appearance of a white spot of light into a red line. This rod is placed in front of one eye and the red line cannot be fused with the unaltered image of the white spot of light which is viewed by the other eye, so that the eyes become dissociated and the extent of the dissociation is measured by obtaining a superimposition of the two images by the use of prisms (with the base of the prism in a direction opposite the direction of the deviation). The Maddox rod may be rotated to make the red line run vertically or horizontally in order to measure latent horizontal and vertical forms of squint, and an abnormal tilting of the line when the Maddox rod is placed correctly in the trial frame indicates a cyclophoria. The Maddox rod test is usually carried out for distant fixation (6 m), but it may be used at other distances of fixation.

The Maddox Wing Test. This is an instrument which dissociates the eyes on near fixation ($\frac{1}{3}$ m); the amount of the horizontal dissociation is indicated by the apparent position of a vertical arrow (seen by one eye) on a horizontal tangent scale (seen by the other eye), and the amount of vertical dissociation is indicated by the apparent position of a horizontal arrow (seen by one eye) on a vertical tangent scale (seen by the other eye). There is also a movable wire which is adjusted by the patient until it appears horizontal and any cyclophoria is detected by an incorrect placement of the wire.

The Synoptophore. This instrument (p. 232) is used to measure the fusional vergence in cases of heterophoria; when the heterophoria is not well compensated the fusional vergence is poor.

Occlusion. The occlusion of one eye for a few days is a useful diagnostic test in cases of heterophoria when it is uncertain if the symptoms of eyestrain are the result of the heterophoria; a disappearance of the symptoms on occlusion is an indication of their association with the muscle imbalance.

Treatment

The treatment of a heterophoria is often limited to a correction of the refractive error and orthoptic treatment, as discussed for a heterotropia. If these measures prove to be inadequate it is necessary to carry out carefully planned surgical treatment on the extrinsic ocular muscle in order to provide a satisfactory degree of control. This must take account of any difference in the extent of the deviation on near as compared with distant fixation; in a convergence excess esophoria a bilateral medial rectus recession, in a divergence weakness esophoria a unilateral (or rarely a bilateral) lateral rectus resection, in a basic esophoria a limited unilateral medial rectus recession and lateral rectus resection, in a divergence excess exophoria a bilateral lateral rectus recession, in a convergence weakness exophoria a unilateral (or rarely a bilateral) medial rectus resection, and in a basic exophoria a limited unilateral lateral rectus recession and medial rectus resection. Sometimes, however, if surgical treatment is contraindicated (as in the very elderly) prisms may be incorporated in the spectacle lenses because these permit the eye to be deviated in the direction of the phoria without producing an awareness of diplopia by causing an appropriate deviation of the light rays before they enter the eye. It should be noted, however, that this method of treatment has two great disadvantages; first, it tends to perpetuate the imbalance by forcing the eye into the deviated position thereby preventing any attempt by the patient to control the imbalance so that there is a further weakening of the fusional vergence, and, second, many forms of heterophoria vary in degree in different positions of gaze so that, although a prism may be able to control symptoms of the deviation in one position of the eyes, it is ineffective in other positions.

In this discussion on manifest and latent squints a distinction has been made between a horizontal type of deviation (esotropia, esophoria, exotropia and exophoria) and a vertical type (hypertropia, hyperphoria, hypotropia and hypophoria). It should be appreciated however, that this distinction is in no way rigid so that the two frequently coexist, and the one may arise from the other. The first association is seen particularly in the *alternating hypertropia* or *alternating hyperphoria* which may accompany an esotropia or esophoria so that, in addition to the convergent deviation, either eye rotates upwards when the other eye is fixing. This vertical element is evident also in the upshoot of each eye which occurs in adduction (where the action of elevation of the inferior oblique is especially effective), and less commonly in the *alternating hypotropia* or *alternating hyperphoria* in which either eye rotates downwards when the other eye is fixing with a downshoot of each eye in adduction (where the action of the superior oblique is especially effective. A vertical element may also be a feature of a divergent squint (exophoria or exotropia) particularly the upshoot which occurs in each eye in a position of abduction.

It is evident that these forms of alternating vertical squint differ from the usual forms of hyperphoria, hypertropia, hypophoria or hypotropia (in which each eye deviates in opposite directions—one eye upwards and the other eye downwards—to more or less equal extents) because each eye deviates in the same direction (upwards or downwards) and quite frequently to unequal extents.

THE A AND V PHENOMENON

Normally when the eyes move from the primary position directly upward (sursumversion) or downward (deorsumversion) there is no significant alteration in the relative positions of the eyes. Sometimes in the presence of a squint this fails to apply so that there is a change in the angle of the squint; the so-called A and V phenomenon.

In an *A-esotropia* (*esophoria*) the angle of the squint (manifest or latent) increases on looking up and decreases on looking down; it follows an underaction of the lateral recti and frequently also an underaction of the inferior obliques.

In an *A-exotropia* (*exophoria*) the angle of the squint decreases on looking up and increases on looking down; it follows an underaction of the medial recti and frequently also an underaction of the inferior obliques.

In a *V-esotropia* (*esophoria*) the angle of the squint decreases on looking up and increases on looking down; it follows an overaction of the medial recti and frequently also an underaction of the superior obliques.

In a *V-exotropia* (*exophoria*) the angle of the squint increases on looking up and decreases on looking down; it follows an overaction of the lateral recti and frequently also an underaction of the superior obliques.

The presence of an A or V element in an esodeviation or exo-deviation necessitates a modification of the usual surgical treatment of the horizontal squint. There are many different procedures, but in general a strengthening operation (resection) of the underacting horizontal muscles (lateral recti in an A-esotropia and medial recti in an A-exotropia) and a weakening operation (recession) on the overacting horizontal muscles (medial recti in a V-esotropia and lateral recti in a V-exotropia) are effective measures, but it is frequently necessary also to carry out a weakening operation (recession) of the overacting oblique muscles (superior obliques in an A-esotropia or A-exotropia, and inferior obliques in a V-esotropia or V-exotropia), that is, of the obliques which are the ipsilateral antagonists of the underacting obliques.

CONVERGENCE INSUFFICIENCY

This implies a failure of both eyes to be directed to a near object in the absence of any true paresis of the medial recti; normally the mechanism of convergence is carried out without any effort of will because it is essentially a reflex phenomenon (p. 220), although there is also a voluntary form of convergence, and symptoms of eye-strain are likely to occur if a conscious effort is required for this movement, as in an exophoria of the convergence weakness type.

Convergence is tested *objectively* by bringing an object (like the examiner's finger) from a distance of about $\frac{1}{3}$ m towards the patient's nose and asking the patient to direct both eyes towards the approaching object; under normal conditions an equal degree of convergence of each eye should be maintained without undue effort until the object is about 7 cm from the eyes, but when there is a convergence insufficiency this position may be achieved with considerable difficulty so that there is a subjective awareness of ocular discomfort, or there may be a failure of one eye (or even both eyes) to carry out the movement adequately. Convergence is tested *subjectively* by an instrument like the Livingston binocular gauge. It is important, however, to distinguish between *reflex convergence* and *voluntary convergence* because a difficulty in inducing the latter does not necessarily indicate any defect of the reflex components.

INCOMITANT SQUINT

This is a condition in which there is a paresis (partial loss of function) or paralysis (complete loss of function) of one or more of the extrinsic ocular muscles so that the squint is an incomitant one in which the angle of the squint is variable (and often even absent) in certain positions of gaze according to the particular muscle (or muscles) involved in the dysfunction so that there are varying degrees of external ophthalmoplegia. The nature of the defect is determined by methods (discussed below) which take account of the facts that two muscles—one from each eye—are concerned primarily in the movements of the eyes in the six main positions of conjugate gaze, and that a paresis of one extrinsic ocular muscle is followed by changes in some of the other muscles: overaction (and often later contractural changes) of the ipsilateral antagonist (the muscle of the same eye which opposes the action of the paretic muscle), overaction of the contralateral synergic muscle (the muscle of the opposite eye which is concerned normally with the paretic muscle in a conjugate movement), and secondary underaction of the antagonist of the contralateral synergist (the muscle of the opposite eye which normally opposes the action of the contralateral synergic muscle). It should be noted that an incomitant seldom remains incomitant indefinitely; many cases recover spontaneously or are relieved by treatment, and those which persist tend ultimately to become concomitant.

An Assessment of the Range of Uniocular and Binocular Movements. This may show the muscles which are underacting and which are overacting (pp. 211–16).

An Assessment of the Nature of the Diplopia. Diplopia is a feature of an incomitant squint, and it is termed *pathological diplopia* in contrast to *physiological diplopia* (p. 225). The separation of the images (the *true image* from the fixing eye and the *false image* from the paretic eye) is in a horizontal direction when one of the horizontally acting muscles is affected and in a vertical direction (often also with some horizontal displacement) when one of the vertically acting muscles is affected; horizontal separation is detected by moving an object like a pencil held vertically into the two main positions of horizontal gaze (to the right and to the left), and vertical separation is detected by moving the object held horizontally into the four main positions of vertical gaze (up and to the right, down and to the right, up and to the left, and down and to the left). The false image is the one which is farther from the eye so that covering the affected eye causes a disappearance of the farther away image; when the paresis is only slight the recognition of the two images is facilitated by the use of red (for one eye) and green (for the other eye) goggles. In a case of multiple pareses or in a case of a single paresis with secondary overaction and underaction of other muscles when diplopia is present in more than one of the six main positions of conjugate gaze, an assessment of the diplopia is made in each position with particular emphasis on the position in which there is a maximum separation of the images. A determination of the affected extrinsic ocular muscle from an assessment of the diplopia is dependent on a knowledge of the main field of action of each muscle (pp. 211–14).

The Cover Test. It is useful to carry out this test (p. 231) in all six positions of conjugate gaze in addition to the primary position to determine the positions in which the deviation is evident. The extent of the deviation differs according to the eye which is used for fixation with the smaller deviation occurring in the affected eye during the fixation of the unaffected eye (the so-called *primary deviation* of the affected eye) and with the greater deviation occurring in the unaffected eye during the enforced fixation of the affected eye (the so-called *secondary deviation* of the unaffected eye) which is the result of the increased innervational effort of the affected eye during fixation being passed also to the unaffected eye by the phenomenon of reciprocal innervation.

The Field of Binocular Fixation. This (p. 215) indicates the area of the field in which the two eyes are unable to function binocularly because of the paresis.

The Hess Screen. This is a projection test in which records are made of the direction of the paretic eye in each of the cardinal positions of gaze when the unaffected eye is fixing these positions (these recordings plot the primary deviation of the affected eye), and of the direction of the unaffected eye in these positions when the paretic eye is fixing (these recordings plot the secondary deviation of the unaffected eye). During the tests the eyes are dissociated by the use of red and green goggles and the cardinal positions (p. 215) are 15° (or 30°) from the primary position.

An Assessment of the Abnormal Head Posture. The nature of the head posture is diagnostic sometimes of a particular paresis (p. 228).

False Projection. In an incomitant squint there is an upset of the normal appreciation of an object in space so that it is incorrectly located by the paretic eye; this is the so-called past-pointing which occurs when the finger points beyond the object of fixation in the direction of the field of action of the paretic muscle during its attempted localization. This occurs because the effort which is made to try to turn the eye into the affected field is interpreted by the brain as evidence that the eye has moved into the desired position so that the subsequent stimulation by the object of a peripheral point on the retina, instead of the fovea, gives the impression that the object is displaced still farther from the eye. The failure of the brain to appreciate the absence of any movement of the eye is explained by the fact that in any *active* (as distinct from *passive*) movement of the normal eye from point A to point B there is no impression of a sensation of movement of the objects between A and B, despite the fact that these objects flit over the retina, as the result of a perceptual adjusting mechanism.

There are two main forms of incomitant squint—*neurogenic* due to some lesion of the complex nervous network which is concerned in the control of ocular movement, and *myogenic* due to some lesion of the muscle or its fascial tissues.

Neurogenic Disorders

There is a wide variety of conditions which may produce neurogenic lesions; only a limited number in each main category is mentioned.

1. Congenital abnormalities (these are very rare)
    (a) Nuclear aplasia
2. Inflammatory conditions
    (a) Encephalitis (septicaemia, poliomyelitis, vaccinia)
    (b) Neuritis (meningitis, herpes zoster)
    (c) Neurosyphilis (meningo-vascular, tabes or general paralysis of the insane)
    (d) Osteoperiostitis (syphilis)
3. Toxic disorders
    (a) Bacterial toxins like tetanus and botulism
    (b) Intoxications like lead, carbon dioxide, alcohol (particularly methyl alcohol), snake venom, spinal anaesthesia

4. Demyelinating diseases
   (a) Disseminated sclerosis
5. Metabolic disorders
   (a) Vitamin B deficiency (beri-beri and pellagra)
6. Vascular lesions
   (a) Intracerebral haemorrhage
   (b) Subarachnoid haemorrhage
   (c) Congenital and acquired intracranial aneurysms
   (d) Vertebro-basilar insufficiency
   (e) Thrombosis
   (f) Embolism
7. Neoplastic diseases

Many different forms of primary and metastatic tumour formations may cause ophthalmoplegia, particularly those involving the
midbrain, the middle cranial fossa and the region of the superior
orbital fissure.

8. Degenerative lesions
   (a) Amyotrophic lateral sclerosis
   (b) Hereditary ataxia
9. Traumatic lesions

Traumatic lesions may cause ophthalmoplegia by a direct involvement of a nerve in the lesion (as in a fractured base of skull), but
the involvement is usually of an indirect nature as the result of a
pressure on the nerve by an associated haemorrhage or oedema.

The diagnostic features of different forms of neurogenic incomitant squint depend on the motor nerves which are involved:

IIIrd Cranial Nerve Involvement. This causes the affected eye to be
maintained in a position of abduction due to the unopposed action
of the intact lateral rectus (innervated by the VIth cranial nerve)
with a failure of the eye to move into positions of adduction, elevation or depression; it might be expected that the intact superior
oblique (innervated by the IVth cranial nerve) would cause the eye
to be somewhat depressed but this is so because it acts as a depressor
mainly when the eye is in an adducted position, although its integrity
is demonstrated by the obvious intorsion of the eye which occurs
on attempting to look down. There are also other features: a drooping of the upper lid caused by a paralysis of the levator muscle, a
dilatation of the pupil (mydriasis) with a failure to respond to light
directly or consensually or to respond to a near stimulus because of a
paralysis of the sphincter muscle of the pupil, and a failure of
accommodation (cycloplegia) due to a paralysis of the ciliary muscle.

Sometimes, however, there is only an external ophthalmoplegia (involvement of the extrinsic ocular muscles and the levator) without an internal ophthalmoplegia (sparing of the sphincter of the pupil and the ciliary muscle), and at other times there is only a partial involvement of the nerve (paresis) so that there is a sparing of the action of some of its muscles.

IVth Cranial Nerve Involvement. This causes a loss of depression in an adducted position, with frequently a latent or manifest upward displacement of the affected eye in the primary position (hyperphoria or hypertropia), and also a defective intorsion of the eye so that it becomes extorted because of the unopposed action of the inferior oblique (the ipsilateral antagonist); the overactions of this muscle and also of the inferior rectus of the unaffected eye (the contralateral synergist) increase the hyperphoria or hypertropia of the affected eye which is increased further by a weakness of the superior rectus of the unaffected eye (the antagonist of the contralateral synergist).

VIth Cranial Nerve Involvement. This leads to an absence of abduction and the affected eye is usually convergent because of the overaction of the medial rectus (the ipsilateral antagonist) which is increased by an overaction of the medial rectus of the unaffected eye (the contralateral synergist) and by a weakness of the lateral rectus of the unaffected eye (the antagonist of the contralateral synergist).

An involvement of all the motor nerves to the extrinsic ocular muscle is associated with a complete external ophthalmoplegia, and the paralysed eye usually assumes the 'position of rest' which is one of divergence because of the forwards and outwards direction of the orbital axis. There may also be an internal ophthalmoplegia (chap. 6) (total ophthalmoplegia).

The proximity of the IIIrd, IVth, and VIth cranial nerves to other nervous structures during their passage from the nuclei to the extrinsic ocular muscles determines the occurrence of certain syndromes.

Brain-stem Lesions. In brain-stem lesions, the following four syndromes are included.

1. *Benedikt's syndrome (tegmental syndrome)* follows a lesion in the dorsal part of the cerebral peduncle in the tegmental part of the midbrain, and it causes involvement of the ipsilateral IIIrd cranial nerve (see above), of the red nucleus (contralateral hemitremor of the face and limbs and sometimes also an impairment or hesitancy of conjugate lateral gaze), and occasionally a lesion of the

medial lemniscus, which represents the ascending sensory fibres to the thalamus after their decussation (contralateral hemianaesthesia).

2. *Weber's syndrome* (*syndrome of the cerebral peduncle or alternating oculomotor hemiplegia*) follows a lesion in the posterior end of the cerebral peduncle, and it causes involvement of the ipsilateral IIIrd cranial nerve (see above) within the brainstem or as it emerges from the brainstem, and of the pyramidal tract in the cerebral peduncle (contralateral hemiplegia of face and limbs).

3. *Foville's syndrome* follows a lesion in the pons, and it causes involvement of the ipsilateral VIth nerve (see above), of the corticofugal fibres from the frontal motor cortex after their decussation in the region of the posterior commissure (loss of conjugate deviation to the side of the lesion), of the VIIth (facial) cranial nerve (ipsilateral facial palsy), and of the pyramidal tract (contralateral hemiplegia).

4. *Millard-Gubler syndrome* follows a lesion in the lower part of the pons and it causes involvement of the VIth and VIIth cranial nerves, as in Foville's syndrome, but with a sparing of the corticofugal fibres so that there is no loss of movement of the contralateral medial rectus on an attempted conjugate movement to the side of the lesion.

Trunk Lesions. This category includes the following five syndromes.

1. *Basal palsy* follows a lesion of the base of the brain and it causes involvement of the IIIrd, IVth, and VIth cranial nerves and often also involvement of the Vth, VIIth and VIIIth cranial nerves.

2. *Gradenigo's syndrome* follows a lesion of the apex of the petrous temporal bone and it causes involvement of the VIth cranial nerve.

3. *Cavernous sinus syndrome* follows a lesion of the cavernous sinus and it causes involvement of the IIIrd, IVth, and VIth, cranial nerves, involvement of the Vth nerve (the ophthalmic division of the nerves when the lesion is placed anteriorly and the maxillary and mandibular divisions when the lesion is placed posteriorly), and sometimes a pulsating type of exophthalmos.

4. *Sphenoidal fissure syndrome* follows a lesion in the region of the superior orbital fissure with progressive involvement of the IIIrd cranial nerve (sometimes only the superior or inferior division* is involved), of the IVth, and VIth cranial nerves, and of the Vth

---

* The *superior division* supplies the levator and superior rectus and the *inferior division* supplies the medial rectus, inferior rectus, inferior oblique, the ciliary muscle and the sphincter of the pupil.

cranial nerve (sometimes only the ophthalmic division but often the ophthalmic and maxillary divisions) causing a combination of anaesthesia and severe neuralgic pain and with an associated proptosis.

5. *Orbital apex syndrome* follows a lesion in the posterior part of the orbit near its apex with involvement of the IInd cranial nerve (papilloedema or optic atrophy) in addition to the features of the sphenoidal fissure syndrome.

Treatment of Neurogenic Ophthalmoplegia. This is directed at the cause of the ophthalmoplegia, although in many conditions (for example, fracture of the skull, disseminated sclerosis) there is often a spontaneous recovery in the absence of any specific treatment; during the waiting period diplopia may be avoided by occlusion of one eye. A persistence of a significant degree of ophthalmoplegia after an interval of six months demands surgical intervention provided repeated examinations confirm that the condition is not in a progressive or regressive phase; the main object is to restore comfortable binocular single vision in the primary position and also in as much of the field of binocular fixation as possible, particularly on depression (because this is the conventional reading position). In complicated forms of paralysis the operative treatment may need to be carried out in several carefully planned stages and there are various methods involved; an increase in the effectiveness of a paretic muscle by its resection, a decrease in the effectiveness of an overacting muscle (ipsilateral antagonist or contralateral synergist) by its recession or by its division—myectomy or tenotomy (usually only of the superior or inferior oblique)—an increase in the range of movement of the eye by a recession of a muscle in a state of contracture (usually the ipsilateral antagonist), and sometimes the restoration of some degree of movement in the paralysed muscle by a transplantation type of operation with slips from unaffected muscles.

The use of prisms may be expedient in cases not suitable for surgical intervention, but they are of limited value (p. 240).

Myogenic Disorders

There are relatively few conditions which produce myogenic lesions except in the congenital category.

Congenital Abnormalities. The majority of cases of congenital ophthalmoplegia are of a myogenic nature and there is a grossly restricted movement of the eye in the direction of action of the affected muscle (or muscles) because of a replacement fibrosis within the muscle, and there is also some abnormality of the movement of the eye in the opposite direction because of a failure of the fibrotic muscle to relax adequately or because of an abnormality of the muscle sheath; in general they are termed *musculo-fascial anomalies*:

1. Duane's Retraction Syndrome. In the typical form the lateral rectus is involved primarily in the fibrotic process with only a minor involvement of the medial rectus (Type A), or sometimes no involvement of the medial rectus (Type B), so that there is a failure of abduction and a defect of adduction with a retraction of the eye on attempted full adduction because of a failure of the lateral rectus to relax; this failure may be confirmed accurately at operation by the resistance which is experienced on attempting to move the globe manually into a position of adduction—the *forced duction test*. The retraction is not simply the result of the mechanical effect of the fibrotic lateral rectus but is produced also by the combined actions of the medial, superior and inferior recti which, in trying to achieve a position of full adduction, produce the effect of retraction (sometimes regarded less accurately as an enophthalmos) with a slight narrowing of the palpebral fissure. There is also a ptosis of the upper lid during the retraction of the eye, but this is simply the result of a failure of the retracted eyeball to support the upper lid. A slight protraction of the eyeball occurs on attempted abduction because the superior and inferior obliques which, in trying to exert their abducting influences following the loss of abduction by the lateral rectus, produce their effects of protraction with a slight widening of the palpebral aperture. In the primary position there is usually only a slight degree of manifest (or latent) convergent squint which is in contrast to the gross loss of abduction; this is characteristic of a myogenic lesion as compared with a neurogenic one (in which there would be an obvious overaction of the ipsilateral antagonist and contralateral synergist particularly on dissociation of the eyes as in the cover test) and it is a feature of great diagnostic significance.

In the atypical form of the syndrome (Type C) the medial rectus is more affected than the lateral rectus by the fibrosis so that adduction is more limited than abduction and a manifest (or latent) divergent squint is present in the primary position; the retraction of the eye on attempted adduction and the protraction of the eye on attempted abduction occur as in the typical form of the syndrome.

Sometimes the features of a Duane's retraction syndrome may occur as the result of a cocontraction of the lateral and medial recti which is motivated by an anomaly of the brain-stem centres controlling ocular movement, so that it is not invariably a musculo-fascial disorder.

Treatment. This is limited to a restoration of comfortable binocular single vision in the primary position, usually by a medial rectus recession of one or both eyes in the typical form of the syndrome, but in many cases treatment is not necessary.

2. Superior Oblique Tendon Sheath Syndrome. In this syndrome there is an abrupt cessation of movement of the affected eye in the field of action of the inferior oblique (elevation in a position of adduction) because of a failure of relaxation of the superior oblique (the antagonist of the inferior oblique) as a result of its abnormal sheath; this is sometimes associated with a sensation of pain in the region of the trochlea (around which the superior oblique hooks) because the sheath may be attached to the pulley. This fascial anomaly is distinguished from a congenital neurogenic palsy of the inferior oblique by the forced duction test which demonstrates the resistance on attempted manual movement of the eye into the field of action of the inferior oblique (that is, away from the field of action of the superior oblique) and also to some extent by the absence of any marked deviation of the eyes in the primary position (often there is no deviation or only a very slight hypotropia) because of an absence of the marked secondary overactions which usually follow a neurogenic lesion.

Treatment. A myectomy of the superior oblique or preferably a removal of the abnormal sheath of the superior oblique is followed by a restoration of some movement of the inferior oblique, but such treatment is usually reserved for cases in which there is a significant deviation in the primary position or for bilateral cases.

Acquired Conditions. There are five acquired myogenic disorders to be considered.

1. Myasthenia Gravis (chap. 11). A paresis of one or more of the extrinsic ocular muscles, which is less common than a paresis of the levator muscle of the lid, is characterized initially by fleeting episodes of diplopia which ultimately become more persistent, particularly towards the end of the day or after periods of fatigue, although they remain variable in extent. The functions of elevation and convergence are most frequently affected and both eyes are seldom involved to equal degrees. The intrinsic ocular muscles are not affected in this condition.

2. Progressive External Ophthalmoplegia (Ocular Myopathy). In this condition there is a gradual and progressive loss of ocular mobility which usually causes a disturbance of elevation before involving the other forms of movement, although a ptosis is often the first feature. The disturbance is bilateral and, although it starts to some extent in adolescence, it is seldom obvious before early adult life or even middle age, except for a few cases which are advanced in childhood. Rarely there may be similar changes in the peripheral skeletal musculature. Its *myopathic* nature accounts for the absence of any involvement of the intrinsic ocular muscles.

3. Ocular Myositis. An acute form occurs in an orbital cellulitis (chap. 14), but there is a rare chronic form with exophthalmos, lid oedema, multiple extrinsic ocular muscle pareses, photophobia and sometimes a disturbance of vision because of a defect of the vascular supply of the optic nerve due to the raised intraorbital pressure with the production of some degree of optic atrophy. It probably represents one of the collagen diseases and this explains the good response sometimes to the use of steroids.

4. Dermatomyositis. A myositis of the extrinsic ocular muscles may occur in association with the other features of the condition (chap. 7).

5. Ophthalmoplegia in Thyrotrophic Exophthalmos. This is discussed under Thyrotrophic Manifestations in Chapter 14.

It should be noted that in addition to the neurogenic and myogenic forms of incomitant squint an abnormality of ocular movement with the features of incomitancy may occur simply as the result of a displacement of the eye or as the result of a limitation of movement for purely mechanical reasons; this type of paresis or palsy is liable to occur in any lesion of the orbit, for example, a fracture of the floor of the orbit, a tumour of the orbit, etc.

Ocular Deviations

The term *ocular deviation* is applied to a supranuclear lesion which causes a disturbance of ocular movement that, unlike a lower motor neuron lesion which causes an incomitant squint, is not capable of being resolved into terms of a disorder of individual muscles because it represents a disorder of one of the combined movements of the eyes; *conjugate movements* (*versions*) or *disjunctive movements* (*vergences*), causing conjugate gaze palsies or *disjunctive gaze palsies*.

A gaze palsy may follow a lesion of the frontal motor centres (or their corticofugal nerve fibres) or of the occipital motor centres (or their corticofugal nerve fibres)

Frontal Lesion Causing a Lateral Gaze Palsy

This shows a diminution or abolition of a conjugate movement to the side away from the lesion (a right-sided lesion causes a failure of laevoversion) when the attempt to carry out the movement is of a voluntary nature or in response to a command, with a slight conjugate movement of the eyes to the side of the lesion because of the unopposed action of the centres in the unaffected side of the brain in the unconscious patient and a slight turning of the head to the side away from the lesion in the conscious patient. There is a retention of the conjugate movements which follow the reflex fixation of an object which may be intensified so that the gaze becomes anchored to the moving object provided it is moved sufficiently slowly. There is also a retention and intensification of the conjugate movements which follow proprioceptive reflexes from the labyrinthine mechanism and neck muscles provided the lesion is above the level of the octavus system; in a right-sided frontal lesion a sudden turning of the patient's head to the right causes the eyes to move conjugately to the left (*the doll's head (or eye) phenomenon*), or the conjugate movement may be induced also by caloric or galvanic stimulation of the labyrinthine mechanism, and a retention of reflex convergence (provided the lesion is above the level of the pons). The condition is not accompanied by any awareness of diplopia because the defective motility is equally represented in each eye.

Paralysis of Vertical Movements (*Parinaud's Syndrome*)

A supranuclear lesion affecting vertical movement is rare and is usually the result of a lesion in the subthalamic region. The persistence of *Bell's phenomenon*—the ability of the eyes to turn up on attempted closure of the lids—is retained. The syndrome is not associated with any awareness of diplopia.

Paralysis of Convergence

A paralysis of convergence in the absence of any defective movement of either eye during ductions or lateral versions is a rare occurrence, and this is in marked contrast to a functional disturbance of the convergence mechanism (p. 242) which is common. The site of the lesion is uncertain (p. 217). It is characterized by persistent diplopia for near objects, but an absence of any diplopia when looking in the distance. There is no satisfactory treatment of the defect, but the diplopia may be avoided on close work by the provision of glasses incorporating prisms (base in).

Spasm of Convergence

A spasm of convergence, usually in association with a spasm of accommodation, is a rare occurrence in children and young adults as the result of some disturbance or of a psychological or hysterical nature. More frequently it is a feature of the convergence excess type of esophoria (p. 238) or intermittent esotropia (p. 237).

Occipital Lesion Causing a Lateral Gaze Palsy

This shows a disorientation of the psychooptical reflex so that there is an inability to turn the eyes conjugately towards an object on the side away from the side of the lesion; the eyes may remain staring ahead or carry out awkward rolling movements. There is a retention of the conjugate movements induced by the frontal centres, and a retention of the conjugate movements which are induced by proprioceptive stimuli from the labyrinthine mechanism and from the neck muscles.

DISSOCIATED PALSIES

These palsies represent a form of supranuclear disturbance which is of an irregular nature so that diplopia is a feature at times. They follow lesions of the medial (posterior) longitudinal bundle which is concerned in providing a link between the various motor nuclei which supply the extrinsic ocular muscles (*internuclear palsy*).

In a bilateral *anterior internuclear palsy* there is a defective movement of the adducted eye and a nystagmus of the abducted eye on attempted movements of lateral gaze on either side, but there is a retention usually of normal convergence except when there is an involvement also of the descending nerve fibres which subserve the convergence reflex. In a unilateral *anterior internuclear palsy* the defective movement of the adducted eye and the nystagmus of the abducted eye occurs on lateral gaze to the side away from the lesion; there may also be a skew deviation on attempted lateral gaze with the ipsilateral eye becoming higher than the contralateral eye. A bilateral internuclear palsy is usually the result of a demyelinating lesion (disseminated sclerosis), and a unilateral palsy may follow a vascular lesion or a brain-stem tumour. (A *posterior internuclear palsy* has been described in which there is a loss of abduction with a retention of adduction but it is doubtful if this is an established entity.)

OVERACTIONS OF THE EXTRINSIC OCULAR MUSCLES

As a general rule an overaction of an extrinsic ocular muscle is secondary to a primary underaction of another muscle, as in the over-action of the ipsilateral antagonist or contralateral synergist of a paretic muscle in an incomitant squint (p. 243). Sometimes a true overaction (spasm) may occur as in a spasm of convergence (see above) or as a conjugate phenomenon in early stages of irritative lesions of the supranuclear centres or pathways. The overaction of one (or more) of the vertical muscles which accompanies a horizontal squint with the production of an hyperphoria, hypertropia, hypophoria or hypotropia has been discussed (p. 241). The following discussion is of the the three conditions in which a overaction appears to be the main event.

Alternating Sursumduction (Dissociated Vertical Divergence)

In this condition when the vision of either eye is embarrassed (as with a tinted glass) the embarrassed eye deviates progressively upwards but reverts to its original position when the embarrassment ceases. Usually there is a symmetrical involvement of each eye, but occasionally it may be asymmetrical even to the extent that it is virtually unilateral. Sometimes the alternating sursumduction may occur spontaneously so that each eye in turn moves up and then down in a slow pendular manner at irregular intervals. In the absence of the upwards movements there may be no deviation (so that there is binocular single vision), but frequently there is a small vertical or even horizontal deviation. The condition is probably the result of some innervational imbalances of the centres controlling vertical movements. Operative measures are seldom warranted because these tend to be ineffective and the condition usually becomes less obvious with age. Diplopia is seldom experienced because it is avoided by suppression.

Skew Deviation

This may follow a destructive lesion of the cerebellum and the eyes at times become deviated in opposite directions; one eye turns up and out whilst the other eye turns down and in.

Oculogyric Crisis

This is liable to occur in paralysis agitans (Parkinsonism) which is a degenerative condition of the corpus striatum. Initially there is a weakness of conjugate and disjunctive movements of the eyes in association with a diminution of movement of the skeletal musculature, but this is followed by a muscular rigidity which is associated with jerky movements of the eyes (*cog-wheel rigidity*) and with a stiffness and tremor of the other muscles. Sometimes marked conjugate spasms of the eyes occur so that they move violently into a certain position (usually upwards) and are maintained there for a variable length of time, the so-called *oculogyric crisis*.

Nystagmus

Nystagmus is a disordered state of ocular posture in which the eyes exhibit involuntary oscillatory movements. There are two main types of rhythm in these movements: *pendular* in which the undulatory movements are equal in speed and in amplitude in each direction, and *jerky* in which a slow movement in one direction (the fundamental movement of the nystagmus) is followed by a rapid jerky movement in the opposite direction (the compensatory movement of the nystagmus to regain fixation)—rarely (except in a form of congenital idiopathic nystagmus) the nystagmus may be *mixed* with a pendular rhythm in one position of gaze and a jerky rhythm in another position of gaze. The nystagmus may occur in different planes: *horizontal, vertical, oblique* or *rotatory*, and in the jerky nystagmus the direction of the nystagmus is designated by the direction of its rapid phase; *right, left, up, down, oblique* (with right or left and up or down components), *clockwise rotatory*, or *anticlockwise rotatory*. Fine degrees of nystagmus which are not detected readily on direct viewing are demonstrated on ophthalmoscopic examination because of the magnification of the movement.

Nystagmus is rarely confined to one eye. The most common form of nystagmus occurs in both eyes in a *conjugate* manner (that is, in position of version), but it may occur also in both eyes in a *disjunctive* manner (that is, in positions of vergence—convergence or divergence—or when one eye turns up and the other eye turns down—the *see-saw nystagmus*), or it may even occur in a *dissociated* manner (that is, the nystagmus of the two eyes is unrelated to one another because each is dissimilar in direction, extent and speed).

Nystagmus is liable to occur in many circumstances, but in

general there are three main aetiological types: ocular, vestibular, and central (or neurological). There is also an idiopathic congenital nystagmus which is not related precisely to any of these three groups:

Ocular Nystagmus

This type of nystagmus is the result of a defective form of central vision which mitigates against a normal type of steady central fixation, perhaps because inadequate visual sensations lead to a failure of the normal tonic control of the extrinsic ocular muscles. An ocular nystagmus is usually of the pendular variety, but it may become jerky on lateral gaze. It should be noted, however, that the occurrence of nystagmus after the loss of central vision depends largely on the age of the patient at the time of the visual failure; in the newborn or young infant nystagmus develops invariably within a few weeks, between the ages of 2 months and 2 years nystagmus usually but not invariably develops, between 2 and 6 years nystagmus seldom develops except for a few irregular unsustained fixation movements, and after the age of 6 years nystagmus is absent.

There are certain distinct forms of ocular nystagmus:

Deviational Nystagmus. This occurs as a normal phenomenon when the eyes are turned conjugately to the limits of the binocular field of fixation (it is described more accurately as *nystagmoid jerks* rather than nystagmus), and it occurs pathologically in the field of action of the affected muscle in an incomitant squint and in certain positions of gaze in a supranuclear lesion.

Latent Nystagmus. This becomes obvious only on dissociation of the eyes so that the binocular visual acuity is significantly better than the uniocular visual acuity. It is sometimes of congenital origin.

Optokinetic Nystagmus. This is a physiological type of nystagmus which is induced by viewing a drum with alternate black and white lines which may be rotated vertically or horizontally; this is sometimes called the *railway nystagmus* because it occurs also in such activities as looking out of the window of a moving train. An optokinetic response may be elicited at an early age of life (certainly after the age of three months) and it forms a reliable method of determining the presence of visual function in an infant with suspected blindness. The integrity of the reflex is disturbed in lesions of the visual cortex or in lesions affecting the association pathways from the region of the visual centres to the motor centres in the brain stem as well as in ocular blindness.

Miner's Nystagmus. This is an acquired type of nystagmus which is due largely to working for prolonged periods in conditions of dim illumination (as in a coal mine), but there are other contributory factors; the crouched attitude of the miner with the persistent adoption of an upward gaze, the repeated exposure to noxious gases, and the mental stress of such work. There may be associated tremor of the head and spasm of the eyelids.

Vestibular Nystagmus

This type of nystagmus is the result of a disturbance of the elaborate labyrinthine mechanism which exerts a proprioceptive influence on the extrinsic ocular muscles. It may be induced in the normal person on causing movements of the fluid within the labyrinth by rotating the subject or by caloric stimulation and it may be induced also by galvanic stimulation. It occurs pathologically in any lesion (congenital or acquired) of the labyrinth or its subcortical pathways and centres. The nystagmus is of the jerky type with fine rapid horizontal and rotatory movements.

Neurological Nystagmus

This type of nystagmus is the result of a disturbance (congenital or acquired) of any part of the complex nervous mechanisms—visual, proprioceptive and motor—which control the posture of the eyes. It is jerky in type.

Idiopathic Congenital Nystagmus

This is a form of nystagmus which is almost certainly present shortly after birth but seldom becomes noticeable until the age of about 3 months when it increases in amount because of increased visual interest. It may be differentiated into two types according to the rhythm of the nystagmus—pendular or jerky.

Pendular Congenital Nystagmus. This is almost invariably the result of some ocular abnormality, so that the prefix *idiopathic* is not appropriate, although the nature of the underlying ocular defect may be difficult to detect, as in congenital tapetoretinal degeneration (p. 140), cone monochromatism (p. 25) and ocular albinism (p. 81) when it is of an inherited nature. The visual prognosis depends on whether the cause of the pendular nystagmus is susceptible to treatment, but almost inevitably the distant vision is restricted because the pendular nystagmus tends to persist even after the elimination of the cause.

Jerky Congenital Nystagmus. This is almost invariably of unknown origin (except when it is of an inherited nature) so that the prefix *idiopathic* is appropriate. It is reasonable, however, to regard it as some form of exaggeration of the fine movements of the normal eyes (high frequency eye tremors, rapid eye flicks—saccades—and slow motion drifts), the fixation movements which occur persistently during steady fixation and which are essential to the maintenance of a clear image of the fixation target; these movements are co-ordinated by the complex centres in the brain stem (p. 217), and presumably a slight derangement of the centres as the result of an inherited factor or some adverse neonatal influence may produce nystagmus in the absence of any other obvious neurological disorder. It is characteristic of this nystagmus that it varies greatly in different positions of gaze, and the position of least nystagmus (the neutral zone) provides the best form of vision so that a compensatory head posture is frequently adopted (unless the neutral zone happens to be to the straight-ahead position). The nystagmus tends to be greatest in the early years of life and then becomes progressively less, but even in adult life it is prone to sudden increases during times of stress and strain; this is of practical significance, for example, during an interview for a job or during an attempt to pass the visual part of a driving test. The close reading vision is usually remarkably good, although it may be necessary for the book to be held fairly near the eyes; this utilizes the reduction in the nystagmus which occurs in a position of marked convergence, and the position also provides magnification.

There are certain other features which may be associated with nystagmus:

1. A sensation of apparent movement of stationary objects is not a feature of nystagmus which develops in early life (congenital nystagmus), but it is a feature sometimes of the acquired forms of nystagmus.

2. An awareness of diplopia is only a feature of nystagmus when it is induced by some lesion of the central nervous system.

3. A head nodding may occur in the ocular type of nystagmus in children, the so-called *spasms nutans*; it seldom occurs before the age of 4 months and usually disappears spontaneously before the age of 3 years, although it may recur to some extent when the child is in dim illumination. This head nodding is not compensatory to the nystagmus because it has a slow and inconstant rhythm in contrast to the nystagmus which is fast and steady.

14 | Diseases of the Orbit

Structure and Function (Fig. 56)

The bony orbit is formed by four walls—roof, floor, lateral wall and medial wall; there is no posterior wall because the roof slopes down to meet the floor and because the lateral wall slopes backwards and medially to meet the medial wall at an angle of about 45°. The medial walls of the two orbits are more or less parallel with another, and this angulation of the lateral and medial walls deter-

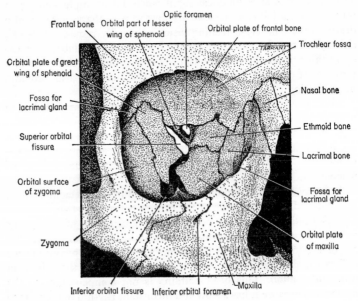

FIG. 56. *The right bony orbit viewed from in front*

mines the forwards and outwards direction of the orbital axis (Fig. 43). There are three spaces in the orbital walls which transmit various structures: the optic canal, the superior orbital fissure, and the nferior orbital fissure.

The Optic Canal

This is the space which is formed by the union of the two roots of the lesser wing of the sphenoid which arise independently from the body of the sphenoid and it transmits the optic nerve with its meningeal coverings (dura mater, arachnoid mater and pia mater), the ophthalmic artery, and some sympathetic fibres from the carotid plexus.

The Superior Orbital Fissure

This is a gap between the posterior part of the roof (lesser wing of the sphenoid) and the lateral wall (greater wing of the sphenoid); part of this is closed by dura mater but its wider part is open and provides a communication between the orbit and the middle cranial fossa for the transmission of several structures—cranial nerves III, IV and VI, the lacrimal, frontal and nasociliary branches of the ophthalmic division of the cranial nerve V, the superior and inferior ophthalmic veins, and sympathetic nerve fibres.

The Inferior Orbital Fissure

This is a gap between the posterior part of the lateral wall (greater wing of sphenoid) and the floor (maxilla and orbital process of the palatine bone) which provides a communication between the orbit and the infratemporal (zygomatic) fossa in front and pterygopalatine (sphenomaxillary) fossa behind for the transmission of several structures—the maxillary division of cranial nerve V, the secreto-motor nerve to the lacrimal gland from the sphenopalatine ganglion, the infraorbital artery, and communications from the inferior ophthalmic vein to the pterygoid venous plexus.

The Orbital Fascia

This consists of six different components:

1. *The bulbar fascia* (*Tenon's capsule*) covers the sclera from the limbus to the exit of the optic nerve from the eye and it provides two potential spaces; a subconjunctival space between the fascia and the overlying conjunctiva and an episcleral space between the fascia and the underlying sclera.

2. *The check ligaments of the extrinsic muscles* are developed to any great extent only in relation to the lateral and medial recti with attachments to the lateral and medial orbital margins, respectively; each check ligament acts by preventing undue freedom of movement of the eye away from the field of action of its associated muscle.

3. *The fascial sheaths of the extrinsic ocular muscles* closely invest each muscle. Superiorly in the orbit there is a close association of the sheaths of the superior rectus and superior oblique muscles with the sheath of the levator muscle which extends medially and laterally to become anchored at the orbital margins (thus forming the *superior transverse fascial expansion*), and inferiorly there is a close association of the sheaths of the inferior rectus and inferior oblique muscles which also extend medially and laterally to the orbital margins (thus forming the *inferior transverse fascial expansion* or *suspensory ligament* of the eyeball); these expansions act as checking mechanisms which prevent undue upwards and downwards movement of the eyes because they become taut by bowing forwards or backwards during such movements.

4. *The periorbital membrane* lines the inner surface of the orbit and is in continuity with the outer layer of the dura mater which lines the inner surface of the cranial cavity and the periosteum which covers the outer surface of the bones of the skull.

5. *The orbital septum* represents a fascial membrane which passes from the upper (and lower) orbital margins to the tarsal plate of the upper (and lower) eyelids so that the orbital space is separated from the lid substance.

6. *The connective tissue of the orbital fat* forms a supporting network within the orbital fat which fills the free space of the orbit.

The other constituents of the orbit—the eye, the optic nerve, the extrinsic ocular muscles and the lacrimal gland—are discussed in other chapters.

Congenital Anomalies

Craniofacial Dysostosis

A dysostosis of the skull is the result of a failure in the development of the primitive mesoderm which is concerned in the formation of the bones of the skull (including the orbit) whereby there is a premature synostosis of one or more of the sutures of the skull at a time when the brain is still expanding (most of this expansion occurs in the first decade of life). It is likely that the condition is determined early in intrauterine life (sometimes as an inherited disorder) so that the defects are evident in the newborn, but the full effects occur in the early years of life. Males are more commonly affected than females. There may be other associated bony defects such as syndactyly and synarthroses.

Oxycephaly (Tower Skull). A premature synostosis of the craniofacial sutures results in a vertical elongation of the head with a shortening of its anteroposterior diameter and, to a lesser degree, of its transverse diameter. The synostosis of the base of the skull determines the upwards expansion of the brain towards the patent anterior fontanelle with the formation of a dome-shaped head which tapers to its summit (and sometimes with the production of a meningocele or even a cerebral hernia) and the associated upwards displacement of the optic nerves is liable to cause optic atrophy; optic atrophy may also follow papilloedema which is the result of an increased intracranial pressure and this also causes headaches. The vertical direction of the forehead is accentuated by the absence of obvious superciliary arches and the face shows characteristic features; prominence of the nose, hypoplasia of the maxillae (flatness of the cheeks), and prognathism (prominence of the lower jaw). The orbits are shallow with a marked loss of the roof so that proptosis (or even a true forwards dislocation of the eye) and a divergent squint are common features; rarely there is an associated narrowing of the optic canals with consequent damage to the optic nerves. Mental retardation is a common feature because of the brain damage. In severe cases the removal of large parts of the bones of the vault of the skull may relieve pressure on the brain and of the roofs of the optic canals may relieve pressure on the optic nerves provided they are carried out sufficiently early.

Dolichocephaly. This represents a variant between *oxycephaly* and *scaphocephaly* (a long narrow head with elongation of the anteroposterior diameter and a narrowing of the transverse diameter) and it is represented characteristically by *Crouzon's craniofacial dysostosis* (*parrot-head*) in which there is a marked frontal bossing, a prominent hooked nose, a very marked recession of the maxillae, a very marked prognathism of the lower jaw with irregularly spaced dentition and persistent salivation, a marked proptosis and a sloping of the palpebral apertures in an outwards and downwards direction.

Hypertelorism. This is characterized by an excessively wide separation of the two eyes with the production of a bovine appearance; the interpupillary distance often exceeds 80 mm (as compared with a normal distance of about 60 mm). It follows a premature ossification of the greater wings of the sphenoid which remain extremely small so that the lateral directions of the orbits which are features of fetal life persist after birth and a divergent squint is a common feature. The optic nerves are not affected. The forehead is extremely shallow and the nose is characteristically upturned (*retroussé*).

Underdevelopment

A small orbit occurs characteristically when the eye is microphthalmic or absent (anophthalmos); it seems likely that the normal growth of the orbit in the child is dependent on an eye of normal size and this is evident also when an eye is enucleated in early childhood because the orbit tends to remain relatively small. A shallow orbit occurs sometimes in hydrocephalus.

Overdevelopment

An enlargement of the orbit is liable to occur in association with the expanding eye in buphthalmos (chap. 15), and in any form of expanding mass in the orbit.

Facial Asymmetry

This may follow undue pressure on the face during a difficult labour, and it is also a feature of the torticollis which occurs as the result of a tautness of the sternomastoid muscle on one side of the neck so that the affected side of the face develops to a lesser extent than the other side; as a rule there are no associated ocular complications.

Dermoid Cyst

This occurs in the orbit as an inclusion cyst and usually in association with the suture lines particularly in the upper and outer part of the orbit with an attachment to the underlying bone. The cyst contains many different tissues, such as sebaceous material, hair and fat. It commonly causes a ptosis of the upper lid, but it may also cause some degree of proptosis when it extends into the orbit. A leakage from a dermoid cyst may lead to the formation of a pseudotumour (see below). The cyst may be removed by simple excision, but sometimes the operation proves to be quite extensive, and a failure to secure complete removal may cause a granulomatous reaction of the surrounding tissues.

Meningo-encephalocele

This represents a herniation of a meningeal sac containing cerebrospinal fluid (*meningocele*) and usually also some brain tissue (*meningoencephalocele*) through a defect in the orbital wall, usually in the upper and inner part of the orbit between the frontal and ethmoid bones; this is readily determined on radiographical examination. Both orbits may be involved in the anomaly. The cystic herniation is usually pulsatile because it contains circulating cerebrospinal fluid; it increases in size when there is an increase in venous pressure, it may transmit a detectable bruit, and it is readily reducible by external pressure although this may cause serious side effects (such as convulsions, decrease in the pulse rate). The pressure of the cyst on the overlying skin is liable to lead to ulceration with an obvious risk of a spreading infection in the meninges (meningitis).

Orbital Varices

Congenital venous malformations may occur in the orbit with the production of a proptosis in childhood which is aggravated by pressure on the neck; there may also be some venous dilatations in the conjunctiva and skin of the affected eye. Sometimes there is a marked increase in the proptosis as the result of a haemorrhage which eventually forms a blood cyst of the orbit. A radiograph may show an enlargement of the orbit and sometimes concentric rings of calcification; *orbital phlebography* provides more detailed information and *ultrasonic examination* is also of localizing value.

Haemangioma

Haemangioma is discussed below under Tumours (p. 275).

Injuries

Orbital Haemorrhage

Severe contusion of the eye or orbit (sometimes in association with a fracture) may produce an intraorbital haemorrhage so that the eye becomes proptosed and there is an associated haemorrhage within the lids (ecchymosis) and the conjunctiva; it may also occur in the sudden venous congestion which follows strangulation. The proptosis of the eye causes a restriction of ocular movement, although this is usually only temporary unless the haemorrhage becomes organized by a process of fibrosis before its absorption is complete.

Perforation

Perforating injuries of the orbit by pointed objects such as a pair of scissors, or a knife, are liable also to cause an orbital haemorrhage, but they may produce more serious effects as the result of damage to other structures in the orbit (nerves, arteries, veins, extrinsic ocular muscles, or optic nerve) or as the result of the introduction of infection (orbital cellulitis), particularly when there is retained foreign material within the orbit. A deep injury may even involve the membranous coverings of the brain with a subsequent leakage of cerebrospinal fluid through the wound.

Treatment. Any infective element is treated by systemic antibiotics; a retained foreign body may be removed by an exploration of the orbit (orbitotomy, p. 277), but sometimes it is expedient (particularly when the foreign material is of a relatively inert metallic nature) to leave it alone unless it produces obvious adverse effects. An antitetanus injection is advisable in perforating injuries of the orbit, particularly when wood or vegetable material is introduced into the tissues.

A depressed fracture of the orbital margins may be widespread in its effect because it may extend into the skull with the occurrence of intracranial and neurological complications, into the nose or into the accessory nasal sinuses.

A fracture of the floor of the orbit (*blow-out fracture of orbit*) is liable to follow a direct blow on the eye which causes a marked increase in the intraorbital pressure during the sudden backward displacement of the eye with a rupture of the floor in the region of its weakest part (the region of the infraorbital groove). Some of the tissues in the lower part of the orbit may become trapped in the fractured area. There is usually a slight hypotropia of the eye when the other eye is looking straight ahead (or even no deviation), but there is a dramatic disturbance of elevation with an abrupt cessation of movement of the eye; this should be relieved by an early exploration of the lower part of the orbit by a subperiosteal approach to free the tethered inferior rectus and to prevent further adhesions by the insertion of a silicone sheet over the fractured area. Sometimes it may be necessary to deal with the fracture through the maxillary antrum.

A depressed fracture of the zygoma is relieved by a direct approach through an incision in the temporal fascia.

In a fracture of the orbit which causes a shattering of bone it is necessary to remove any bony fragments (together with any retained foreign material) and to attempt to restore the bony contours later.

A radiographic examination of the orbit is necessary in any form of suspected orbital fracture.

Inflammatory Conditions

Orbital Cellulitis

This is an acute inflammatory condition of the orbital fascia which is becoming relatively uncommon in modern times; the chronic form is discussed as a 'pseudotumour of the orbit'. The infection may spread directly into the orbit from a periostitis (of the periorbital membrane) or from a paranasal sinusitis. It may also reach the orbit indirectly by the bloodstream from some neighbouring or remote source of infection, or it may be introduced into the orbit in association with a perforating wound (particularly when there is a retained foreign body) or during an intraorbital operation. There is marked swelling and redness of the eyelids, chemosis of the conjunctiva, a tense form of proptosis, severe pain and restricted ocular movement. The increased intraorbital pressure causes oedema of the optic disc, congestion of the retinal veins, and sometimes obstruction of part of the vascular supply to the optic nerve with a consequent visual field defect. Infection of the exposed eye is liable to occur and may lead to a panophthalmitis. There is an associated pyrexia. Sometimes the infection may spread backwards with the production of the orbital apex syndrome or the sphenoidal fissure syndrome (chap. 13), a meningitis or a cavernous sinus thrombosis (see below).

A more localized form of orbital cellulitis occurs when the inflammatory process is limited largely to Tenon's capsule (*tenonitis*), although this condition is more commonly secondary to a severe inflammatory change of the eye (panuveitis or panophthalmitis).

Treatment. The condition may be relieved by intensive systemic antibiotics, but the formation of an abscess demands its incision and drainage.

Pseudotumour of the Orbit

This term is applied to a group of different clinical conditions which present in a manner similar to an orbital neoplasm but in the absence of any neoplastic change, hence the term *pseudotumour*. It seems likely that most of these conditions are forms of chronic orbital granulomata in association with some other disease like tuberculosis, sarcoidosis, syphilis, Wegener's granulomatosis (chap. 7), leakage from a dermoid cyst, fungal or parasitic disorders, or after trauma. There is evidence also that a pseudotumour may follow the release of lipids in the orbital tissues following a focus of fat necrosis, and it may also occur as a tissue reaction to an underlying adenocarcinoma of the lacrimal gland or to one of the reticuloses particularly a lymphosarcoma (chap. 12). It should be noted that a unilateral form of endocrine exophthalmos (see below), an ocular myositis (chap. 13), or an orbital cellulitis (see above), may simulate a pseudotumour. The usual feature is proptosis, but other features— pain, swelling of the lids, chemosis of the conjunctiva, and limitations of ocular movement with diplopia—are also inconstant manifestations. The proptosis may be sufficienctly severe to cause papilloedema or exposure keratitis. Radiological examination of the orbit shows an absence of any bony abnormality, but a soft tissue orbital shadow is sometimes evident. The diagnosis is only possible after the histological examination of a biopsy specimen, but as mentioned above such changes may mask the presence of an adenoma of the lacrimal gland with malignant tendencies or lymphosarcomatous deposits.

Treatment. Surgical removal usually necessitates exploration of the orbit by a lateral approach, but this is liable to be followed by postoperative scar tissue and extensive surgical interference is seldom worth while. The administration of systemic steroids is of value in many cases in reducing the proptosis, although the condition may recur on discontinuing the drug; sometimes a small maintenance dose may be sufficient to prevent this. Systemic antibiotics are unlikely to be of value, and irradiation is helpful only in the cases in which the cellular element is much greater than the fibrotic one in the biopsy specimen. Obviously an underlying malignant element demands extensive surgical treatment (exenteration) or irradiation of the whole orbit.

Cavernous Sinus Thrombosis

This usually results from an infection which spreads directly to the sinus by the bloodstream from various sources—the face, orbit, middle ear, mouth or paranasal sinuses—or which occurs in association with a generalized infection (pyaemia or septicaemia). There is usually some proptosis of the globe with loss of all movement as the result of an involvement of the motor cranial nerves (III, IV and VI) to the extrinsic ocular muscle; the involvement of the IIIrd cranial nerve determines also the fixed dilated pupil and the absence of accommodation. The cornea is anaesthetic because of the involvement of the ophthalmic division of the Vth cranial nerve. There is usually, but not invariably, an engorgement of the retinal veins and an oedema of the optic disc. The patient is generally acutely ill. The condition is liable to become bilateral because of the vascular communication which exist between the two cavernous sinuses.

Treatment. Intensive treatment with antibiotics and anticoagulants usually prevent a fatal termination to the disease which is becoming rare.

Mucocele of the Paranasal Sinuses

This follows a blockage of the accessory nasal sinuses by a polypus or by catarrhal inflammatory changes. It may enlarge sufficiently to extend into the orbit with a gradual displacement of the eye in a particular direction depending on the situation of the affected sinus; a sphenoidal sinusitis is liable to involve the optic nerve.

Lipodystrophies

Hand-Schüller-Christian Syndrome

In this disorder of lipid metabolism, which is one of the reticuloendothelial granulomatoses, xanthomatous deposits may occur in the orbits (sometimes within the sheaths of the optic nerve). Similar deposits may occur in the membranous bones of the skull (showing radiologically as large deficient areas) and less commonly in the long bones. Pituitary disorders (diabetes insipidus, dwarfism, etc.), pressure effects on the optic nerves or optic chiasma, and ophthalmoplegia may also occur in some cases.

The rare *eosinophilic granuloma* represents a related condition.

The deposits respond to irradiation with frequently a restoration of bony contours.

Vascular Disorders

Orbital Haemorrhage

This may occur after trauma and in severe blood dyscrasias such as leukaemia and chloroma.

Caroticocavernous Fistula

A severe head injury may cause a rupture of the internal carotid
artery **as** it lies within the cavernous sinus (a venous chamber) with
the formation of an arteriovenous communication (caroticocavernous
fistula) although the rupture may be delayed for several weeks
because it is preceded usually by the formation of an aneurysm;
such an aneurysm may occur also spontaneously. There is a pulsating form of proptosis which is synchronous with the pulse beat and
accompanied by a rhythmical throbbing within the head because of
the disruption of the orbital venous drainage which passes predominantly to the cavernous sinus; the conjunctival (and even
the retinal) veins are darkened and dilated, and the optic disc
may be oedematous. A secondary optic atrophy may develop later.
The condition is often self-limiting because the free arteriovenous
communication becomes obliterated by the development of a
thrombosis, but a more speedy resolution may be obtained by a
ligation of the ipsilateral internal (or common) carotid artery in
the neck.

Orbital Varices

This is discussed in congenital anomalies (p. 265).

Bony Disorders

Osteopetrosis (Albers-Schönberg Disease)

In this condition, which may become evident in early life, there
is an excessive formation of osseous tissue (osteosclerosis) so that
radiographically the bones appear unduly thickened and this is
liable to produce various defects—pareses (or palsies) of the extrinsic
ocular muscles as the result of compression of the motor cranial
nerves and optic atrophy as the result of its compression. Other
general abnormalities may occur such as hydrocephalus.

Osteitis Deformans (Paget's Disease)

In this condition, which usually becomes evident in later life, there
is a progressive enlargement of the bones. The vault of the skull is
particularly affected (the presenting feature may be an elderly
person's need for a larger hat size); similar changes are liable to
occur in the vertebral column and in the long bones. The progressive narrowing of the foramina of the skull leads to a compression

of the cranial nerves—the optic nerve is particularly liable to be affected—and headaches are common.

Exophthalmos and Proptosis

These terms are applied to an eye which is more prominent than normal; there is no precise distinction between them but there is a tendency to reserve the term *exophthalmos* for the prominence which is the result of an endocrine disorder and to apply *proptosis* to all other forms of prominence.

Diagnostic Methods. It is difficult to diagnose the presence of proptosis (or exophthalmos) on straightforward examination particularly as a marked difference in the width of the palpebral fissures of the two eyes gives a false impression but viewing the apices of the corneae from above by looking over the patient's head gives an accurate assessment of the relative prominence of one eye (or of the relative recession of the other eye). There are various forms of instruments (exophthalmometers) which measure the degree of prominence of each corneal apex from the lateral margin of the orbit.

ENDOCRINE EXOPHTHALMOS

In an understanding of the occurrence of exophthalmos (and its related phenomena—lid retraction and ophthalmoplegia) in thyroid dysfunction it is expedient to consider the manifestations which are associated directly with thyrotoxicosis (thyrotoxic manifestations) and those which are only indirectly associated with thyrotoxicosis (thyrotrophic manifestations).

Thyrotoxic Manifestations

In thyrotoxicosis an excessive amount of thyroid hormone (thyroxine) is responsible for two main effects:

First, an increased excitability of the sympathetico-adrenal system (sympathicotonia) probably as a result of a sensitization of the tissues by thyroxine to the circulating adrenaline; this accounts for many of the general features of the disease—tremor, increased excitability, increased sweating, tachycardia—and also perhaps for the lid retraction following an overaction of the well-developed smooth muscle in the upper lid and of the less well-developed smooth muscle in the lower lid; this concept is endorsed by the temporary decrease which occurs in the degree of lid retraction following the administration of a sympatholytic drug like hexamethonium and more recently by guanethidine which even when administered in the form of drops has a dramatic effect on lid retraction. The occurrence of lid retraction has led to the description of several clinical signs; a staring and frightened appearance of the eyes (Dalrymple's sign) which is particularly marked on attentive fixation (Kocher's sign), and a lagging of the upper eyelid on downward movement of the globe (von Graefe's sign).

Second, a generalized weakness of the striated muscles which accounts for some degree of ophthalmoplegia and even possibly for some degree of exophthalmos on the assumption that the weakness of the recti muscles which normally exert a retracting influence on the eye may allow the increased activity of the smooth muscle fibres of the periorbital and peribulbar tissues to exert a slight protracting influence on the eye); it should be noted, however, that ophthalmoplegia mainly and exophthalmos almost invariably are of a thyrotrophic nature, as discussed below.

It has been suggested that lid retraction in thyrotoxicosis is the result of an overaction of the levator muscle because the retraction is found essentially in the upper lid alone. It is difficult, however, to reconcile an overaction of the levator muscle (a striated muscle similar to the extrinsic ocular muscles) with a weakness of the other striated muscles, and the apparent confinement of the retraction to the upper lid is not necessarily against a sympathetic overaction because the greater effect of the smooth muscle of the upper lid masks any effect of the smooth muscle of the lower lid except in the early stages of lid retraction.

Thyrotrophic Manifestations

These may occur at any stage of a thyrotoxicosis, but sometimes they arise or become intensified after various forms of antithyroid treatment (surgical, medical or irradiational), and in other cases they may develop without any preceding general manifestations of the disease. There is some evidence that the changes are related to the activity of thyrotrophic hormone (TSH), a product of the basophile cells of the anterior pituitary body. Under normal conditions there is a close relationship between the pituitary and thyroid glands, the so-called pituitary-thyroid axis, and, therefore, between the thyrotrophic and thyroid hormones, whereby TSH stimulates the production of thyroid hormone (thyroxine) which is utilized by the tissues so that there is a gradual fall in the thyroxine level of the blood until a critical point is reached when there is a resumption of TSH secretion. It follows, therefore, that the ocular complications may be attributed to the unrestrained influence of TSH which occurs spontaneously or as a result of a reduction in circulating thyroid hormone following therapeutic measures, although it is more likely that the pituitary secretes an exophthalmos-producing substance (EPS) which is distinct from TSH. There is also a possible sex hormone factor because of the greater frequency of the condition in males despite the higher incidence of thyrotoxicosis in females. It is suggested that the production of exophthalmos is related to the activity of long acting thyroid stimulator (LATS), but evidence for this is inconclusive and the suggestion that the severe exophthalmos which sometimes follows thyroidectomy can be avoided by ensuring a total removal of thyroid tissue has found little acceptance. On the other hand, LATS seems to be associated with pretibial myxoedema which has similar pathological features to the orbit in thyrotrophic exophthalmos.

The thyrotrophic manifestations follow pathological changes within the orbit including the extrinsic ocular muscles; an increase of mucin, the hydrophilic nature of which induces oedema so that there is an increase in the bulk of the orbital contents with a further increase because of a secondary circulatory disturbance. Later a widespread fibrosis develops in the mucinous and oedematous tissue unless there is a speedy resolution. There is also some increase in lymphocytosis of the affected tissues. Clinically there are two main features—exophthalmos and ophthalmoplegia—and this form of endocrine exophthalmos may be termed *thyrotrophic exophthalmos* which relates TSH (probably incorrectly) to the exophthalmos, *progressive exophthalmos* which denotes the active nature of the exophthalmos, *malignant exophthalmos* which emphasizes its grave nature in certain cases, *exophthalmic ophthalmoplegia* which indicates the characteristic association of ophthalmoplegia with the exophthalmos, or the *hyperophthalmopathic form of Graves' disease* which defines the fact that the ocular manifestations sometimes predominate over the general signs. The extent of the exophthalmos is determined by simple inspection and the degree of retroocular resistance, which is a measure of the intraorbital pressure, is determined by attempting manually to retroplace the eye in the orbit or to move the eye from side to side or up and down in the absence of any rotation (*translatory movements*); often this may provide more important information than an assessment only of the degree of exophthalmos. The changes in the orbit are reflected in the surface

tissues of the eye with a marked oedema of the lids and chemosis of
the conjunctiva. A retraction of the swollen eyelids may follow the
protrusion of the eye, but this form of lid retraction is purely mechanical and is unrelated to the retraction which occurs in thyrotoxicosis. A superficial keratitis is liable to develop in the exposed eye
and this may lead to a severe hypopyon keratitis. Sometimes a
visual field defect may arise from an occlusion of one of the nutrient
vessels to the optic nerve because of the increased intraorbital
pressure. The ophthalmoplegia varies considerably in extent because certain muscles may be markedly affected (particularly the
elevating muscles) whereas other muscles may be relatively unaffected and even within one muscle the pathological changes may
assume a patchy distribution; this explains the failure sometimes of
a single biopsy specimen to provide a truly representative picture.
The squint usually shows obvious vertical and horizontal elements
because the impaired movement of the affected muscles is accompanied by gross overactions of the ipsilateral antagonist and contralateral synergic muscles (unless they are also affected) and a
subsequent fibrosis with contracture of an affected muscle decreases
the ocular mobility still further.

  Treatment. The main aim is to correct the underlying endocrine
dysfunction, and there is evidence that carefully planned treatment
may avoid severe thyrotrophic exophthalmos in certain cases; for
example, it may be unwise to relieve the thyrotoxic state too rapidly
when a moderate degree of thyrotoxicosis is associated with advanced thyrotrophic manifestations. An attempt may be made to
depress the progress of the exophthalmos by the use of hormones
(thyroxine, oestrogen, cortisone and ACTH) which damp down
the influence of the pituitary on the ocular tissues, or by the use of
direct pituitary irradiation, but the effects of these measures are
often unpredictable. The integrity of the cornea must be maintained
by the use of local antibiotics and by a large central tarsorrhaphy if
the cornea is exposed unduly; sometimes an orbital decompression
(lateral or transfrontal) may be necessary to relieve the pressure of
the orbital contents. Finally, when the condition is static the diplopia which follows a persistence of varying degrees of ophthalmoplegia may be relieved by surgical treatment (chap. 13).

PROPTOSIS

Proptosis may occur in a wide variety of conditions—congenital
(craniofacial dysostosis, meningo-encephalocele), traumatic (orbital

haemorrhage, orbital fracture), inflammatory (orbital cellulitis, pseudotumour of the orbit, cavernous sinus thrombosis, mucocele of the paranasal sinuses), and vascular disorders (orbital haemorrhage, caroticocavernous fistula, orbital varices), discussed above. It also occurs in a wide variety of tumour formations.

Tumours

There are various forms of orbital tumour which may be primary, secondary (by direct spread from an adjacent structure) or metastatic (by indirect spread from a distant source).

PRIMARY TUMOURS

Dermoid cyst. This type is discussed above (p. 264).

Haemangioma. This represents a collection of abnormally formed vessels and is essentially of congenital origin, although its full effect may not be apparent in the early weeks of life. The proptosis increases during any rise in the venous congestion, for example, when the infant cries. It seldom causes any interference with the other structures in the orbit and is often best left alone particularly as it may become slowly less marked. Irradiation is of limited value, and attempted surgical excision may prove unwise because of the difficulty of removing the whole mass without endangering the integrity of the many structures in the orbit and because of the liability to postoperative fibrosis. Sometimes a ligature of feeding vessels may be indicated following angiography.

Lacrimal Gland Tumours. Pleomorphic adenoma and adenocarcinoma (chap. 12).

Optic Nerve Tumours. Glioma, meningioma and fibroma (chap. 8).

Neurofibroma. This may develop in one of the peripheral nerves in the orbit, sometimes in association with other manifestations of Von Recklinghausen's disease (chap. 7).

Reticuloses. This term comprises several related tumours of the haemopoietic system—*lymphoma, lymphosarcoma, lymphadenoma (Hodgkin's disease),* and *reticulum cell sarcoma.* Occasionally the tumour may occur as an isolated mass, but usually similar deposits occur elsewhere because of their multicentric nature or because of an associated blood dyscrasia (leukaemia). These tumours almost invariably respond to irradiation, but if the condition is widespread it is necessary to attempt systemic treatment with anticancer drugs.

Chloroma. This is a malignant tumour of the haemopoietic system which is liable to involve the bones of the orbit (and skull) with usually an associated myelogenous leukaemia. It is more common in young children, particularly males. It spreads rapidly and almost invariably ends fatally despite a temporary response to irradiation.

Multiple Myelomatosis. This is a tumour which arises in many different parts of the myeloblastic tissue of the bone marrow in association with a severe anaemia.

Sarcoma. This primary malignant tumour occurs particularly in young people especially in males; the round-celled sarcoma has a higher degree of malignancy than the fibrosarcoma. It may occur rarely as a long-term complication of extensive irradiation for retinoblastoma.

Embryonal Sarcoma (Rhabdomyosarcoma). This tumour usually occurs in the orbit in early childhood (rarely after the age of 10 years) and it may start in the eyelid or in the region of one of the conjunctival fornices before spreading to the orbit with a rapid proptosis, chemosis of the conjunctiva and oedema of the eyelids so that it may be difficult to observe the eye. Irradiation of the orbit usually effects a fairly rapid resolution, but this is followed by a recurrence in the majority of cases (about 70 per cent); this recurrence usually becomes evident within six months of treatment and is very rare after an interval of two years. Exenteration of the orbital contents may be attempted in the cases which recur, or as a primary procedure, but the prognosis is very poor, even when it is followed by perfusion of the orbit with an antimetabolite like methotrexate or a biological alkylating agent like nitrogen mustard. The prognosis is most grave in those presenting in the first two or three years of life.

Endothelioma. This primary malignant tumour arises from the endothelium of the blood vessels or lymph vessels and they are sometimes extremely vascular so that the term *haemangioendothelioma* may be used. A variant of this tumour is the *perithelioma.*

Melanoma. This is a rare primary tumour of the orbit.

SECONDARY TUMOURS

From the Nasal Sinuses. This is usually a carcinoma.

From the Nasopharynx (Postnasal Space). This, too, is usually a carcinoma, but sometimes a sarcoma, a plasma-cell tumour or rarely a chordoma. The orbit may be invaded directly with the development of proptosis and with an involvement of the structures in the posterior part of the orbit with the features of the sphenoidal fissure syndrome (chap. 13) or the orbital apex syndrome (chap. 13), or it may be invaded indirectly after an intracranial extension so that the proptosis is preceded by a disturbance of one or more of the cranial nerves (the hypophyseo-sphenoidal syndrome or the petrosphenoidal syndrome).

From the Cranial Cavity. For example, a meningioma, glioma, or chordoma.

From the Ocular Tissues. For example, a uveal melanoma or a retinoblastoma.

METASTATIC TUMOUR

These are rare—a neuroblastoma from the adrenal gland or from the abdominal ganglia in early childhood, or a carcinoma from the breast, bronchus, etc. in the adult.

A form of false proptosis occurs when the eyeball is unduly large (high axial myopia, buphthalmos, staphyloma) and this is particularly obvious when it is unilateral.

Orbitotomy

The orbit may be explored from three different directions:

Anterior Orbitotomy. An incision through the eyelid and orbital septum along the upper (or lower) orbital margin is appropriate for lesions which are readily palpable through the eyelids and which are unlikely to extend deeply into the orbit.

Lateral Orbitotomy (Krönlein's Operation). An incision through the skin along the lateral orbital margin with an extension from the centre of this incision laterally to permit the removal of a quadrilateral part of the bone of the lateral orbital wall after reflection of the periosteal covering of the bone allows good exposure of the lateral and posterior parts of the orbit; sometimes a skin incision alone may be sufficient.

Transfrontal Orbitotomy (Naffziger's Operation). A removal of a portion of the orbital roof after exposure of the frontal lobe of the brain (which is then elevated) through the quadrilateral opening in the frontal bone is sometimes necessary in extensive lesions of the upper and posterior parts of the orbit.

Sometimes when the lesion which is responsible for the proptosis lies within the core of the extrinsic ocular muscles, an approach to this region by a *subconjunctival approach* is sufficient for diagnostic (biopsy) purposes.

Exenteration

This involves the removal of the entire orbital contents (including the eye and the orbital part of the optic nerve) within their peri-orbital coverings by an incision with cutting diathermy through the skin, muscle and periosteum around the entire orbital margin. The exposed bony orbit may be covered by a split skin graft from the medial surface of the thigh, but this is not essential and spontaneous epithelialization of the orbital surface occurs from the skin edges within a few months; it is usually expedient to omit the skin graft when there has been previous (or liable to be subsequent) irradiation of the area.

Enophthalmos

This term is applied to an eye which is less prominent than normal. It occurs when the eye is unduly small (microphthalmos, phthisis bulbi, or atrophia bulbi) or when a fracture of the floor of the orbit leads to a displacement of some of the orbital contents into the underlying antrum. A form of enophthalmos occurs when the eyeball is retracted in Duane's retraction syndrome (chap. 13) but the enophthalmos which is described in Horner's syndrome is a misnomer (chap. 11).

15 | Glaucoma

Glaucoma is a condition in which there is a rise of intraocular pressure (ocular tension) above the normal level. There are certain aspects of the structure and function of the eye to be considered before discussing the clinical features.

The Aqueous Humour

This is a clear fluid which passes from the capillary vessels within the processes of the ciliary body into the posterior chamber by a complex process which involves the mechanisms of dialysis, ultra-filtration and secretion. The aqueous passes forwards from the posterior chamber into the anterior chamber through the pupillary opening and percolates also backwards through the vitreous. It is concerned with the metabolic requirements of the cornea and the lens which are avascular structures and contributes to the maintenance of the intraocular pressure. The aqueous leaves the eye through the filtration angle (see below).

The Posterior Chamber

This is the narrow space which lies between the anterior surface of the lens and the posterior surface of the iris; it contains aqueous.

The Anterior Chamber (Fig. 57)

This is the space in the anterior segment of the eye which lies between the posterior surface of the cornea and the anterior surface of the iris and lens and which is bounded laterally by the filtration angle; it contains aqueous.

The Filtration Angle (Fig. 57)

The angle of the anterior chamber is bounded by a sieve-like structure (the trabecular tissues) through which the aqueous passes to a canal (the *canal of Schlemm*) within the sclera immediately behind the corneoscleral junction (the *limbus*); from this canal the aqueous passes to the episcleral veins on the surface of the eye by way of small veins, some of which contain only aqueous (*aqueous veins*) and others contain a mixture of blood and aqueous. The angle of the anterior chamber is not visible on straightforward examination

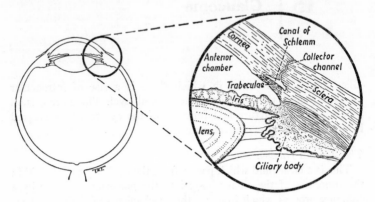

FIG. 57. *Section of the anterior segment of the eye to show the anterior chamber, the trabeculae of the filtration angle, the canal of Schlemm and a collector channel*

because it lies under the sclera beyond the limits of the cornea, but the use of a special corneal contact lens (a *gonioscope*) which incorporates an angled mirror provides an indirect view of the angle. The detailed inspection of this region is facilitated by the use of the slit-lamp microscope, and the following structures are visible in sequence: the root of the iris, the recess of the angle (this lies beyond the entrance and is wider than the entrance which is the narrowest part of the anterior chamber), a faint line which represents the scleral spur, the inner surface of the trabecular meshwork of the filtration area (the canal of Schlemm may be visible beyond this when filled with blood, but invisible when filled with aqueous), the terminal edge of Descemet's membrane (*Schwalbe's ring*) and the inner surface of the cornea.

The Intraocular Pressure (IOP) (Ocular Tension)

This is dependent on the influences of the vitreous which fills the posterior part of the eye and of the aqueous which fills its anterior part, but the aqueous is concerned primarily with the variations which may occur in this pressure because the volume of the vitreous tends to remain fairly constant except in gross intraocular disease or after a perforating injury involving the posterior segment of the eye. The influence of the aqueous is determined by two main considerations; the rate of entry of aqueous into the eye from the ciliary body and the rate of exit of aqueous from the eye through the filtration angle.

The intraocular pressure is measured indirectly by assessing the resistance of the sclera or of the cornea to compression; a manometric method involving the insertion of a needle into the anterior chamber would provide a direct and more accurate measurement, but it is obviously unsuitable for routine clinical use. The following methods are in use:

Digital Measurement. This is assessed by placing the tips of both forefingers on the surface of the upper lid, with the patient looking down, and then pressing the sclera through the lid with each forefinger in turn so that the resistance of the sclera to indentation is assessed in much the same way as the determination of fluctuation within an abscess. This is obviously only a comparative method whereby the tension of the eye is compared with the tension which is found in the average eye and it requires considerable experience before becoming even remotely reliable, but it provides a more accurate assessment of the differences in the tension between the two eyes.

Tonometric Measurement. This involves the use of an instrument termed a *tonometer* (for example, the *Schiötz tonometer*), the lower end of which is curved so that it may be applied to the outer surface of the cornea after surface anaesthesia with amethocaine 1 per cent drops. A metal plunger passes down the central part of the tonometer and impinges on the anterior pole of the cornea thereby causing a certain amount of indentation which is recorded by a lever on a scale; the weight of the plunger may be altered in some types of tonometer so that different readings on the scale are obtained in the same eye. The results of these readings are then translated into terms of intraocular pressure by graphic readings which have been obtained experimentally. This method is fairly accurate in most cases but it assumes, incorrectly sometimes, that the rigidity of the outer coat of the eye (cornea and sclera) has a more or less uniform value in all persons. More recently the *applanation tonometer*, which measures the amount of pressure which is required to cause a flattening of a small area of the normally curved cornea, has come into use and has a much greater degree of accuracy. Ideally the recording of the intraocular pressure of each eye by the applanation method should be a routine procedure in an examination of the eyes, certainly over the age of 40 years.

The normal intraocular pressure is between 16 and 22 mmHg, but is not maintained at a constant level in any one individual because of the variations (up to 3 to 5 mmHg) which occur during each 24 hours, the so-called *diurnal variations*; the highest pressure usually occurs in the early hours of the morning during sleep.

Tonographic Measurement. This is a more elaborate form of tonometry whereby the *coefficient of the facility of aqueous outflow* (*C*) is estimated by a measurement of the change which occurs in the pressure of the eye from its initial level (Po) during the application of the tonometer to the eye for a given length of time (usually 4 minutes). It is difficult, of course, to obtain values of C which are strictly comparable between individuals because the method does not take into account the variability of the rigidity of the outer coat of the eye, and a more accurate value is obtained by the applanation tonometer. Furthermore, it is obvious that any pressure on the eye produces modifications in its entire hydrodynamic system so that the significance of this method as a measurement simply of the ease with which aqueous is able to leave the eye must be regarded with some caution. Under normal conditions the value of C, as derived mathematically, should be more than 0·18, although values between 0·12 and 0·18 may be considered sometimes as within normal limits, or the value of C may be considered in relation to the initial intraocular pressure (Po/C) which should be less than 100, although values between 100 and 200 may be considered sometimes as within normal limits.

Anterior Chamber Cleavage Syndrome

This is a generic term applied to a number of morphologically distinct abnormalities which are the result of a faulty cleavage between the cornea and iris during embryonic development; in normal development at about the seventh week a split appears in the solid mass of undifferentiated mesenchymal cells which fill the anterior segment and this split extends laterally so that the cornea becomes separated from the trabecular meshwork and the iris with the formation of the anterior chamber. There are various anomalies which comprise this syndrome: *posterior embryotoxon* which represents an undue prominence of Schwalbe's ring which lies on the inner surface of the cornea near the filtration angle; *Axenfeld's anomaly* in which prominent iris processes span the anterior chamber angle and become adherent to Schwalbe's ring; *Rieger's anomaly* in which there are varying degrees of dysgenesis of the iris stroma; *Rieger's syndrome* in which Rieger's anomaly is associated with other forms of mesodermal dysgenesis particularly skeletal defects, hypodontia and partial anodontia; *congenital anterior synechiae* or *congenital leucoma adherens* in which the collarette of the iris is adherent to the pericentral corneal endothelium and stroma—this mimics the leucoma adherens which follows a perforating corneal ulcer (p. 55), and in the past many such cases have been regarded incorrectly as following an intrauterine kerato-uveitis. All these conditions are liable to be associated with the development of an infantile glaucoma (see below).

The Different Forms of Glaucoma

The term *glaucoma* indicates a diseased condition of the eye which follows an abnormal increase in the level of the intraocular pressure and covers many different conditions which may be *primary* or *secondary*.

Primary Glaucoma

Infantile Glaucoma (Buphthalmos)

This is a form of glaucoma which is determined congenitally as a result of a developmental anomaly of the tissues of the filtration angle, although the obvious effects of the condition are usually not apparent until some months or even a few years after birth. Sometimes only one eye is affected, but usually the condition involves both eyes although often to varying degrees. It is more common in boys than in girls. There may be a hereditary factor, and rarely it is part of the rubella syndrome (chap. 9).

A progressive enlargement of the eye is often the presenting feature because the immature outer coat of the infantile eye is unable to withstand the increased intraocular pressure. This causes an increase in the anteroposterior diameter of the eye with an increased curvature of the expanding cornea so that the anterior chamber becomes deep, and the eye becomes red and irritable with considerable photophobia. The eye becomes progressively myopic, but this is often unrecognized because of the other changes in the eye. The cornea often remains remarkably clear despite its enlargement,

K*

but eventually it becomes hazy as a result of oedematous changes in the epithelium and in the stroma following localized ruptures of Descemet's membrane. The increased intraocular pressure also exerts its effect on the optic nerve head so that the optic disc becomes progressively atrophic and cupped with severe and permanent loss of vision so that eventually blindness may ensue in the absence of effective treatment.

Treatment. Many forms of drainage operation (trephine, flap sclerectomy with iris inclusion, etc.) have been attempted in this condition, but a goniotomy is the most satisfactory procedure; this consists of stripping away the abnormal tissues from part of the filtration angle with a goniotomy knife which is inserted at the limbus into the anterior chamber and directed across the anterior chamber to the angle on the opposite side of the point of insertion under direct view through a gonioscopic lens which lies on the surface of the cornea, aided by the magnification which is provided by special operating glasses or the operating microscope and by an intense focal illumination. This operation may be repeated several times if necessary in a different or in the same part of the filtration angle. It is desirable for the goniotomy to be carried out at a reasonably early stage before the development of advanced degenerative changes in the eye.

Chronic Simple Glaucoma (Open-angle Glaucoma)

This is a form of glaucoma, the mechanism of which is inadequately understood, but it seems likely that the defect lies in the region of the filtration angle: perhaps as the result of abnormal changes in the tissues of the filtration angle (for example, of a mucinous nature) which gradually impede the passage of aqueous; as the result of a failure of the action of cells in the trabecular meshwork which normally produce an adjustment to changes of osmosis; as the result of sclerotic changes in the fine vessels which drain the aqueous from the canal of Schlemm; or as the result of an anomaly of the sympathetic (or parasympathetic) nerve complexes of the region. It is essentially a disease of the middle aged or elderly—only a few cases occur before the age of 40 years—although isolated cases may occur at any age even in childhood (*juvenile glaucoma*). It is almost invariably bilateral, but both eyes are seldom affected equally at any one stage.

Clinical Features. In contrast to most other forms of glaucoma this type is practically free from all symptoms (no pain, except perhaps a very occasional ache, no haloes, etc.), except for an insidious and progressive visual loss which usually only affects the peripheral part of the vision to any marked degree until the later stages so that it may remain unnoticed by the patient until it encroaches on the fixation area. This lack of awareness is also explained by the fact that the visual fields of the two eyes have a large amount of overlap (the binocular field of vision, chap. 16, Fig. 60) so that extensive loss of vision of one eye, even with involvement of the central vision, may be masked by the less affected visual field of the other eye.

There are, however, many objective findings in the disease:

1. *Visual field loss.* Characteristically there is a progressive loss of the peripheral visual field, as demonstrated on the perimeter (chap. 16), particularly in the nasal part of the field and often in the upper nasal quadrant before the lower one, with a gradual spread towards the fixation area so that ultimately there is a permanent loss of central vision. It is important, however, to appreciate that other subtle changes are present in the more central parts of the visual field, as demonstrated on the tangent (for example, Bjerrum) screen (chap. 16), at a much earlier stage. For example, there is a restriction of the peripheral limit of the field using a very small white target (1 mm in diameter) at a distance of 2 m in the region of the blind spot which becomes isolated (or 'bared') outside the distorted circle (Fig. 58); normally this target would provide a circular field of 25° to 30° so that the blind spot which lies about 13° to 18° from the fixation point would lie within the field. There are also sometimes small scotomata within a narrow zone extending in an arcuate form above (Fig. 58) and below the blind spot—when these scotomata become confluent they are termed *arcuate scotomata.* These changes in the central field are of vital importance in the early recognition of the disease but they are detected only by careful quantitative methods of perimetry.

2. *Increased intraocular pressure.* A characteristic feature is a raised intraocular pressure, but the extent of this is variable in different patients—in some it may be only slightly raised whereas in others it may be high—and it is also variable in any one patient over a period of 24 hours when there is an exaggeration of the normal diurnal variation so that recordings of the pressure every 4 hours over a period of 24 (or even 48) hours are sometimes necessary to ascertain the true extent of the pressure. An isolated reading may even be normal in some cases.

3. *Abnormal facility of aqueous outflow.* Tonographic measurements show a diminished outflow of aqueous—C less than 0·18 (or in certain cases 0·12) and Po/C more than 100 (or in certain cases 200)—in a significant number of cases.

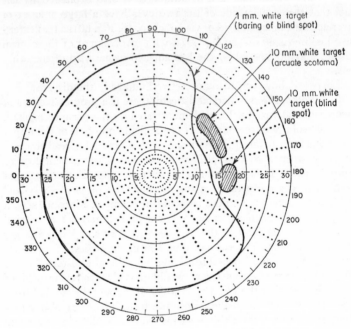

FIG. 58. *Visual field chart to show 'baring' of the blind spot and an arcuate scotoma*

4. *Pathological cupping of the optic disc* (Fig. 59). The effect of the increased intraocular pressure is noted particularly in the optic disc with a gradual enlargement of the optic cup due to a progressive degeneration of the optic nerve fibres within the optic disc; this degeneration is the result of an interference with the capillary bood supply of the nerve fibres rather than a direct pressure effect on the fibres. In advanced glaucoma the cup extends to the disc margin so that the retinal vessels dip markedly on crossing it, but it is important to recognize earlier forms of cupping. It is not possible to define the size of the abnormal cup because the size of the normal cup varies in different individuals and in different types of refraction, but there

are certain features which should be considered during any ophthalmoscopic examination:

It is rare for the size of the cup to occupy more than 70 per cent
of the area of the disc. This measurement applies only to the cross-
sectional area of the cup; the depth of the cup is of much less significance and the ability to observe the lamina cribrosa which lies
beyond the floor of the cup may be a feature even of a relatively
small cup.

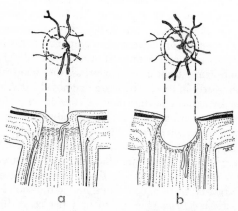

FIG. 59. *(a) Physiological cupping and (b) pathological cupping of the optic disc
as seen on section of the optic nerve head and as seen ophthalmoscopically*

It is usual for the cups of the two discs in any one individual to
be similar in size, except when the two eyes have a marked difference
in refractive error so that ophthalmoscopic examination inevitably
provides a misleading impression.

The development of pathological cupping is associated with an
accentuation of the normal nasal shift of the retinal vessels as they
pass through the cup.

Note: There is evidence that cupping of the optic disc may occur
rarely in the absence of any increased intraocular pressure (the so-
called *cavernous optic atrophy* or *low-tension glaucoma*); it is possible
that the susceptibility of the optic nerve-head to the effects of a
normal intraocular pressure is the result of obliterative sclerosis of
the nutrient vessels.

5. *Abnormalities of the filtration angle.* Gonioscopic examination
usually shows an open angle in chronic simple glaucoma with no

demonstrable pathological features, but in advanced cases there are sometimes areas of angle closure because of the formation of peripheral anterior synechiae particularly in cases where the angle is not uniformly wide.

6. *Provocative tests.* The water-drinking test (1 litre of water after 12 hours of fasting) produces a significant rise in the intraocular pressure and a decreased facility of aqueous outflow in the majority of cases.

Treatment: Medical. The treatment of open-angle glaucoma by the topical application of various drugs has been in force since the later part of the nineteenth century, but in recent years the emergence of new drugs has provided a fresh emphasis of the importance of medical treatment and indeed it seems possible that it may eventually supplant surgical treatment as the main therapeutic method, particularly in cases which are diagnosed early.

The ocular hypotensive drugs may be considered in four groups according to their pharmacological characteristics:

1. *The anticholinesterase drugs.* These drugs which potentiate the effects of acetylcholine at the myoneural junctions as the result of an inhibition of the cholinesterase which normally destroys it, form a large group of pressure-lowering drugs which act primarily by lowering the resistance to aqueous outflow (and also act as miotics and cyclospastics). *Eserine* ($\frac{1}{4}$ per cent or $\frac{1}{2}$ per cent) drops have a maximum effect during a period of about 6 hours, but this is somewhat variable in certain eyes and their prolonged use is liable to cause irritation and even intolerance after a time. DFP (di-isopropyl fluoro-phosphonate) 0·025 per cent, 0·05 per cent, or 0·1 per cent) and phospholine iodide (0·06 per cent, 0·125 per cent or 0·25 per cent) are powerful drugs which retain their effects for 24 or even 48 hours but they are also liable sometimes to cause congestion, discomfort and even pain.

2. *Pilocarpine* (1 per cent, 2 per cent, 3 per cent or 4 per cent) drops. This drug has a pressure-lowering effect which is limited to about four hours, although its miotic and cyclospastic effects persist for a longer time. It acts directly on the muscle fibres unlike the anticholinesterase drugs. It causes a lowering in the resistance to aqueous outflow and also a diminution in the secretion of aqueous; the contraction of the ciliary muscle reduces the arterial supply to the ciliary processes so that there is a reduction of aqueous formation and opens up the choroidal veins so that there is an increase of aqueous removal.

3. *The epinephrine drugs.* Laevo-epinephrine is the most potent pressure-lowering drug of this group and is used in the form of drops. It lowers the resistance to aqueous outflow and acts as an inhibitor of aqueous function for at least 24 hours. It has no miotic effect and indeed causes some dilatation of the pupil so that it is useful in glaucoma associated with central lens opacities, although it is contraindicated if there is any element of angle closure. It has no cyclospastic effect. Unfortunately it may have certain side effects; cardiac arrhythmias, increased pigmentation of the skin, vasospastic degenerative macular lesions, etc.

4. *Carbonic anhydrase inhibitors.* The administration of Diamox (for example, 125 mg 6 hourly) by mouth causes a diminution of the entry of aqueous into the eye from the ciliary body because it inhibits the action of carbonic anhydrase which is concerned in the transference of aqueous across the blood-aqueous barrier; it is of great value in reducing the intraocular pressure for short periods, but is liable to cause complications when used for prolonged periods—loss of appetite, general malaise, paraesthesia, and renal colic.

Treatment: Surgical. Most of the operations for chronic simple glaucoma are designed to promote drainage of the aqueous humour from the eye into the subconjunctival tissues thereby preventing an excessive rise of the intraocular pressure. The drainage area is formed at the limbus and consists of a circular hole (*trephine*), a flap opening (*sclerotomy*) or the formation of a flap (*sclerectomy*), and these procedures are combined usually with the removal of the underlying part of the iris (*peripheral iridectomy*) to prevent the iris from sealing the opening; in this way the aqueous drains freely into the subconjunctival tissues. Sometimes part of the iris may be left projecting through the sclerotomy (*iris inclusion* or *iridencleisis*), although care is taken to ensure that the iris is completely covered by the overlying conjunctival flap because exposed iris tissue might lead to the development of a uveitis, perhaps even a sympathetic ophthalmitis (chap. 6); this operation is of particular value in cases showing areas of angle closure. In another type of operation the aqueous is drained into the choroidal circulation along a channel which is formed in the suprachoroidal space (*cyclodialysis*); this operation is of particular value in aphakic eyes. More rarely an attempt is made to diminish the production of aqueous by the application of diathermy to parts of the ciliary body (*surface or perforating cyclodiathermy*) or the application of intense cold (*cryotherapy*); such an operation is

seldom indicated in an uncomplicated case of chronic simple glaucoma, except perhaps in Negroes in whom excessive amounts of
pigment greatly prejudice the permanent patency of any drainage
operation.

Closed-angle Glaucoma (Congestive Glaucoma)

This form of glaucoma is caused by a narrowing of the entrance
to the angle of the anterior chamber; it is found particularly in the
small hypermetropic eye which has a shallow anterior chamber (it is
very rare in the myopic eye with a deep anterior chamber), and this
shallowness occurs sometimes as a familial characteristic. The narrow
angle by itself, however, is not sufficient to produce glaucoma so
that many such eyes remain normal indefinitely, and various other
factors play significant contributory roles:

1. A swelling of the root of iris as the result of some vascular
change which may be induced by a nervous stimulus perhaps of
hypothalamic origin. Certainly there is often an emotional factor in
congestive glaucoma.

2. A crowding of the angle of the anterior chamber by a dilatation of the pupil—after the use of a mydriatic or sometimes merely
on exposure to darkness—or by an increase in the bulk of the lens in
an elderly person.

3. A state of relative pupillary block which causes a lifting forwards of the iris against the trabecular meshwork by the pressure of
the aqueous which accumulates behind the iris in the posterior
chamber.

These changes may produce an area of iridocorneal contact at
the entrance into the angle so that the passage of aqueous is impeded;
the subsequent absorption of the residual aqueous in the angle
through the filtration meshwork obliterates the entire angle and, in
the absence of effective treatment, leads to the formation of peripheral anterior synechiae.

Clinical Features. The subjective symptoms of closed-angle glaucoma are usually strikingly evident. In a mild subacute attack there
is discomfort of the eye (because of a sudden rise of intraocular
pressure) and some degree of generalized mistiness of the vision
often with an awareness of rainbow-like haloes (resulting from the
development of corneal oedema); these attacks may be only transient
(the *prodromal attacks*), but usually they tend to become more prolonged and severe so that an acute attack occurs with intense pain
in and around the eye, photophobia, lacrimation, marked loss of

vision, and sometimes even vomiting; if not relieved intractable blindness is inevitable (*absolute glaucoma*).

The objective signs of closed-angle glaucoma are also strikingly evident:

Redness of the eye particularly in the circumcorneal region (*ciliary injection*) which varies in intensity according to the severity of the attack; this type of redness may occur also in acute irido-cyclitis or even to some extent in intense conjunctivitis.

Steamy haze of the cornea caused by varying degrees of corneal epithelial oedema with eventually an oedema also of the corneal stroma.

Shallowness of the anterior chamber; this is a basic characteristic of the condition which is accentuated by the oedematous state of the iris. The angle of the anterior chamber is obliterated, but it is usually not possible to examine the angle in detail because of the corneal haze.

Partial dilatation of the pupil which becomes elongated vertically so that it assumes an oval shape. The direct and consensual reactions of the pupil to light are diminished and even absent in severe cases.

Swelling of the eyelids in a severe and persistent attack.

Raised intraocular pressure often to extremely high levels.

The optic disc is seldom cupped except in the very advanced stages of the condition, although it is usually impossible to obtain an adequate view of the fundus during the course of a congestive attack because of the corneal haze, and this is in contrast to chronic simple glaucoma when cupping occurs early in the disease. It follows that visual field changes are also only late features.

Provocative tests: The *mydriatic test* (confinement to a dark room or the instillation of a mydriatic like homatropine) causes a signifi-cant rise in the intraocular pressure in the majority of cases of con-gestive glaucoma so that it may be used to confirm the diagnosis in doubtful cases; the significance of vague congestive symptoms may be difficult to determine otherwise because the eye remains normal in appearance except for the narrowness of the angle of the anterior chamber.

Treatment : Medical. A subacute closed-angle glaucoma may re-spond rapidly to the use of a miotic like eserine ¼ per cent and sub-sequent attacks may be avoided, at least for a reasonable period of time, by the routine use of a miotic like pilocarpine 1 per cent al-though it is best to avoid the possibility of later complications by surgical intervention (see below). An acute congestive glaucoma demands rapid and energetic treatment; oily eserine 1 per cent every 15 minutes for 2 hours and then less frequently, the application of heat to the eye in the form of hot spoon-bathings or by the use of an electrically heated eye pad (*Maddox heater*), and the use of Diamox (usually by intramuscular injection to promote a speedy effect) to reduce the formation of the aqueous, or the use of osmotic agents like urea or glycerol. The mechanism of miotics in reducing the intraocular pressure has been discussed in relation to chronic simple glaucoma, but in congestive glaucoma their main effect is in pulling the iris away from the filtration angle.

Treatment : Surgical. In cases which respond to medical treatment subsequent attacks may be avoided by the performance of a *peripheral iridectomy* to prevent the occurrence of iridocorneal contact, although it is important to ascertain that there is no impairment of the facility of aqueous outflow (at a time when there is no congestive attack) otherwise the peripheral iridectomy should be combined with some drainage procedure as in chronic simple glaucoma. In cases which fail to respond completely to medical treatment within a reasonable period (about 6 hours) a basal iridectomy should be performed.

Congestive glaucoma should always be regarded as a potentially bilateral disease, so that treatment of the affected eye must also include the use of a simple miotic like pilocarpine in the apparently unaffected eye to prevent any risk of angle closure if there is any form of narrow angle, with subsequently a peripheral iridectomy even in the absence of any previous congestive symptoms.

Secondary Glaucoma

Mechanism

Secondary glaucoma may occur in a wide variety of conditions (which are discussed elsewhere) usually as a result of a mechanical interference of the circulation of the aqueous humour.

Obstruction of the Filtration Angle by an Accumulation of Abnormal Materials. This would include:

1. *Haemorrhage* as the result of trauma (perforating or nonperforating), following some intraocular operation, particularly involving the iris, or as the result of some lesion of the anterior uvea (for example, an angioma or a leiomyoma) which is liable to bleed.

2. *Inflammatory material* (cells or exudate) as the result of an irido-cyclitis—sometimes in the acute stage of the disease but more commonly in the later stage after several recurrences.

3. *Vitreous* as the result of the extension of vitreous into the anterior chamber after injury or after a cataract extraction.

4. *Lens material* as the result of the liberation of lens particles into the anterior chamber following a perforating injury involving the lens, following an extracapsular cataract extraction or discission, or following a phaolytic glaucoma (chap. 9).

5. *Abnormal material from the ciliary body*. In this condition the filtration angle becomes embarrassed by the accumulation of white particles which collect also on the anterior lens capsule and on the pupillary margin where they give the impression of representing ex-foliations of the lens capsule, but it is now known that this material, which is of a mucinous nature, arises from the inner surface of the ciliary body and that its occurrence on the pupillary margin is purely coincidental; hence the term *pseudocapsular glaucoma* (or *pseudoexfoliation of the lens capsule*). The condition usually occurs in the elderly.

Obliteration of the Filtration Angle by the Formation of Peripheral Anterior Synechiae. This is a result of:

1. The subsequent organization of the abnormal materials discussed above.

2. The delayed reformation of the anterior chamber after its partial or total loss following a perforating injury or operation or following an anterior dislocation of the lens.

3. The occurrence of new vessel formations on the anterior sur-face of the peripheral part of the iris (*rubeosis iridis*), a complication liable to follow conditions of severe retinal damage; central retinal vein thrombosis, diabetic retinopathy, old-standing retinal detach-ment, retrolental fibroplasia, etc. It is suggested that the neovascu-larization is the outcome of an abnormal stimulus from the anoxic retina.

Obstruction of the Passage of the Aqueous from the Posterior Cham-ber to the Anterior Chamber through the Pupillary Aperture. This is a result of:

1. The occurrence of an *iris bombé* (total adherence of the pupil margin to the lens) after severe uveitis (see chap. 6). This may be termed *seclusion of the pupil* and it may occur also as the result of an adhesion between the iris and the prolapsed intact vitreous face following an intracapsular cataract extraction (pupil block).

2. The occurrence of an *occlusion of the pupil* following a severe anterior uveitis (p. 85).

3. The occurrence of a pupil block may result from a congenital abnormality of the shape of the lens (spherophakia) (chap. 9) or from a hernia of vitreous through the pupil in the aphakic eye.

Note : There is recent evidence that the persistent use of topical steroids may cause some increase in the intraocular pressure in normal (nonglaucomatous) eyes particularly when there is a family history of glaucoma, so that in a few cases a chronic simple form of secondary glaucoma is liable to follow their use. Fortunately the glaucoma usually subsides after the withdrawal of steroids or following the use of pilocarpine drops.

Prevention

It is essential to try and prevent secondary glaucoma by the adequate treatment of the conditions which predispose to its occurrence, for example, full mydriasis in iridocyclitis, the restoration of the anterior chamber after its loss by the use of air, the removal of an extensive hyphaema, etc.

Treatment. In general treatment should be directed to the cause of the secondary glaucoma, but Diamox is of value in obtaining a temporary reduction in the intraocular pressure before the general measures become effective. In intractable cases operation is necessary—an iridectomy may be of value in certain cases when there is an obstruction in the filtration angle or in the pupillary area, but sometimes a drainage operation or a procedure to reduce the production of aqueous is necessary.

16 | The Afferent Visual Pathway

Each component of the afferent visual pathway is discussed with regard to the disposition of the visual fibres, their blood supply, the characteristics of the visual field defects which follow their involvement, and the nature of the lesions which cause such defects, thus providing an opportunity to describe various neuro-ophthalmological conditions instead of including them in a separate chapter.

Structure and Function

Retina and Optic Nerve Head

The visual fibres arise from the retinal ganglion cells and are divided into four main groups by a vertical line which bisects the macula,* so that there is a temporal hemiretina (including a temporal hemimacula) and a nasal hemiretina (including a nasal hemimacula), and by a horizontal line which bisects the macula, so that there is an upper (or dorsal) hemiretina (including an upper hemimacula) and a lower (or ventral) hemiretina (including a lower hemimacula) so that there are four different retinal quadrants—upper temporal, lower temporal, upper nasal and lower nasal—with fibres subserving central vision (from part of the macula) and peripheral vision (from the rest of the retina) in each quadrant. It should be noted that all the macular fibres and most of the peripheral fibres have corresponding fibres in the other eye (chap. 13) which are concerned with the binocular field of vision, but the most peripheral fibres of the upper and lower nasal quadrants have no corresponding fibres in the other eye and are concerned with the peripheral uniocular

---

* The term *macula* is used to denote the part of the retina which is concerned with central vision; it embraces the fovea and parafovea.

field of vision which forms a small extension on each temporal side of the binocular visual field (Fig. 60).

All the retinal fibres converge on the optic nerve-head as though it lies at the junction of the nasal and temporal parts of the retina and not, as it is, within the nasal part, so that some of the fibres run

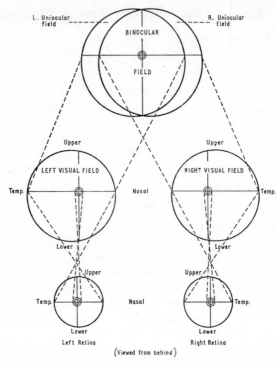

FIG. 60. *Diagram to show the projection of the visual field from each retina, and the relation of the binocular visual field to the right and left uniocular visual fields*

a complex course (Fig. 61). The nasal peripheral fibres pass more or less directly to the nasal border of the disc, except those arising from the retina above and below the temporal side of the optic disc which curve slightly in passing to the upper and lower aspects of the nasal border of the disc; this curve is accentuated markedly by the nasal fibres from the small portion of the retina between the temporal side of the optic disc and the macula (the *juxtapapillary* *fibres*) which pass to the extreme upper and lower aspects of the nasal border of the disc. The temporal peripheral fibres pass by a curved course from their origins above and below the horizontal raphe* to the upper one-fifth and lower one-fifth of the temporal border of the optic disc; this curved course is dictated by the presence of the large papillomacular bundle of fibres on the temporal side of

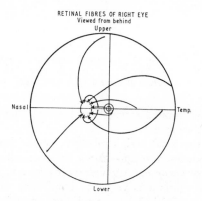

RETINAL FIBRES OF RIGHT EYE
Viewed from behind
Upper

Nasal

Temp.

Lower

FIG. 61. *Diagram to show the direction of the visual fibres on passing from the different areas of the retina to the optic disc (right eye viewed from behind)*

the disc. The nasal macular fibres pass directly in closely related upper and lower groups to the temporal aspect of the optic disc in association with temporal macular fibres which curve sharply from their origin to form with the nasal macular fibres a large compact oval-shaped bundle which occupies three-fifths of the temporal margin of the disc (the *papillomacular bundle*).

In all quadrants the more peripheral fibres lie deeply in the nerve fibre layer of the retina and peripherally in the optic nerve-head, whereas the less peripheral fibres lie superficially in the retina and centrally in the optic nerve-head (Fig. 62).

The blood supply of the retina has a dual nature; the inner part, including the nerve fibre layer, is supplied by the central retinal artery, and the outer part, including the visual receptors, is supplied by the underlying capillary layer of the choroid (the choriocapillaris), except for the macular area which is nourished

* The horizontal raphe extends from the macula to the temporal periphery of the retina and separates the temporal peripheral fibres into upper and lower groups.

only by the choriocapillaris. The terminal branches of the central
retinal artery function as end arteries so that each branch supplies
a clear-cut bundle of visual fibres. The blood supply of the optic
nerve-head is derived almost exclusively from the ciliary circulation
with some contributions also from the adjacent choroid, and it is

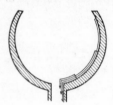

FIG. 62. *Diagram to show the relative positions of the
peripheral, equatorial and central visual fibres in the
retina and in the optic nerve-head*

doubtful to what limited extent branches from the central retinal
artery share in the process.

A lesion of the nasal peripheral fibres on the nasal side of the
optic disc produces a sector-shaped scotoma which lies in the
temporal field of vision and expands as it passes to the periphery;
the scotoma is continuous with the blind spot when the lesion
borders on the disc (Fig. 63a), it extends to the peripheral limit of the

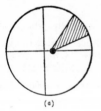
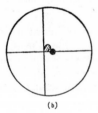

(a)   (b)

FIG. 63. *Diagrams to show the scotomata which occur in the temporal part of the
visual field following isolated lesions of the nasal visual fibres in the retina (right
eye)*

temporal field when all the nerve fibres in the affected area are involved, it is broad when the affected area is large, and it is narrow
when the affected area is small. A lesion of the nasal peripheral
fibres which lies between the optic disc and the macula produces a
markedly arcuate scotoma which is adjacent to the blind spot (juxtapapillary scotoma) (Fig. 63b). A lesion of the temporal peripheral
fibres produces an arcuate scotoma which extends from the region
of the blind spot around the fixation area towards the horizontal

meridian in the nasal part of the field (Fig. 64a). Sometimes there may be arcuate scotomata in both the upper and lower parts of the field although these are often of unequal size so that they produce a characteristic nasal step on the horizontal meridian (Fig. 64b). The arcuate scotoma often fails to reach the blind spot even when the lesion directly involves the upper or lower temporal borders of the

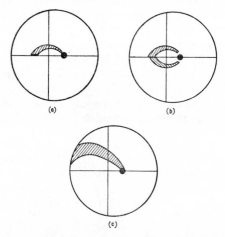

FIG. 64. *Diagrams to show the scotomata which occur in the nasal part of the visual field following isolated lesions of the temporal visual fibres in the retina* (*right eye*)

disc, and this results from the failure of such a lesion to involve the nasal retinal fibres which lie between the temporal border of the disc and the macula because these fibres terminate in the upper and lower parts of the nasal border of the disc. The greater frequency of an arcuate scotoma in the upper than the lower part of the visual field in chronic simple glaucoma may be related to the increased crowding of the fibres in the lower part of the optic nerve-head as a result of its slightly asymmetrical division into upper and lower parts. A localized lesion of the retina from behind, for example a patch of choroiditis, produces an isolated scotoma in the visual field corresponding to the area which suffers a destruction of its visual receptors, but this is followed by an extension of the scotoma towards the periphery due to a subsequent involvement of the nerve fibre layer; at a certain stage there is sometimes a small area of sparing of the visual field between the two defects because of a temporary sparing of the fibres from the retina immediately peripheral to the affected area which lie superficially in the retina.

The lesions which affect the retina and optic nerve-head are discussed in Chapters 7 and 8.

Optic Nerve

In the distal part of the optic nerve the visual fibres maintain to a large extent the distribution which they assume in the optic nerve-head; the upper retinal fibres lie in the upper half of the nerve and the lower retinal fibres in the lower half, the nasal peripheral fibres lie in the upper and lower regions of the medial part with the most peripheral fibres (uniocular fibres) lying superficially, the temporal peripheral fibres lie in the upper and lower regions of the lateral part, and the macular fibres lie in the central region of the lateral part so that they extend to the surface on the nerve

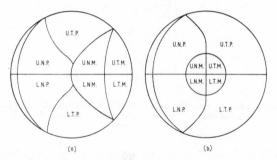

(a)   (b)

FIG. 65. *Diagrams to show the distribution of the visual fibres in the right optic nerve (viewed from behind)—(a) near the optic nerve-head, and (b) midway between the optic nerve head and the optic chiasma).* $U = upper$, $L = lower$, $T = temporal$, $N = nasal$, $P = peripheral$, $M = macular$)

(Fig. 65a). In the main part of the optic nerve the different groups of fibres maintain similar positions except for the macular fibres which pass to the central region so that the temporal peripheral fibres occupy the whole of the lateral part of the nerve (Fig. 65b), and this distribution is continued until the proximal part of the nerve near the optic chiasma where the temporal peripheral fibres move from a lateral position to a ventrolateral one (Fig. 66a), the nasal peripheral fibres move from a medial position to a dorsomedial one (Fig. 66b), and the macular fibres move from a central position to a dorsocentral one (Fig. 66c).

The blood supply of the optic nerve is derived from two sys-tems—a peripheral vascular system of the pial sheath which is formed by various branches from the orbital arteries (ophthalmic, ciliary and lacrimal arteries), and an axial vascular system which is formed by the central retinal artery and its branches. There is evidence that the peripheral and axial vascular systems form anasto-moses with one another within the nerve.

Lesions of the optic nerve tend to produce field defects which are similar to those which follow retinal lesions, although there is a predilection for the macular fibres to suffer damage. This may be the result of an involvement of the axial circulation within the nerve, and it is important to remember that atrophy of a nervous tissue is usually the result of a defect of blood supply rather than a direct pressure effect; this may account for the visual field defects which occur sometimes in severe cases of endocrine exophthalmos when there is a marked increase in intraorbital pressure.

The lesions which affect the optic nerve are discussed in Chapter 8.

Optic Chiasma

In the optic chiasma there is a partial decussation of the nerve fibres so that the fibres from the temporal hemiretina (peripheral and macular fibres) pass to the optic tract of the same side, thus constituting the *uncrossed* fibres, and the fibres from the nasal hemiretina (peripheral and macular fibres), pass to the optic tract of the opposite side, thus constituting the *crossed* fibres.

The temporal peripheral fibres (Fig. 66a) from both eyes traverse the lateral parts of the optic chiasma as two widely separated com-pact masses, and in each mass the fibres from the upper temporal retina lie dorsal and slightly medial to those from the lower tem-poral retina with the most peripheral fibres lying superficially and the most central fibres lying deeply. It is evident, therefore, that these fibres maintain the same relative positions as in the main part of the optic nerve, although they turn slightly dorsally near the caudal end of the chiasma to enter the dorsolateral part of the ipsi-lateral optic tract.

The nasal peripheral fibres (Fig. 66b) from both eyes traverse the central part of the optic chiasma and there is a considerable intermingling of the fibres from the two eyes although with a distinct separation of the upper and lower groups of fibres from each eye. The upper nasal peripheral fibres lie in the more dorsal part of the chiasma and travel towards the ipsilateral optic tract

before crossing in the posterior part of the optic chiasma to enter
the upper dorsomedial part of the contralateral optic tract, whereas
the lower nasal peripheral fibres lie in the ventral part of the optic
chiasma and, after crossing in the anterior part of the chiasma,
travel towards the contralateral optic nerve before looping back to

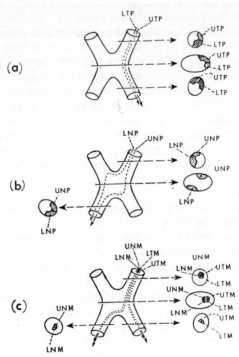

FIG. 66. *Diagrams to show the distribution of (a) the temporal peripheral, (b) the*
nasal peripheral, and (c) the macular fibres in the optic chiasma viewed from above
through the central part of the chiasma and also in cross-section). Key to lettering
as in Fig. 65)

pass to the lower ventromedial part of the contralateral optic tract.
Sometimes a few fibres of this anterior loop enter the terminal part
of the optic nerve and these are from the most peripheral part of
the lower nasal retina. It should be noted that the most peripheral
nasal fibres, which lie on the superficial medial aspect of the optic
nerve, maintain this superficial medial position in the optic tract,
and this necessitates a single spiral twisting of all these fibres rela-

tive to one another during their passage through the central part of the chiasma.

The temporal macular fibres (Fig. 66c) from both eyes traverse the lateral parts of the optic chiasma as two distinct compact masses on the inner aspects of the temporal peripheral fibres and they enter the ipsilateral optic tracts in that situation. The nasal macular fibres (Fig. 66c) from both eyes pass through the chiasma on the outer aspects of the nasal peripheral fibres and cross in the posterior part of the chiasma where the fibres from both eyes mingle with one another. In this situation they lie near the surface of the chiasma but, as they enter the contralateral optic tracts, they are covered on their inner aspects by the nasal peripheral fibres so that they become adjacent to the temporal macular fibres in the central part of the commencement of the optic tract.

The optic chiasma is supplied by a complex series of arteries which comprise the internal carotid artery with its branch—the lateral or inferior chiasmal artery—which passes to the inferolateral aspect of the chiasma, the anterior cerebral artery with its branch— the superior chiasmal artery—which passes to the superoanterior aspect, the anterior communicating artery which sends branches to the superoanterior aspect, the anterior hypophyseal artery which sends a recurrent branch to the inferior aspect with ramifications which extend to the posterior aspect, the posterior communicating artery which sends branches to the inferoposterior aspect, and possible contributions from the middle cerebral artery, the anterior choroidal artery and the ophthalmic artery which sometimes sends a prechiasmal branch to the anteroinferior aspect. These branches form a dense network of capillaries; in the lateral region the capillaries run in an anteroposterior direction, in the more central areas the capillaries pass across the midline and in the median plane they form a free anastomosis so that the capillaries appear to follow the distribution of the groups of nerve fibres through the chiasma.

Median pressure on the ventral surface of the optic chiasma from an expanding intrasellar lesion gives rise eventually to a bitemporal hemianopia, with an involvement of the upper temporal quadrants before the lower ones (Fig. 67), and in both quadrants the visual field defects remain sharply limited by the vertical meridian although after an interval the lower nasal and the upper nasal quadrants may be affected ultimately. The involvement of the lower nasal quadrant before the upper nasal one is the result of the more medial position of the upper temporal fibres as compared with the lower temporal ones so that the upper fibres are affected first by an expanding lesion despite their more dorsal situation. In contrast median pressure on the dorsal surface of the optic chiasma from a purely suprasellar lesion, although it also causes a bitemporal hemianopia, changes the sequence of the involvement of these two quadrants so that the lower quadrant is affected before the upper one. In the event of the later development of a binasal hemianopia, however, the sequence of the involvement of the two quadrants, lower before upper, is retained.

It should be noted, however, that the visual field changes in chiasmal lesions are not confined to depression of the peripheral parts of the fields because central or paracentral changes may occur at any stage, even before the peripheral ones, in the progress of the lesion. Involvement of the anterior chiasmal angle (the junction of one of the optic nerves with the optic chiasma) is liable to produce an arcuate scotoma which curves in a paracentral position in the upper or lower temporal quadrant as far as the vertical meridian in addition to the peripheral field changes (Fig. 67). Similarly involvement of the posterior chiasmal angle (the junction of one of the optic tracts and the optic chiasm) is liable to produce changes in the central parts of the visual fields because of the presence of the macular fibres in the posterior part of the chiasma.

There are many lesions which produce chiasmal defects.

Injuries

Injury is rare except in a penetrating wound which is usually rapidly fatal because of the associated damage to the surrounding great vessels. Sometimes, however, the optic chiasma may be damaged by a violent frontal blow as the result of a disruption of the small chiasmal vessels which follows a sudden displacement of the brain relative to the skull.

Inflammatory Conditions

Basal Meningitis
This form of meningitis is often of an acute nature as the result of a primary infection or as the result of a secondary infection from some neighbouring source (nasal sinusitis, otitis media or cerebral abscess) so that the grave general manifestations predominate, but when it is of a chronic nature the ocular manifestations predominate.

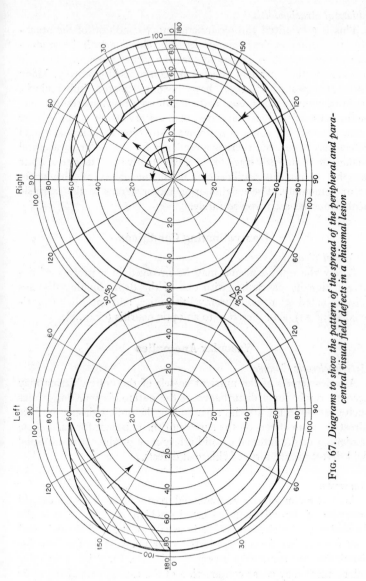

FIG. 67. Diagrams to show the pattern of the spread of the peripheral and para-central visual field defects in a chiasmal lesion

Chiasmal Arachnoiditis

This is a localized chronic inflammatory condition of the arachnoid membrane in the region of the optic chiasma with the production of hyperplastic changes so that the visual fibres of the optic chiasma (or their nutrient vessels) are compressed gradually. Many different types of infection have been postulated (tuberculosis, syphilis, actinomycosis, etc.) and sometimes a previous trauma may be the cause of the local adhesive inflammatory changes, but in most cases the exciting agent is unknown. Any type of chiasmal visual defect may occur, but there is a tendency for central or paracentral changes to be an early stage feature. Eventually some degree of optic atrophy occurs, but papilloedema is an unusual event. Headaches occur commonly. The neighbouring motor nerves to the extrinsic ocular muscles are involved rarely.

Demyelinating Conditions

Chiasmal Neuritis

Rarely the optic chiasma may be involved in a process of demyelination in association with one of the demyelinating diseases (disseminated sclerosis, neuromyelitis optica, and encephalitis periaxialis diffusa), akin therefore to an optic neuritis (chap. 8).

Vascular Anomalies

Arteriosclerotic Changes

Arteriosclerosis of the nutrient vessels of the optic chiasma may account rarely for a disturbance of the optic chiasma. Sometimes such changes in the arteries surrounding the optic chiasma produce direct pressure effects on the surface of the chiasma; for example, a hardening of the internal carotid artery may produce a nasal visual field defect (a rare form of chiasmal defect).

Aneurysm

An aneurysm of the supraclinoid part of the internal carotid artery or of the neighbouring arteries which are concerned in the formation of the circle of Willis is usually of congenital origin and may remain free from complications for many years (or even indefinitely), but sometimes it produces defects. First, its progressive enlargement may cause compression of the caudal part of the optic nerve or of the optic chiasma with the production of typical visual field defects or it may cause compression of the IIIrd cranial nerve with the production of an ophthalmoplegia (chap. 14). Second, it may permit a gradual or intermittent leakage of blood through its attenuated wall into the subarachnoid space with various forms of ophthalmoplegia which may be transient, but often recurrent, with usually an associated headache (the *ophthalmoplegic migraine*). Third, it may rupture suddenly with the formation of a massive subarachnoid haemorrhage; this is associated with severe headache, vomiting, ophthalmoplegia, and coma. Death occurs rapidly in about 50 per cent of cases.

An aneurysm of the infraclinoid part of the internal carotid artery within the cavernous sinus may enlarge sufficiently to produce the pressure effects of a supraclinoid aneurysm, but more commonly it is associated with the formation of a caroticocavernous fistula (chap. 14).

Tumours

Craniopharyngioma

This is a congenitally determined tumour which arises in the epithelial remnants concerned in the formation of Rathke's pharyngeal pouch, the anterior lobe of the pituitary body or the hypophyseal duct. It may become evident at any age but occurs commonly in the early years of life. The general manifestations vary greatly but are often of a hypothalamic nature; headaches, generalized weakness, progressive mental deterioration, drowsiness sometimes with transient periods of unconsciousness, dystrophia adiposogenitalis, diabetes insipidus. Visual defects occur usually fairly early, but in the child are often ignored until they reach an advanced stage when there is obvious optic nerve atrophy, usually bilateral. The suprasellar situation of the tumour is demonstrated radiographically by ventriculography but a simple radiographic examination of the skull is also of great importance because, although an enlargement of the sella turcica is not common, other features such as decalcification of the clinoid processes, shortening of the dorsum sellae, or suprasellar calcification are frequently evident. Sometimes it is not possible for the neurosurgeon to remove the entire tumour without sacrificing the optic chiasma (or the caudal part of one of the optic nerves), although an aspiration of any cystic part of the tumour is of great value in relieving its immediate pressure effects; postoperative supervoltage X irradiation may eradicate the tumour and prevent its recurrence.

Chromophobe Adenoma

This pituitary tumour becomes evident usually in early adult life or in middle age. The general manifestations are varied: headaches, generalized weakness, loss of libido, loss of body hair, amenorrhoea, mental sluggishness, fits of extreme temper, diabetes insipidus. Visual defects occur almost invariably after a suprasellar extension and are quite frequently early although they tend to be ignored by the patient because of their trivial nature (a fluid appearance of the outlines of distant objects, transient attacks of misty vision, a slight impairment of reading vision), or disregarded by the examiner who considers them to be simply the result of some uncorrected error of refraction despite the fact that the provision of glasses fails to relieve symptoms. The true nature of these visual defects is determined only by careful examination of the visual fields, particularly with coloured targets, except in the later stages when optic nerve atrophy is apparent. Some form of ophthalmoplegia due to involvement of the IIIrd, IVth or VIth cranial nerves may occur rarely when the tumour spreads laterally. Simple radiographic examination of the skull reveals the enlargement of the sella turcica which follows the intrasellar expansion of the tumour; it may also show thinning of the dorsum sellae or of the posterior clinoid processes or undermining of the anterior clinoid processes, but the full extent of any suprasellar expansion is only demonstrated by more complicated methods (ventriculography or carotid angiography). The treatment may be neurosurgical (craniotomy with a hypophysectomy) or radiotherapeutic (supervoltage X irradiation) or a combination of both procedures.

Chromophile Adenoma

This pituitary tumour usually becomes evident in early adult life with gigantism or in middle age with acromegaly (in the acidophil type) or with Cushing's syndrome (in the basophil type). There is marked enlargement of the sella turcica (except in the basophil type), but visual field defects are not invariable features because the tumour tends to remain intrasellar.

Meningioma

This tumour affects the chiasma in different ways depending on whether it arises in a presellar, suprasellar or parasellar situation:

Presellar Meningioma. A meningioma of the olfactory groove (causing anosmia due to pressure on the olfactory nerve) affects the caudal part of the optic nerve with the development of an optic atrophy before causing a backwards and downwards displacement of the optic chiasma. This chiasmal involvement leads to various forms of visual field defect, but sometimes it produces bilateral central scotomata.

Suprasellar Meningioma. A meningioma arising from the region of the chiasmatic sulcus or tuberculum sellae tends to affect the caudal part of the optic nerve (or sometimes both optic nerves) before causing a backwards and upwards displacement of the optic chiasma with the production of characteristic chiasmal defects involving the peripheral or central parts of the visual fields. In the later stages signs of a pituitary defect (see above) of a hypothalamic disturbance, or of an internal hydrocephalus may become evident.

Internal Hydrocephalus. This is the result of a distortion of the third ventricle which leads to a blockage of the foramen of Monro by an extraventricular tumour like a suprasellar meningioma or by an intraventricular tumour like a glioma or ependymoma, or the result of a blockage of the aqueduct of Sylvius or the fourth ventricle by the extension of a tumour from the brain stem (midbrain and pons), pineal body, vermis of the cerebellum, or VIIIth cranial nerve; it follows that a tumour of the posterior fossa, quite apart from causing papilloedema, is liable also to produce signs of chiasmal compression.

Parasellar Meningioma. A meningioma from the region of the lesser wing of the sphenoid causes involvement of the adjacent optic nerve (characteristically with the production of an upper altitudinal hemianopic defect of the ipsilateral visual field before leading to blindness of the eye) and then involvement of the optic chiasma. A spread laterally produces the sphenoidal fissure syndrome (chap. 13).

Glioma

This tumour may occur as a primary event in the optic chiasma or as a glioma of the frontal lobe which spreads downwards to implicate the optic nerves and optic chiasma (suprasellar involvement).

Tumours of the Sphenoid Bone

An osteoma, osteochondroma, haemangioma, chordoma or sarcoma may cause pressure on the optic chiasma and sometimes also proptosis, ophthalmoplegia and trigeminal neuralgia.

Tumours of the Basal Meninges

A primary tumour of the basal meninges is rare, but a metastatic carcinoma may spread rapidly with involvement of the optic nerves, optic chiasma, IIIrd, IVth, Vth and VIth cranial nerves, pituitary body and hypothalamus; death follows after a short interval.

Optic Tract and Its Defects

In the most distal part of the optic tract the visual fibres maintain the same relative positions as in the posterior part of the chiasma; the temporal peripheral fibres lie dorsolaterally with the upper

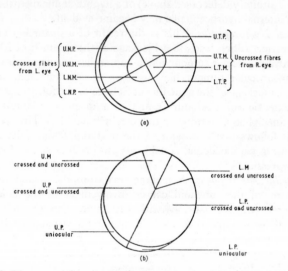

FIG. 68. *Diagrams to show the distribution of the visual fibres in the optic tract—* (a) *at the optic chiasma, and* (b) *midway between the optic chiasma and the lateral geniculate body* (right optic tract viewed in cross-section from behind). (*Key to lettering as in Fig. 65*)

ones above the lower ones, the nasal peripheral fibres lie ventromedially with the upper ones above the lower ones and with the uniocular peripheral fibres in a superficial position, and the macular fibres lie centrally with the temporal fibres lateral to the nasal ones and the upper fibres above the lower ones (Fig. 68a). There is, however, a rapid redistribution of the fibres in the tract so that the fibres from corresponding areas of each retina tend to be associated with one another; the upper peripheral binocular fibres (uncrossed and crossed) lie dorsomedially, the lower peripheral binocular fibres (uncrossed and crossed) lie ventrolaterally, the peripheral uniocular fibres (crossed only) lie on the superficial aspect of the ventromedial border, and the macular fibres (uncrossed and crossed) lie dorso-laterally with the upper fibres dorsal to the lower ones although it is uncertain if the macular fibres extend as far as the surface of the optic tract (Fig. 68b). It is evident that there is some tilting of the main part of the optic tract whereby its upper border lies more laterally than its lower border.

In this way the horizontal meridian of the retina is represented by a line which passes from a dorsolateral position to a ventromedial one, the upper and lower halves of the vertical meridian of the retina are probably represented in the region of the junctions between the upper peripheral and macular fibres and the lower peripheral and macular fibres, the upper and lower halves of the circumferential meridian of the retina are represented by a line which passes round the dorsomedial and ventrolateral borders and the fixation point in the retina is represented in the dorsolateral region.

The optic tract is supplied by the peripheral pial vascular net-work which is formed by branches from the anterior choroidal artery (usually a branch of the internal carotid artery), the middle cerebral artery, the posterior communicating artery and the posterior cere-bral artery.

The optic tract is the first part of the visual pathway in which lesions consistently produce homonymous field defects, as the result of the involvement of the visual fibres from corresponding areas of the retina of both eyes within a single lesion, although these are seldom congruous. In a complete hemianopia (loss of the nasal half field of the ipsilateral eye and temporal half field of the contralateral eye) the fovea is bisected vertically.

There are many lesions which produce optic tract defects—basal meningitis, demyelinating conditions, infraclinoid aneurysms (of the internal carotid artery, posterior communicating artery, middle cerebral artery or posterior cerebral artery), and rarely supraclinoid aneurysms which extend backwards—but the usual lesion is a tumour; the anterior part of the optic tract by a pituitary tumour which spreads backwards or by a parasellar meningioma, the pos-terior part of the optic tract by a tumour of the third ventricle or a tumour of the basal ganglia, and the lateral aspect of the optic tract by an expanding tumour of the temporal lobe. The associated involvement of neighbouring structures produces other features; hemiplegia and hemianaesthesia (the internal capsule), dissociated gaze palsies (the posterior longitudinal bundle) or defective pupillary reactions (the region of the superior colliculus).

Lateral Geniculate Body

The dorsal nucleus of the lateral geniculate body serves as a relay station in the projection of the visual fibres from the retina to the striate area of the visual cortex with the formation of synaptic junctions. The majority of the fibres from the optic tract enters the nucleus through its convex anterior surface, but some fibres enter through the hilum which lies in a concavity on the ventral surface of the medial part of the nucleus. The visual fibres terminate in different parts of the nucleus according to their positions of origin in the retina: the crossed and uncrossed fibres from the hemimacula of each eye pass to a large median sector which lies in a dorsocentral position in the caudal two-thirds of the nucleus with a rounded caudal margin for the foveal fibres—the upper macular fibres terminating medially, and the lower macular ones laterally—the crossed and uncrossed fibres from the peripheral binocular hemiretina of each eye pass ventrally on the medial and lateral aspects of the macular area—the upper retinal fibres terminating medially in the medial tubercle and in the rostral one-third of the nucleus and the lower fibres terminating laterally in the lateral horn, and the crossed fibres from the peripheral uniocular retina pass to a narrow area on the ventral aspect of the rostral part of the nucleus—the upper fibres terminating medially and the lower fibres terminating laterally (Fig. 69). The fibres terminate in the nucleus in different grey laminae (composed of nerve cells) which are separated from one another by white laminae (composed of medullated nerve fibres); in the macular and main binocular peripheral areas there are 6 grey laminae—laminae 1, 4, and 6 for crossed fibres and laminae 2, 3, and 5 for uncrossed fibres, in the rest of the binocular peripheral areas there are only 4 grey laminae—lamina 1 and a lamina composed of laminae 4+6 for crossed fibres and lamina 2 and a lamina composed of laminae 3+5 for uncrossed fibres, and in the uniocular peripheral area there are only 2 grey laminae both for crossed fibres. There is evidence that corresponding retinal areas are represented in adjacent parts of all the laminae in a linear manner along a radius which passes through the nucleus in the direction of the centre of the hilum so that there is a point-to-sector representation of the retina. The optic radiation emerges from the nucleus through its dorso-caudal surface.

In this way the horizontal meridian of the retina is represented by a plane which is more or less vertical through the lateral genicu-late body in a rostrocaudal direction, the vertical meridian of the

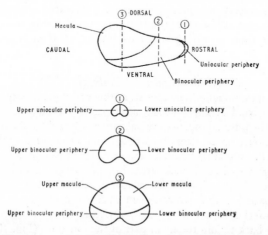

FIG. 69. *Diagrams to show the distribution of the visual fibres in the dorsal nucleus of right lateral geniculate body (viewed from the side and in cross-section through (1) the rostral part; (2) the central part; and (3) the caudal part of nucleus*

retina is represented by a plane which lies along the posterior border of the lateral geniculate body with the upper part of the vertical meridian extending extending medially and the lower part of the vertical meridian extending laterally, the circumferential meridian of the retina is represented by a plane which lies along the anterior border of the body with the upper part of the meridian extending medially and the lower part of the meridian extending laterally, and the fixation point of the retina is represented in the central part of the most caudal region.

The function of the dorsal nucleus of the lateral geniculate body is not clearly understood, but it appears to serve largely as a relay station with possibly an ability to exert integrating and modulating influences on the visual impulses. The suggestions that it is con-cerned with a distinction between the perceptions of light and colour with a trichromatic form of colour vision or with an appreciation of spatial relationships are not established with any certainty. It should be noted, however, that this is the first structure in the afferent visual pathways which emphasizes anatomically the functional importance of the macula by devoting such a large area to its fibres. The lateral geniculate body is supplied mainly by the posterior cerebral artery or its posterior choroidal branch, but the anterior choroidal artery also plays some part. There are no specific visual field changes in lesions of the lateral geniculate body and they tend to mimic those occurring in lesions of the optic tract or optic radiation.

Optic Radiation (Geniculo-calcarine Pathway)

The optic radiation emerges from the lateral geniculate body as a compact band of fibres which, after passing through the posterior part of the internal capsule, spreads out as a broad band covering the outer surface of the lateral ventricle to its termination in the striate area of the visual cortex. The upper fibres of this broad band pass more or less directly backwards, but the lower fibres turn downwards before passing backwards and some of these fibres pass forwards as well as downwards so that they form a loop in the region of the inferior horn of the lateral ventricle (the loop of Meyer) before turning back to join the main part of the radiation (Fig. 70).

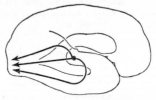

FIG. 70. *Diagram to show the optic radiation from the dorsal nucleus of the lateral geniculate body to the striate cortex (viewed from the lateral side). Note the relation of the lower fibres to the inferior horn of the lateral ventricle*

There is evidence that the distribution of the visual fibres in the optic radiation has a uniform pattern throughout most of their course with a fairly precise point-to-point arrangement according to their origins from corresponding areas of the retina of each eye, but it is likely that there are certain unusual features of the anterior part of the radiation, particularly within the loop of Meyer.

In the anterior part of the optic radiation it is likely that the visual fibres maintain to a large extent the disposition which they have in the lateral geniculate body, with the exception that all the groups of fibres are rotated through 90°, so that the upper retinal fibres (macular, and peripheral, crossed and uncrossed) lie dorsally, and the lower retinal fibres (macular and peripheral, crossed and uncrossed) lie ventrally. The macular fibres lie in the lateral part of the intermediate area, the binocular peripheral fibres lie in the medial part of the immediate area and in the whole of the upper and lower areas except for the most medial part of these areas in which lie the uniocular peripheral fibres (Fig. 71a). In this way the horizontal meridian of the retina is represented by the horizontal line which separates the radiation into its dorsal and ventral halves, the upper and lower halves of the vertical meridian of the retina are represented by the upper and lower halves of the lateral border of the radiation, the upper and lower halves of the circumferential meridian of the retina are represented by the upper and lower halves of the medial border of the radiation, and the fovea is represented by the central part of the lateral border (Fig. 71a).

In the main part of the optic radiation the upper retinal fibres (macular and peripheral, crossed and uncrossed) lie dorsally and the lower retinal fibres (macular and peripheral, crossed and uncrossed) lie ventrally, as in the anterior part of the radiation, but within these areas the grouping of fibres is different. The macular fibres occupy the whole of a large intermediate area, the binocular peripheral fibres lie above and below this intermediate area with the upper and lower extremities for the uniocular peripheral fibres (Fig. 71b). In this way the horizontal meridian of the retina is represented by the curved medial border, the upper and lower halves of the vertical meridian of the retina are represented by the upper and lower halves of the curved lateral border, the upper and lower halves of the circumferential meridian of the retina are represented by the upper and lower extremities of the radiation and by the upper and lower margins of the binocular peripheral areas, and the fovea is represented by the central part of the lateral border (Fig. 71b). It has been suggested, however, that the representations of the different retinal areas in the radiation may not be in a rigid series but rather in a system of layering so that there is some overlap of the fibres from adjacent retinal areas with the more peripheral area lying on the medial side of the more central one.

The loop of Meyer represents the lower fibres of the optic radiation which turn forwards in the region of the inferior horn of the lateral

ventricle in the temporal lobe although the exact relation of the fibres
to the horn is in doubt; it is suggested that they sweep round the
lateral side of the tip of the horn, that they cap the anterior surface
of the horn, or that they turn backwards a short distance behind the
horn, and this last description is the most likely one because field

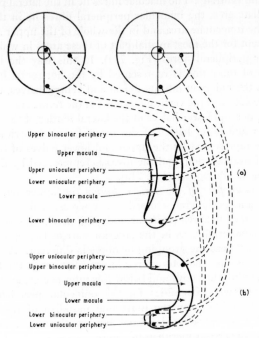

Upper binocular periphery

Upper macula

Upper uniocular periphery
Lower uniocular periphery

Lower macula

Lower binocular periphery

(a)

Upper uniocular periphery
Upper binocular periphery

Upper macula

Lower macula

Lower binocular periphery
Lower uniocular periphery

(b)

FIG. 71. *Diagram to show the distribution of the visual fibres in (a) the anterior
part, and (b) the posterior part of the optic radiation (right optic radiation viewed
in cross-section from behind)*

defects are not common after opening the tip of the inferior horn by
an anterior approach. It is suggested that the loop of Meyer, in
contrast to the rest of the radiation, contains a greater proportion of
uncrossed than crossed fibres, but it is more likely that there is an
equal number of uncrossed and crossed fibres although the uncrossed
ones lie more superficially than the crossed ones.

The optic radiation is supplied anteriorly by the anterior choroidal artery and posteriorly by the posterior cerebral artery; the intermediate part is supplied also by the middle cerebral artery.

As a general rule a lesion of the optic radiation produces a congruous type of homonymous visual field defect (Fig. 72a), but some times when the lesion involves the anterior part of the radiation the field defects are of an incongruous type with the larger defect in the ipsilateral field. This incongruity occurs when the lesion approaches the radiation from a lateral direction because in this position the ipsilateral fibres are more superficial than the contralateral ones, and it occurs also when there is an associated involvement of the nearby optic tract or lateral geniculate body by direct involvement or by an interference with its blood supply, although sometimes the incongruity may be more apparent than real because it may be the result

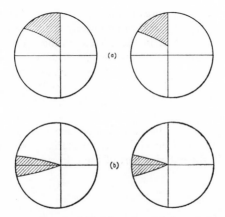

FIG. 72. *Diagrams to show the field defects due to lesions of the optic radiation :* (a) *upper homonymous congruous partial quadrantic defects ; and* (b) *homonymous sector-shaped defects in the horizontal meridians*

simply of a sparing of the crossed uniocular peripheral fibres suggesting a reduction of the field defect in the contralateral eye. The additional involvement of some other part of the optic pathway is the only likely explanation of the more rare cases of incongruity in which the contralateral defect is larger than the ipsilateral one.

Lesions of the upper or lower parts of the optic radiation usually cause a precise quadrantopia thereby suggesting that the upper and lower peripheral areas are separated by an anatomical interval. In lesions of the anterior part of the radiation, however, this precise quadrantopia is often absent because of the contiguity of the upper and lower peripheral areas in that region, and when the lesion is limited to this area only the field defect consists of sector-shaped homonymous defects immediately above and below the horizontal meridians (Fig. 72b).

There are many lesions which affect the integrity of the optic radiation: encephalitis, cerebral abscess, demyelinating conditions, vascular lesions (intracerebral haemorrhage caused by a rupture of an atheromatous artery, intracerebral thrombosis due to atheromatous occlusion or syphilitic endarteritis, or embolism), and tumours of the temporal, parietal or occipital lobes—primary (glioma, meningioma) or metastatic (carcinoma).

Visual Cortex

The optic radiation fibres terminate on the medial aspect of the occipital cortex (striate area) in an orderly sequence with regard to their positions of origin in the corresponding areas of the retina of each eye so that the point-to-point arrangement of the optic radiation is maintained in the visual cortex. The upper retinal fibres (macular and peripheral, crossed and uncrossed) lie dorsally and the lower retinal fibres (macular and peripheral, crossed and uncrossed) lie ventrally. To a large extent this separation of upper and lower fibres is fairly clear-cut because they are separated from each other by the deepest part of the cleft in the posterior part of the calcarine fissure, but, in the anterior part of the calcarine fissure beyond the

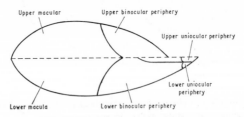

FIG. 73. *Diagram to show the distribution of the visual fibres in the striate area (right striate area viewed medially)*

level of the parieto-occipital fissure, both groups of fibres lie in the lower half of the fissure although the dorsoventral arrangement of the two groups of fibres is maintained. The macular fibres terminate in a large portion of the more caudal part of the striate area with the foveal fibres terminating in the extreme caudal region and extending usually on to a small part of the lateral surface of the occipital lobe, the binocular peripheral fibres terminate in the central part of the striate area with the most peripheral of these fibres extending beyond the level of the parieto-occipital fissure, and the uniocular peripheral fibres terminate in the most rostral part of the striate area below the calcarine fissure (Fig. 73). In this way the horizontal meridian of the retina is represented by the horizontal line which lies in the floor of the posterior part of the calcarine fissure which separates the striate area into its dorsal and ventral parts and by the line which forms the junction between the dorsal and ventral parts of the striate area below the anterior part of the calcarine fissure, the upper and lower halves of the vertical meridian of the retina are represented by the upper and lower borders of the striate area, the upper and lower halves of the circumferential meridian are represented by the rostral extremity of the striate area and by the rostral border of the part for the binocular peripheral fibres, and the fovea is represented by the caudal extremity of the striate area (Fig. 74).

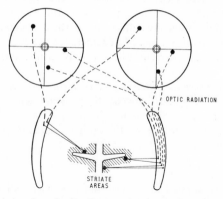

FIG. 74. *Diagram to show the distribution of the visual fibres in the striate areas (viewed in cross-section) with regard to their origin from the horizontal and vertical meridians of the retinae (right and left striate areas viewed in cross-section from behind)*

The main blood supply of the striate area is from the calcarine branch of the posterior cerebral artery, but the terminal branches of the middle cerebral artery also supply the caudal part of the area so that the macular region has a dual blood supply. Nutrient vessels arise from the vascular network which covers the striate area; short vessels pass to the grey matter of the cortex and longer vessels pass to the white matter and there is evidence that these two types of vessels maintain some degree of independence.

Lesions of the striate area produce field defects which are characterized by their homonymous and congruous natures and also very often by the phenomenon of macular sparing even in the presence of a hemianopic field defect. There is no conclusive evidence that macular sparing is the result of any bilateral representation of the macula in each striate area or of any link between the macular zones of the two striate areas through the corpus callosum, and it is likely that it is largely the result of the failure of a lesion to involve the entire macular zone because of its large extent within the striate area. In some cases, however, macular sparing is present despite the known total destruction of one striate area, and it is suggested that this sparing is the result of a slight shift of fixation so that it is more apparent than real.

The lesions which affect the visual cortex are similar to those which affect the optic radiation with the addition of trauma which is liable to disrupt the visual cortex, particularly the part concerned with macular function because of its position at the posterior part of the brain. The injury is usually a direct one in the occipital region (penetrating wound, fracture, etc.), but sometimes the effect may be of a contrecoup type as the result of a severe blow in the frontal region.

Encephalitis Periaxialis Diffusa (Schilder's Disease)

This is a widespread demyelinating disease which is discussed here because its main effect is usually in the visual cortex, although it may involve the optic nerve, the optic chiasma, the optic tract, or the optic radiation.

Cortical Blindness

This term is applied to a severe defect of vision of both eyes, or even complete blindness, as the result of a lesion of the visual cortex, and the suprageniculate situation of the lesion determines the absence of any ophthalmoscopic evidence of optic atrophy and the presence of normal pupillary responses to light (unless there is an accompanying infrageniculate lesion). It occurs in a variety of conditions; encephalitis periaxialis diffusa (see above), vertebrobasilar insufficiency, uraemia, and encephalopathy (chap. 7).

THE DETERMINATION OF THE VISUAL FIELD

This may be achieved by different methods.

The Confrontation Test. This is a simple and rapid method and, although it is sometimes not capable of detecting subtle abnormalities, it is a most useful form of routine examination. The examiner stands opposite to and at arm's length from the patient so that the patient's right eye is fixing the examiner's left eye (and the patient's left eye is fixing the examiner's right eye); the patient closes each eye in turn and the examiner brings a moving object (his finger or preferably a white target) from the periphery inwards until the patient is just aware of the object. This determines the peripheral limit of the visual field and is compared with the examiner's (normal) visual field. It is possible also to detect defects (scotomata) within the visual field.

The Perimeter. This instrument is placed on a table and contains an adjustable chin rest so that the patient is able to place his head

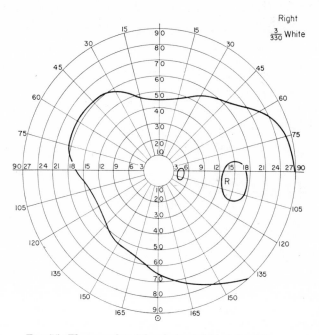

Fig. 75. *The normal peripheral visual field of the right eye*

in an upright position with each eye (in turn) directed to a fixed target in the centre of a movable curved semicircular arc which is 330 mm from the eye. The arc is moved into 6 different positions for each quadrant of the visual field (with 15° between each position)

and with one eye fixing the central target (the other eye being
occluded) a target is moved along the arc from a position beyond
the extent of the visual field until it is just apparent; this point
determines the extent of peripheral visual field in each position for
the particular object. At this distance of 330 mm a white object of
3 mm in diameter provides a measure of the full extent of the peripheral visual field and in the normal subject this is about 45° in the
upper vertical meridian, 90° in the temporal horizontal meridian,
65° in the lower vertical meridian and 55° in the nasal horizontal
meridian (the contours of the face, particularly the nose, determine
the difference in these measurements in different meridians)—the
peripheral extent of the normal visual field in the right eye (Fig. 75)
and in the left eye (Fig. 76) are shown. The visual field to colour

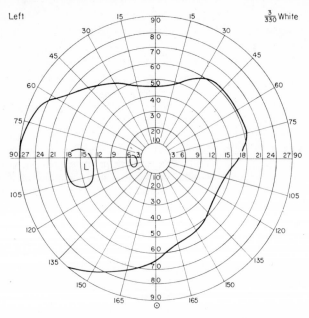

FIG. 76. *The normal peripheral visual field of the left eye*

targets is similar in outline to that with white targets except that it is
less in extent (green less than red and red less than blue) provided
the point is recorded at which the colour (and not merely the movement) of the target is recognized by the observer.

The Bjerrum Screen. This flat screen provides detailed information of the state of the visual field within 30° of the fixation point; there are two sizes of Bjerrum screen, a smaller one with the patient seated 1 m (1,000 mm) from the central fixation target and a larger one when the patient is 2 m (2,000 mm) from the screen. Its main value is the determination of scotomata in the central or paracentral parts of the visual field which are so small as to be overlooked on the perimeter. The patient (with one eye occluded) fixes a central target on the screen and indicates the disappearance of a target which is moved over the screen. The normal blind spot (which is produced by the optic nerve-head) is plotted on the Bjerrum screen as an oval area (5·5° in the horizontal diameter and 7·5° in vertical diameter) the centre of which lies about 15° on the temporal side of the fixation point and just below the horizontal meridian (Figs. 75 and 76); this is determined first because its accurate appreciation confirms that the patient is cooperating in the test. The central visual field is then examined carefully for any central and paracentral defects and it is essential to employ targets of different sizes and different colours (the method of quantitative scotometry) in order to determine areas of the visual field in which there is a relative (as distinct from an absolute) loss of visual function; small white targets and coloured targets (red and green) may reveal scotomatous areas which are not determined by other means particularly in such conditions as retrobulbar neuritis, chiasmal lesions, and toxic amblyopia.

It is apparent that a careful assessment of the significance of any visual field defect which has been determined accurately is of great value in the localization of many forms of ocular and intracranial disease. The appearance of the optic disc is also of localizing importance because an infrageniculate lesion of the afferent visual pathway is usually followed within a period of about 6 weeks with some degree of optic atrophy, whereas a suprageniculate lesion is not accompanied by any alteration in the appearance of the optic disc.

THE HIGHER VISUAL MECHANISMS

The striate area of the visual cortex is the terminal sensory area for the fibres of the afferent visual pathway; but there are other related areas—the parastriate area (which surrounds the striate area) and the peristriate area (which surrounds the parastriate area) which are concerned in the higher visual (visuopsychic) functions with an elaboration of the straightforward visual impressions into patterns which have meaning and which are interpreted in relation to past experience. Lesions in these visual association areas do not cause true blindness but rather a form of mind blindness (visual object agnosia) in which objects are observed but remain meaningless. The supramarginal gyrus (which is part of the parietal lobe) and the angular gyrus (which extends from the parietal lobe into the temporal lobe) also serve as important association areas which link the visual sensations with other sensory modalities (such as touch, hearing); lesions of these areas produce various forms of visual agnosia—colour agnosia (an inability to recognize colours), visual spatial agnosia (an inability to orientate different objects in space) and corporeal agnosia (an inability to identify the different parts of the body).

17 | Injuries

The limited scope of this book precludes any detailed account of ocular injuries, although in many chapters an account is given of the more common forms of injury. In this chapter brief mention is made of perforating injuries of the eyeball.

The cornea or sclera may be perforated in different ways; directly by a sharp pointed instrument (knife, scissors), directly by small particles (metal, glass), or indirectly by a severe contusion which leads to a rupture of the globe. There are several aspects in the management of such injuries:

The Restoration of the Integrity of the Eyeball

This involves a careful suturing of the wound after the removal of any devitalized tissue and after the abscission of any prolapsed uveal tissue. When the cornea is perforated by the injury this suturing is of great importance because the achievement of an air-tight wound permits the restoration of the anterior chamber by the injection of air at the end of the operation so that any subsequent adhesion of the underlying iris to the region of the wound or any development of adhesions between the iris and the cornea in the region of the filtration angle (peripheral anterior synechiae) are avoided thereby reducing the likelihood of the development of a subsequent uveitis or secondary glaucoma.

The Avoidance of Infection

The use of antibiotics (by topical application, by subconjunctival injection or systemically) reduces the risk of a septic type of inflammation of the eye (endophthalmitis, panophthalmitis) which is liable to lead to a rapid loss of the eye. A nonseptic type of inflammation (uveitis) is not avoided by the use of antibiotics, but is less likely to occur when the integrity of the eye is achieved rapidly after the injury so that prolapsed uveal tissue is not present within the wound, and it may be controlled by the use of topical or systemic steroids. The danger of a sympathetic ophthalmitis after an injury is discussed in Chapter 6.

The Removal of Any Retained Foreign Body

All forms of perforating injury of the eyeball should be subjected to careful radiographic examination in order to determine the presence of one or more intraocular foreign bodies and there are various specialized methods (for example, stereoscopic radiography) which permit an accurate localization of the position of each foreign body; this is of particular value when a detailed view of the structures within the eye is prevented by a disorganization of the cornea, by a traumatic cataract, or by haemorrhage within the anterior chamber or vitreous. Other specialized methods of detection (the Roper-Hall foreign body detector which works on the principle of the land-mine detector, or the use of ultrasonics) are of value in certain cases.

There are many different substances which may enter the eye and their effects are variable:

Metallic Particles. These commonly enter the eye at great speed and the heat which is generated at their liberation is retained until they enter the eye so that they seldom lead to any sepsis; the introduction of copper, however, may lead to the production of a sterile type of pus. The extent of the damage to the eye depends on the size of the foreign body, the tissues which are disrupted by its passage through the eye and the site of its final termination. A retained particle of iron or steel gives rise, after an interval of several months (or even years), to widespread deposits of ferrous material on the lens capsule, in the uveal tract and in the retina with progressive degenerative changes and ultimately loss of vision; the affected tissues assume a characteristic rusty brown discoloration (*siderosis*). A retained particle of copper gives rise to similar deposits (*chalcosis*) which in the early stages are evident beneath the anterior lens capsule with a sunflower distribution, but eventually the deposits become more widespread with the production of a panophthalmitis. A retained particle of brass causes similar changes to copper. Sometimes, however, these effects are avoided if the particle of iron, steel, copper or brass becomes encapsulated or if it becomes lodged in the lens where it is divorced from the circulation.

Other metallic particles—lead, aluminium, gold, silver and zinc—are less likely to cause reaction within the eye so that they may remain relatively inert for an indefinite period.

Nonmetallic Particles. Stone and glass particles tend to remain relatively inert, but vegetable materials such as wood splinters are likely to lead to sepsis.

A magnetic metallic particle (iron and steel) may be removed by a magnet; when it lies in the anterior part of the eye it is removed readily by opening the anterior chamber at the limbus (the anterior approach), but when it lies in the posterior part of the eye it is removed best by a posterior scleral incision (the posterior approach) because of the disruption of the tissues of the eye which would follow any attempt to bring it forward into the anterior chamber; the opening in the underlying retina is sealed by the application of surface diathermy or cryotherapy. When the magnetic metallic particle lies in the lens it may be left alone, but if the lens becomes cataractous (sometimes after a considerable delay) the foreign body is eliminated simply by removing the lens.

A nonmagnetic particle is only susceptible to removal by forceps under direct view through an opening in the sclera or using an ophthalmoscope, a procedure which is usually fraught with difficulty and with a liability to cause damage to the structures within the eye (retina, vitreous, etc.). It follows that an inert particle should be left alone as a general rule.

Artificial Eyes

These are made of glass or of a plastic material; a plastic eye has certain advantages—it does not break, it is less likely to become rough and it is more durable. It is natural for an artificial eye to cause a certain amount of discharge from the socket because the conjunctival lining of the socket is a mucous surface; it follows that the artificial eye and the socket should be cleansed routinely each day.

Contracted Socket

Sometimes a socket may become contracted when the conjunctiva has been the site of some previous disease (trachoma, ocular pemphigus, etc.) or more commonly when the artificial eye has not been worn for a prolonged period. An attempt may be made to enlarge the socket and then to line it with a skin graft which is retained by a mould of dental wax (although this lining of skin may produce a somewhat offensive discharge). Sometimes a satisfactory method is simply to enlarge the socket by dividing the adhesions and to maintain it by the insertion of a plastic mould at the time of the operation.

There is evidence that the growth of the orbit in early childhood is dependent to some extent on the presence of the eye, so that the removal of an eye in early childhood or the absence of an eye (anophthalmos) from birth, or a gross degree of microphthalmos creates problems in later life in retaining a cosmetically satisfactory prosthesis. It is essential, therefore, to fit a sufficiently large prosthesis as soon as possible, and in the case of microphthalmos the prosthesis may be incorporated in a contact shell which fits over the eye provided there is no useful visual function of the microphthalmic eye.

The Removal of an Eye

It may be necessary to remove the eye after severe injury, particularly when there is a risk of the development of a sympathetic ophthalmitis, although the operation may be carried out for many other reasons; a blind painful eye, an eye harbouring a malignant melanoma, etc.

There are two main forms of the operation:

Enucleation. This involves the removal of the whole eye with a small portion of the optic nerve but with the retention of the conjunctiva and the bulbar fascia (to provide a lining for the socket) and the extrinsic ocular muscles which are sutured to a buried implant to provide a fair degree of movement of the overlying prosthesis.

Evisceration. This involves the removal of the contents of the eye with a retention of the posterior part of the sclera so that there is no section of the optic nerve. An evisceration is the method of choice when the eye has been the site of a septic inflammation (panophthalmitis) because an enucleation in such a case might cause a contamination of the cut end of the optic nerve with the development of a spreading meningitis, but the use of antibiotics in recent years has reduced the indications for an evisceration.

18 | Care of the Blind

The statutory definition for the purposes of registration as a blind person is that the person is 'so blind as to be unable to perform any work for which eyesight is essential'; the test is not whether the person is unable to pursue his ordinary occupation or any particular occupation, but whether he is too blind to perform *any work* for which eyesight is essential, and only the visual conditions are taken into account, other bodily or mental infirmities are disregarded.

The principal factor to be considered is the corrected visual acuity of each eye separately or with both eyes together. The person examined may be classified in one of three groups:

Groups 1—Below 3/60 *Snellen*
In general a person with visual acuity below 3/60 Snellen may be regarded as blind. In many cases, however, it is desirable to test the vision at one metre and not to regard a person having acuity of 1/18 Snellen as blind unless there is also considerable restriction of the visual field.

*Group 2—*3/60, *but less than* 6/60 *Snellen*
A person with visual acuity of 3/60 but less than 6/60 Snellen may be regarded as blind if the field of vision is considerably contracted but should not be regarded as blind if the visual defect is of long standing and is unaccompanied by any material contraction of the field of vision, for example, in cases of congenital nystagmus, albinism, myopia, etc., particularly if there is a reasonable level of close reading vision.

*Group 3—*6/60 *Snellen or more*
A person with a visual acuity of 6/60 Snellen or better should ordinarily not be regarded as blind. He may, however, be regarded

as blind if the field of vision is markedly contracted in the greater part of its extent, and particularly if the contraction is in the lower part of the field; but a person suffering from homonymous or bi-temporal hemianopia retaining central visual acuity of 6/18 or better should not be regarded as blind.

Note: (*a*) The question whether a defect of vision is recent or of long standing has a special bearing on the certification of blindness. A person whose defect is recent is less able to adapt himself to his environment than is a person with the same visual acuity whose defect has been of long standing. This is specially applicable in relation to Groups 2 and 3.

(*b*) Another factor of importance, particularly in relation to Group 2, is the age of the person at the onset of blindness. An old person with a recent failure of sight cannot adapt himself so readily as can a younger person with the same defect.

(*c*) On rare occasions cases will arise which are not precisely covered by the foregoing observations, and such cases must be dealt with according to the judgement of the certifying ophthalmic surgeon.

(*d*) In a person up to and including the age of 16 years other factors may influence the local education authorities regarding the need for special educational facilities (p. 335).

The Blind Child

Special consideration must be given to blindness in children and the definition of blindness in a child is related essentially to the educational methods which are going to prove to be necessary for his upbringing; in this way the blind child is one who is dependent on a form of education which does not involve the use of sight. It follows that children who are classified as blind by this definition have different degrees of blindness. Some may have true blindness— the total absence of light perception in either eye—but others may have an awareness of light, an awareness of movement, or even an ability to discern to some extent large objects in the distance or near at hand. It is obvious that a blind child who has retained a certain amount of visual awareness has distinct advantages over a completely blind child, such as the ability to move more easily and more confidently in strange surroundings, but this ability in no way alters the necessity for him to be educated as a truly blind child.

The Determination of Blindness

This is a matter of great importance because it involves a decision that the child is going to be incapable of benefiting from a normal form of visual education or even from a modified form of education involving the use of special visual methods which is appropriate for the partially sighted, as distinct from the blind, child. It is also of great importance because it involves a decision that the blindness is incapable of being relieved to any significant extent by appropriate medical and surgical procedures. It is therefore essential for each case to be scrutinized with extreme care by an ophthalmic surgeon who is experienced in the diagnosis and treatment of the conditions which lead to blindness in childhood. The main difficulty occurs in the infant when it is not possible to determine the vision objectively. In such cases an indirect assessment may be made by observing the reaction of the child to a bright light because it is usual for a child, even when only a few days old, to be attracted to such a stimulus although the gaze may be directed to the light only momentarily. The behaviour of the infant's eyes during feeding is also of significance because, despite the fact that the eyes generally remain closed, at certain times there is a tendency for the eyes to open and be directed to the mother's face, and provided the mother continues to gaze at the child the child's eyes may move when she moves; a persistent absence of this phenomenon over a period of time is certainly suggestive of blindness. However, failure to be attracted to a light or to gaze at the mother may be due to mental retardation rather than the presence of any organic visual disturbance, so that a final decision is possible only after careful observation of all the relevant facts.

The most common causes of blindness in children are congenital or developmental anomalies which may be present at birth or may become apparent some time after birth. Sometimes these anomalies are confined to the eyes alone but at other times they are associated with widespread changes in other parts of the body. A knowledge of the transmission of these inherited diseases may reduce their incidence by appropriate eugenic measures, but their elimination must await an elucidation of their basic mechanisms. Fortunately, many other forms of blindness following such conditions as ophthalmia neonatorum, infantile glaucoma, congenital cataract, etc., have been combated to varying extents by improved methods of prevention, diagnosis and treatment.

It is essential that the child be registered as blind whenever the determination of blindness has been made in order to allow him to benefit from the excellent facilities which are available. The management of the blind child varies according to his age.

The First Two Years of Life

The baby and the infant up to the age of 2 years are the concern of the welfare department of the local authority, as an integral part of the National Health Service, which authorizes a qualified health visitor to supervise the child in his own home. This implies that unless there are exceptional circumstances the blind child continues to live at home and the brunt of the responsibility for his initial progress is quite rightly imposed on the parents. It is generally recognized that during the early and formative years of the life of any child there is nothing to replace an upbringing within the family because the love and affection which he receives there foster a sense of security which enables him to become established subsequently as an individual who is self-reliant and yet part of the community. This integration within the family is even more important for the blind infant, who is unduly dependent upon the influence of his parents because of his impaired means of communication which of necessity prolong and make more difficult the early period of training.

It is, of course, necessary for the parents to adapt themselves as quickly as possible to the vital part which they have to play in the early years of their blind child. Initially it is often difficult for them to overcome the emotional stress which quite naturally surrounds them after the final realization that the child is blind, but the happiness of the parents, of the blind child and of the whole family is dependent upon a rapid period of adjustment and an important factor in delaying this period is the failure of some parents to accept the verdict that the blindness is inevitable. In such circumstances it is the responsibility of the ophthalmic surgeon to show that his opinion is based on sound judgement which has been reached only after a careful and detailed examination of the patient. In many cases it is desirable for the surgeon to obtain confirmation of his diagnosis from a colleague, but every effort should be made to save the parents the needless anxiety which is produced by trailing the poor child unnecessarily from clinic to clinic, and sometimes even from country to country, in the forlorn hope of finding some miraculous cure.

It is the task of the parents, and particularly of the mother who is with him most of the time, to see that the blind child is allowed to progress as far as possible in a normal way: undue protection and excessive pampering are barriers to his progress and must be avoided at all costs. It is, of course, necessary to modify the approach to the child's development so that an effort is made to cultivate his other senses (the appreciation of touch, of changes in temperature, of hearing and of smell) which are usually unimpaired and which are indeed capable of much greater development than in the sighted child, in order to provide a compensation for the loss of sight.

Normally, a child's visual awareness plays a large part in his increasing appreciation of his surroundings. It follows therefore that the blind baby should be handled much more than usual, although the initial contact with the child must always be very gentle so as not to startle him unduly. Also the blind baby should be spoken to frequently and be made conscious of the noises around him, otherwise there is a tendency for him to adopt a trance-like attitude because he feels so excluded from the outside world. It is important at a very early stage to name the objects with which he is in contact and in this way he learns to recognize them readily by touch and by name. Speaking to the child also helps to develop his powers of speech which often are late in development because the absence of sight prevents the young blind child from making spontaneous comments which characterize the sighted child who is constantly aware of his surroundings. There are obviously special problems in teaching a blind child to feed himself, but these can be overcome by patience and by care in seeing that he is provided with food which can be manipulated fairly easily. Similarly there are problems in learning to walk because he requires more guidance and support than the sighted child.

Later, when the child is beginning to move around, he must be taught to become self-reliant so that he is able to move around a room by himself and then to move around the whole house, including the staircase. It is necessary, of course, to protect him from undue danger (but this applies also to a sighted child of that age), and it is a great help to him if his toys and the different articles of furniture are kept in constant positions so that he becomes adapted to his surroundings as quickly as possible with increasing assurance and self-confidence.

There is a tendency for the blind child to develop certain mannerisms, such as poking the eyes with the fingers or rocking to and fro when sitting down, and these often occur because he is bored and feels isolated from his surroundings. It is desirable to prevent these mannerisms from becoming persistent and this is best achieved by diverting him to some form of useful activity: a further example of the necessity for constant care of the blind child. Unfortunately this poking of the eyes may be carried out in such a vigorous way in the older blind child (it is suggested that it is motivated because it induces pleasurable sensations), that it may lead to a rupture of fibres in the corneal stroma or even of Descemet's membrane with the development of a bullous keratopathy (chap. 4), and the eye becomes painful as well as blind; this may necessitate the removal of the eye.

The Third to Fifth Years of Life

When the conditions in the parental home are suitable it is ideal that the blind child should continue to live there until he reaches his fifth birthday so that he is able to maintain his close connection with the family. In these circumstances the parents often require special advice and guidance on the management of their child and a Parents' Unit at Northwood in Middlesex is designed to cater for this need. In this Unit, which is run by the Royal National Institute for the Blind (RNIB—an organization with unique knowledge and experience of the problems of the care of the blind) the parents and their child are able to stay for a short period to learn the practical aspects of the task which lies ahead. Unfortunately at present there is only one unit of this kind, but its scope is extended by a home counselling service so that a member of the staff visits the parents and child in the home. Sometimes, however, if the home is over-crowded or if the parents have insufficient time to devote to the welfare of the blind child, it is better for him to be transferred after his third birthday to a residential nursery school for blind children (for example, the Sunshine Home Nursery Schools for Blind Children which also are run by the RNIB), and the child returns home during the holidays as in a normal boarding school. These homes are situated in 6 counties of England and Wales (Lancashire, Middlesex, Shropshire, Sussex, Warwickshire and Glamorgan) and the child is accommodated in a home which is situated as near as possible to his parents' house so that he is able to maintain contact with his family. The homes are also of particular value to a child who has an additional form of handicap which requires special methods of care and treatment.

A Sunshine Home provides the perfect substitute for the parental home because it creates the atmosphere of the family. In each home there are about 20 children who are divided into small groups each of which is in the charge of an experienced nursery nurse who is responsible for all the different aspects of the welfare of the child. The homes are situated in pleasant surroundings so that the child has freedom to play in the garden with complete safety and in this way to increase his awareness of the outside world. The homes also function as schools which provide the early education of the child, with particular emphasis on handicraft, music, story-telling and nature studies. The radio and the gramophone are important substitutes for the picture books of the sighted young child.

After the Age of Five Years

When the blind child reaches the age of 5 years it is necessary for the parents to arrange for his education. This usually entails his admission to a residential primary school for blind children which is under the control of the local authority, although the child may be admitted in the first place to a Sunshine Home and then transferred to the primary school on reaching his seventh birthday; it is, of course, possible for the parents to make their own arrangements for his education but these must have the approval of the educational authorities. Naturally, particular stress is laid on the learning of Braille, which is the medium for reading and writing. Sometimes the blind child has an additional handicap, such as deafness or mental deficiency, and there are special schools which cater for the blind and deaf child and for the blind and educationally subnormal (ESN) child.

Thereafter the blind child's education may continue at a grammar school (for example, Worcester College for Boys and Chorleywood College for Girls) and every opportunity is given for the child subsequently to enter a university. The less gifted child proceeds to a secondary technical college which provides a further education which is designed to prepare him for a career in such activities as typing, piano-tuning or music. The blind child remains the responsibility of the local education officer during the school and university period, but thereafter the blind person enters the care of the Department of Employment which is concerned with maintaining him in suitable employment. In all the different stages of the education of the child an important person is the home teacher of the blind who is an officer of the welfare department. She maintains contact with the blind child throughout the period of training, and her experience is valuable in fostering progress and in helping the parents to appreciate the ways in which they are able to contribute to the child's well-being.

The Blind Adult

The blind adult who has been blinded in childhood will pass automatically into a sphere of employment which is suitable for his capabilities, but the normally sighted adult who becomes blind as the result of some injury or disease faces entirely different problems. There are, however, facilities which are available through the Department of Employment in cooperation with the Blind Persons Settlement Officer at certain Local Employment Exchanges. This officer covers a specified group of Employment Exchanges, which may embrace two counties in certain country areas, and he assists the registered blind adult to reenter employment with confidence and courage. In England, a third of the blind of working age are employed and more than half of these are in normal competitive occupations. As a general rule a course at a residential rehabilitation centre which provides instruction in the basic requirements of the blind person (Braille, typewriting, etc.) is followed by some form of specialized training in light engineering at a Government Training centre, or in shorthand typewriting, telephone switchboard operating or physiotherapy at the Royal National Institute for the Blind. Special facilities are available for the ex-Service blind at St. Dunstan's Hospital.

The National Library for the Blind provides a comprehensive selection of books of all kinds (technical, classics, novels, etc.) in Braille which are sold or loaned at low cost. More recently a talking library is available with books on records or tapes for those who are too old to learn Braille because of intellectual difficulties or frequently because their fingers are not sufficiently sensitive to achieve any degree of fluency. In such cases the simpler MOON books are more readily mastered and have proved a great comfort to the lonely and elderly, although the method is less versatile than Braille because it can only be read not typed. The MOON system avoids the use of the small dots which constitute each letter in the Braille method. The letters of the MOON alphabet which have clear bold outlines are of three main types: 8 letters of unaltered roman form

(C I J L O U V Z); 13 characters which are based on parts of roman letters (A B D E F K M N P Q S T X); and 5 new forms which replace the remaining roman letters (G H R W Y).

The blind person receives certain benefits: welfare services provided by the Local Authority, pension at the age of 40 years, supplementary benefits when applicable through the Department of Health and Social Security, and certain income tax concessions.

Sometimes the facilities which are available for the blind child and for the blind adult fail to meet the peculiar needs of the person who becomes blind during the adolescent period, and there is now a Voluntary Assessment Centre for the Adolescent Blind in Surrey run by the RNIB.

PARTIAL SIGHT

There is no statutory definition of partial sight, but the Department of Health and Social Security has advised that a person who is not blind within the meaning of the Act but who is, nevertheless, substantially and permanently handicapped by congenitally defective vision or in whose case illness or injury had caused defective vision of a substantial and permanently handicapping character is within the scope of the welfare services which the local authority provides for handicapped persons, and is entitled to a supplementary benefit when applicable through the Department of Health and Social Security, but not to a pension before the usual age and not to income tax concessions.

The following criteria should be used as a general guide when determining whether a person falls within the scope of the welfare provisions for the partially sighted, as well as in recommending, where the person is under 16 years of age, the appropriate type of school for the particular child concerned:

1. For registration purposes and the provision of welfare services the following persons may be regarded as partially sighted:

those with visual acuity:

(*a*) 3/60 to 6/60 with full field;

(*b*) up to 6/24 with moderate contraction of the field, opacities in media, or aphakia;

(*c*) 6/18 or even better if there is a gross field defect, e.g. hemianopia, or there is marked contraction of the field as in tapetoretinal degeneration, glaucoma etc.

2. For children whose visual acuity will have a bearing on the appropriate methods of education:

(a) severe visual disabilities—to be educated in Special Schools by methods involving vision—3/60 to 6/24 with glasses;

(b) visual impairment—to be educated at ordinary schools by special consideration—better than 6/24 with glasses.

It should be emphasized that a determination of the level of close reading vision is essential in all children because in certain conditions (congenital nystagmus, Marfan's syndrome, etc.) this may be remarkably good so that the child is able to cope with an ordinary school, provided he has a sufficient degree of intelligence, despite a marked restriction of the distant vision.

It is obvious that the classification of a child as partially sighted creates certain difficulties which are resolved only when the child is sufficiently old to permit an accurate assessment of the visual acuity (uniocular and binocular, for distance and for near); indeed, it is recommended that any infant with a congenital anomaly causing a visual defect should be registered as partially sighted, unless obviously blind. It follows that any infant or young child who is classified in this way should be reexamined every 12 months (or more frequently if necessary) in order to make an alteration in the category (to normally sighted or to blind) as early as possible. This also applies to the adult who is registered as partially sighted because the category may change if sight is restored following successful medical or surgical treatment of the condition or if sight becomes worse following an inevitable deterioration of the condition.

The reading vision of a partially sighted adult may be sufficiently good to permit the use of books with a reasonable size of print, and a selection of books with specially large print is available in most Public Libraries and the talking library is also available to the partially sighted on special certification.

Index